Stroke: A Case-Based Approach

Stroke: A Case-Based Approach

Editor: Conor Russell

AMERICAN
MEDICAL PUBLISHERS
www.americanmedicalpublishers.com

AMERICAN
MEDICAL PUBLISHERS
www.americanmedicalpublishers.com

Cataloging-in-Publication Data

Stroke: a case-based approach / edited by Conor Russell.
p. cm.
Includes bibliographical references and index.
ISBN 979-8-88740-658-9
1. Cerebrovascular disease. 2. Cerebrovascular disease--Pathophysiology.
3. Cerebrovascular disease--Diagnosis. 4. Cerebrovascular disease--Treatment.
5. Brain--Diseases. I. Russell, Conor.
RC388.5 .S77 2023
616.81--dc23

American Medical Publishers,
41 Flatbush Avenue,
1st Floor, New York,
NY 11217, USA

ISBN 979-8-88740-658-9 (Hardback)

Contents

Preface

The main aim of this book is to educate learners and enhance their research focus by presenting diverse topics covering this vast field. This is an advanced book which compiles significant studies by distinguished experts in the area of analysis. This book addresses successive solutions to the challenges arising in the area of application, along with it; the book provides scope for future developments.

Stroke is a medical emergency that occurs when blood flow to the brain is disrupted, resulting in damage to brain cells. Rapid diagnosis and treatment are essential to minimize brain damage and improve outcomes. Strokes are broadly divided into ischemic strokes and hemorrhagic strokes. The strokes which are caused due to the blockage of an artery are known as ischemic strokes. Hemorrhagic strokes are caused by the rupturing and bleeding of a blood vessel which supplies blood to the brain. The diagnosis of a stroke can be done by studying the medical history and conducting a physical examination. It can also be done through imaging tests such as CT scan, MRI scan and angiography. From theories to research to practical applications, case studies related to all contemporary topics of relevance to strokes have been included in this book. It will serve as a valuable source of reference for graduate and postgraduate students.

It was a great honour to edit this book, though there were challenges, as it involved a lot of communication and networking between me and the editorial team. However, the end result was this all-inclusive book covering diverse themes in the field.

Finally, it is important to acknowledge the efforts of the contributors for their excellent chapters, through which a wide variety of issues have been addressed. I would also like to thank my colleagues for their valuable feedback during the making of this book.

Editor

1

Low-Molecular-Weight Heparin use in a Case of Noncardiogenic Multifocal Perinatal Thromboembolic Stroke

Matthew A. Saxonhouse,[1] Dan Tarquinio,[2] Paul R. Carney,[3] Jeff Bennett,[4] Amy Smith,[5] Stephen P. Hunger,[6] and James D. Geyer[7]

[1] *Division of Neonatology, Department of Pediatrics, University of Florida, Gainesville, FL 32610-0296, USA*
[2] *Division of General Pediatrics, Department of Pediatrics, University of Florida, Gainesville, FL 32610-0296, USA*
[3] *Division of Neurology, Department of Pediatrics, University of Florida, Gainesville, FL 32610-0296, USA*
[4] *Department of Radiology, University of Florida, Gainesville, FL 32610-0296, USA*
[5] *Division of Hematology/Oncology, Department of Pediatrics, University of Florida, Gainesville, FL 32610-0296, USA*
[6] *Section of Pediatric Hematology/Oncology/Bone Marrow Transplantation and Center for Cancer and Blood Disorders, The Children's Hospital, University of Colorado, Denver School of Medicine, Aurora, CO 80045, USA*
[7] *Division of Neurology and Sleep Medicine, Department of Internal Medicine, College of Community Health Sciences, University of Alabama, Tuscaloosa, AL 35487, USA*

Correspondence should be addressed to Matthew A. Saxonhouse, saxonma@peds.ufl.edu

Recommended by Charles S. Greenberg

A full-term neonate suffered multifocal cerebral infarctions due to multiple large vessel thrombi. Thrombophilia and cardiovascular assessments were negative, but due to the severity of the lesions and the concern for expansion of the thrombi or future embolic events, treatment with low-molecular-weight heparin (LMWH) was initiated. No complications from treatment were experienced. We present this severe case in order to highlight difficult management decisions for newborns with multifocal perinatal thromboembolic stroke and to stress the need for further practice guidelines and research in this area.

1. Introduction

Perinatal stroke, occurring between 20 weeks' gestation through the 28th postnatal day [1–3], has a prevalence ranging from 17.0 to 43.4 per 100 000 live births [4–6]. The majority (80%) of these events is ischemic in nature and most abnormalities occur in the left hemisphere within the distribution of the middle cerebral artery (MCA). Rarely, multifocal cerebral infarctions can occur and these tend to be embolic in origin [7, 8].

Despite the prevalence of perinatal stroke, no randomized clinical trials exist to address acute management or prevention [1, 8, 9]. Current guidelines from the American College of Chest Physicians (ACCP) suggest anticoagulation or aspirin therapy only for neonates with a first perinatal stroke with a documented ongoing cardioembolic source (Grade IB) or recurrent arterial ischemic stroke (AIS; Grade 2C) [9]. However, recent recommendations from the American Heart Association (AHA) suggest that anticoagulation may be selected in neonates with multiple cerebral emboli (Class IIb, Level of Evidence C) [1].

We present a neonate who suffered multifocal cerebral infarctions due to thrombosis of five vessels. No evidence suggested cardiac disease or a prothrombotic disorder. Due to the severity, size, and locations of the thrombi, plus the multifocal presentation of the cerebral infarctions, we decided to anticoagulate the patient with low-molecular-weight heparin (LMWH) in an attempt to decrease the risk of extension of the thrombi and/or secondary emboli. This case of multifocal thromboembolic perinatal stroke represents the most severe end of the spectrum and highlights the difficulties inherent in management of these types of patients.

2. Case Report

A 40-week, 2884 g, female infant was delivered via cesarean section to a 41-year-old primigravida after arrest of descent and failed vacuum extraction. Complications of the pregnancy included a history of infertility, gestational diabetes (glyburide controlled), prolonged rupture of membranes, and chorioamnionitis. Apgar scores were 1, 7, and 8. Umbilical artery and venous pH were 6.94 and 7.06, respectively. Initial blood testing was nonspecific. Physical examination was significant for a large left caput succedaneum with a soft and flat anterior fontanel. Neurological examination demonstrated mild hypotonia. At approximately 36 hours of age, the patient had seizure activity consisting of eye fluttering, bilateral clonic movements of the upper extremities, and tongue thrusting. Two separate events occurred, each lasting less than three minutes.

Repeat blood testing revealed a normal glucose level, no significant electrolyte abnormalities, a white blood count of $9.8 \times 10^3/\text{mm}^3$, and hematocrit of 46.8%. The platelet count had decreased from 155 (initial) to $119 \times 10^3/\text{mm}^3$ with subsequent drop to $109 \times 10^3/\text{mm}^3$ twenty four hours later. Cerebrospinal fluid evaluation revealed (traumatic lumbar puncture) $115\,000/\text{mm}^3$ red blood cells, $50/\text{mm}^3$ white blood cells with 87% polys and 12% lymphs. The patient was given a loading dose of phenobarbital, and ampicillin and gentamicin had been started shortly after birth.

Magnetic resonance imaging (MRI) of the brain (Figure 1) demonstrated bilateral multifocal regions of increased signal on diffusion-weighted imaging in the left pons, left occipital lobe, left thalamus, left and right frontal lobes, and left and right frontoparietal regions. No evidence indicated hemorrhage, and all of the lesions were dark on apparent diffusion coefficient of water (ADC) mapping indicating that they were acute in nature (within 1 week). A transthoracic echocardiogram demonstrated normal cardiac anatomy with no intracardiac thrombus or vegetation. Magnetic resonance angiography (MRA) of the head and neck without contrast (Figure 2) demonstrated occlusion of the right internal carotid artery (ICA) at its origin without distal reconstitution. Collateral flow directed blood through the anterior communicating artery to the right anterior cerebral artery (ACA) and right middle cerebral artery (MCA). The vertebral arteries were diminutive and the basilar artery was occluded. The posterior communicating arteries and PCAs were not visualized. With this extent of vessel occlusion, even more widespread brain infarction might be expected. However, the complex distribution of the infarcts demonstrated on diffusion-weighted images can be explained by the relative robustness of the patient's leptomeningeal collateral vessels. EEG evaluation demonstrated left parieto-occipital spike wave discharges with associated slowing, excessive subtransients for age, and mild slowing and suppression of background activity.

Bacterial and viral studies were negative. Placental pathology demonstrated a third trimester placenta with acute necrotizing chorioamnionitis and a three-vessel cord with acute funisitis (inflammation of the umbilical cord). Extensive thrombophilia evaluation performed on day of life

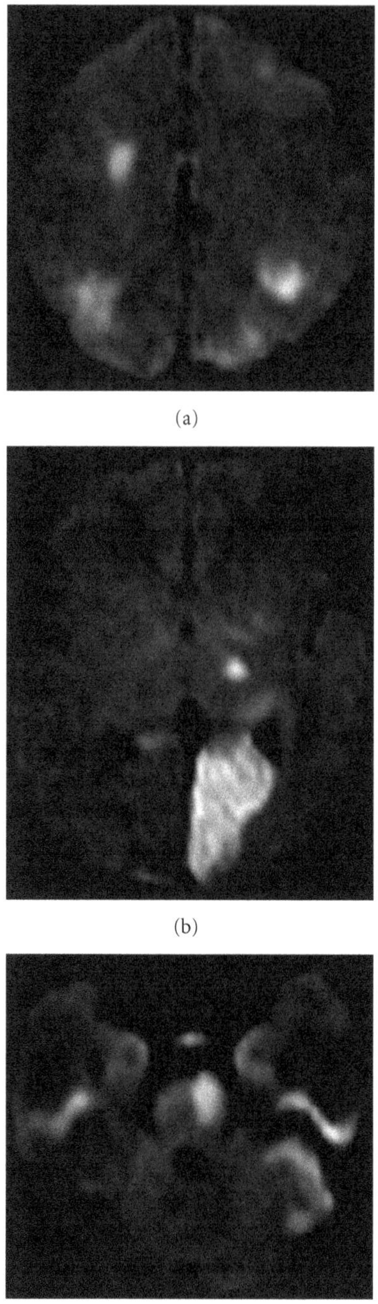

(a)

(b)

(c)

Figure 1: (a)–(c): Axial diffusion-weighted images, $b = 1000$, demonstrate multiple areas of high signal in bilateral frontal and parietal lobes, left occipital lobe, left thalamus, and left pons.

four (Table 1) failed to identify any inherited or acquired prothrombotic risk factors. However, other than negative DNA mutation analysis, definitive protein abnormalities could not be ruled out until repeat evaluation performed at 3–6 month of life [10]. State metabolic screening through the State of Florida was negative.

Prior to the results of the thrombophilia evaluation, we decided to anticoagulate the patient with LMWH. We based

Table 1: Thrombophilia Evaluation Performed [10, 11].

Test	Performed	Test	Performed
PT	*1 and *2	Anti-B2 glycoprotein IgG	1 and 2
INR	1 and 2	Anti-B2 glycoprotein IgM	1 and 2
aPTT	1 and 2	Anti-phosphatidylserine IgG	1 and 2
Fibrinogen	1 and 2	Anti-phosphatidylserine IgM	1 and 2
Factor V Leiden	1	Heparin cofactor 2	1 and 2
Prothrombin 20210	1	Homocysteine	1 and 2
MTHFR	1	Lipoprotein (A)	1 and 2
Protein C activity	1 and 2	Antithrombin	1 and 2
Protein S activity	1 and 2	Factor VIII activity	2
Anticardiolipin IgG	1 and 2	Lupus anticoagulant	2
Anticardiolipin IgM	1 and 2	Factor XII activity	2
Plasminogen	2		

PT: prothrombin time; aPTT: activated partial thromboplastin time; INR: international normalized ratio; MTHFR: methylenetetrahydrofolate reductase.
*1 Test performed at day of life no. 4; *2 Test performed at four months of age.

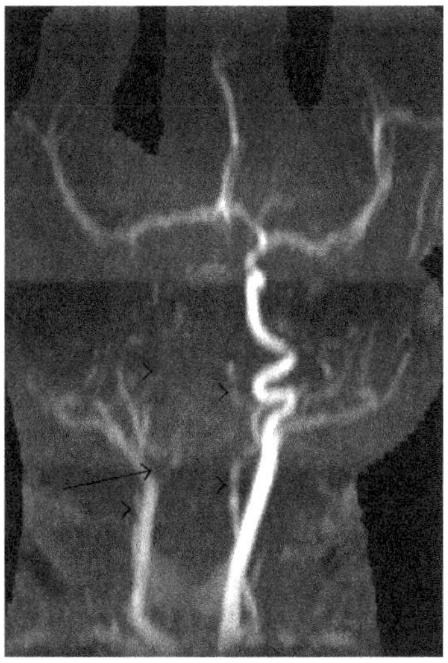

Figure 2: 3D maximum-intensity projection (MIP) image from a 3D time of flight MRA demonstrates occlusion of the right internal carotid artery at its origin (arrow). The vertebral arteries are diminutive (arrowheads) and the basilar artery is not visualized.

this decision on the occlusion of multiple large blood vessels with evidence of multifocal cerebral infarctions, a pattern indicative of an embolic process. Our rationale for choosing LMWH was to decrease the risk of clot extension, which was suggested by the progressive thrombocytopenia. LMWH was initiated, using a therapeutic antifactor Xa level of 0.5–1.0 IU/mL.

The patient had no further seizure activity, and gradually improved during her admission. The platelet count increased after starting therapy to $156 \times 10^3/mm^3$ and then $253 \times 10^3/mm^3$, at 48 hours and 96 hours, respectively. She was discharged home on day of life 13 from the neonatal intensive care unit taking full oral feedings, and her family was instructed to continue phenobarbital and LMWH with scheduled follow-up.

MRI evaluation at four months of age demonstrated bilateral encephalomalacia in areas of prior infarction with no evidence of current or prior hemorrhage. Mild encephalomalacia was also seen in the right PCA territory, which was not ischemic on the initial MRI. This likely reflected an additional infarct which most likely occurred during or soon after the initial scan, possibly before the initiation of LMWH. MRA evaluation (Figure 3) revealed resolution of the right ICA thrombus with overall decreased caliber of the vessel compared to the left, and residual irregularity and narrowing at the superior cervical segment. The intracranial vessels were all patent, although the right PCA was diminutive. Repeat thrombophilia assessment at four months of life was negative (Table 1).

We discontinued LMWH treatment after obtaining the results of the repeat MRI, MRA, and thrombophilia evaluations. Neurological evaluation at 4.5 months of age demonstrated asymmetric tracking and blinking to confrontation which was worse on the left, mildly increased flexor tone of the left upper extremity, normal lower extremity tone and reflexes bilaterally, and age appropriate milestones for gross motor, fine motor, and social interaction. No seizure activity has been observed or suggested on EEG evaluation, and phenobarbital has been weaned. Neuro-ophthalmological examination at 6 months of age demonstrated normal visual acuity for age and normal blinking to confrontation. The patient continues to thrive and develop at home.

3. Discussion

Multifocal cerebral infarction is a rare type of perinatal stroke that tends to be embolic in origin [8]. Despite the multiple risk factors ascribed to perinatal stroke, little evidence exists to inform management of these infants after initial stabilization [1, 9]. Previous studies of perinatal stroke have been limited due to small sample size or lack of adequate control groups [6, 8].

Current ACCP guidelines suggest that only neonates with proven cardioembolic arterial ischemic stroke or those with

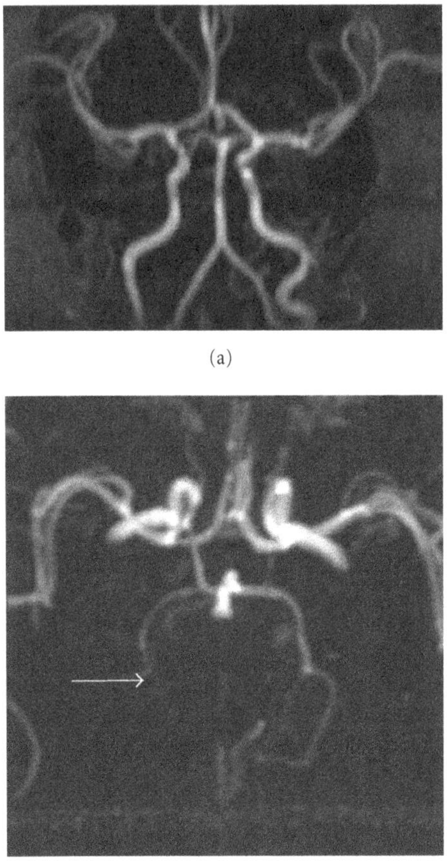

(a)

(b)

Figure 3: 3D MIP images from a noncontrast 2D time of flight MRA demonstrate restoration of flow in the right internal carotid artery and posterior circulation. Residual occlusion of the distal right PCA persists (arrow).

recurrent arterial ischemic stroke should receive treatment with anticoagulation or aspirin therapy [9]. Recommendations from a special writing group of the AHA stroke council and the council on cardiovascular disease in the young [1] suggest that anticoagulation may be considered in neonates with multiple cerebral emboli. Both of these recommendations are based on expert opinion and case series/reports. However, they leave the clinician with difficult treatment decisions to make when faced with a neonate with severe multifocal perinatal thromboembolic stroke (such as our case report).

Recent research has demonstrated increasing evidence that LMWH may play a pivotal role in perinatal stroke [12]. Studies in pediatric patients have shown efficacy and safety of LMWH similar to that observed in adults, and they have demonstrated that LMWH prevents progression of stroke, development of new symptomatic thrombi, and extensions of existing thrombi [12–14]. Punzalan et al. present two children with internal carotid artery thrombi who had either complete or partial resolution of thrombi while being treated with LMWH [13]. One of the largest neonatal studies involving LMWH demonstrated that with careful monitoring and laboratory evidence of therapeutic LMWH effect, complete or partial resolution of thromboembolism was achieved in the majority of cases [15]. Significant bleeding occurred in four of the 62 infants, but none of the events resulted in severe sequelae or death. Other studies and case reports have not only demonstrated similar efficacy, but also decreased clot extension and prevention of embolic phenomenon [16]. One limitation with applying these reports to perinatal stroke is that only four patients in these studies had clots in the central nervous system [15]. Although LMWH does appear to be a safe medication for treatment and prophylaxis of neonates with perinatal stroke, individual judgment (for now) should be applied to specific cases.

This case is characteristic of the severe end of the spectrum of perinatal stroke and emphasizes the difficult acute management decisions regarding such neonates. The comprehensive ACCP guidelines provide recommendations that facilitate the standardized use of antithrombotic and thrombolytic therapy in neonates and children. We appreciate that extreme cases, such as the one presented, are not routinely encompassed by such guidelines, and in these situations optimal treatment may fall outside the recommendations provided. Other sources (such as those of the AHA) can be referred to in order to provide some guidance but the physician may ultimately have to make a balanced decision.

We decided to treat the neonate described above with LMWH based on the severity of the thrombus in the right internal carotid artery and the multifocal nature of the arterial ischemic stroke. Although the probable source of the initial thrombus was the placenta, we believed that there was a high risk for extension of the internal carotid thrombus and/or further embolic complications. We felt that the potential risk associated with bleeding was significantly less than the devastating ramifications of further central nervous system insult. Our patient suffered no complications from the treatment and had resolution of the thrombi, thus supporting the safety and efficacy of LMHW in neonates.

We cannot prove definitively that LMWH resulted in clot resolution without a similar control patient and a timeline involving serial imaging studies. Serial MRA/MRI was not performed due to the extreme cost and the potential morbidity associated with repeated sedation. The patient's thrombocytopenia and clinical condition improved after initiation of LMWH, suggesting that LMWH halted clot extension. Moreover, the follow-up MRI/MRA after four months of LMWH treatment demonstrated almost complete recanalization of the cerebral vessels. This MRI did demonstrate encephalomalacia in the right PCA territory which was not predicted from the original infarct pattern. However, based on consistent clinical improvement, we strongly feel that this infarct occurred in close proximity to the initial MRI, most likely before the initiation of LMWH. In addition, it suggests that LMWH may have prevented further infarcts. Therefore, we feel that this case supports the recommendations provided by the AHA for LMWH treatment in complex cases of multiple cerebral emboli. While we recognize that one case study does not represent strong evidence, we propose that when the ACCP guidelines are again updated, the authors consider review and inclusion of a subset of patients with severe multifocal noncardioembolic stroke who may benefit from anticoagulation. This case also highlights the need for controlled clinical trials to address the management of the broad spectrum of perinatal stroke [2].

References

[1] E. S. Roach, M. R. Golomb, R. Adams, et al., "Management of stroke in infants and children: a scientific statement from a Special Writing Group of the American Heart Association Stroke Council and the Council on Cardiovascular Disease in the Young," *Stroke*, vol. 39, no. 9, pp. 2644–2691, 2008.

[2] T. N. K. Raju, K. B. Nelson, D. Ferriero, and J. K. Lynch, "Ischemic perinatal stroke: summary of a workshop sponsored by the national institute of child health and human development and the national institute of neurological disorders and stroke," *Pediatrics*, vol. 120, no. 3, pp. 609–616, 2007.

[3] K. B. Nelson, "Perinatal ischemic stroke," *Stroke*, vol. 38, no. 2, pp. 742–745, 2007.

[4] Y. W. Wu, J. K. Lynch, and K. B. Nelson, "Perinatal arterial stroke: understanding mechanisms and outcomes," *Seminars in Neurology*, vol. 25, no. 4, pp. 424–434, 2005.

[5] S. Schulzke, P. Weber, J. Luetschg, and H. Fahnenstich, "Incidence and diagnosis of unilateral arterial cerebral infarction in newborn infants," *Journal of Perinatal Medicine*, vol. 33, no. 2, pp. 170–175, 2005.

[6] J. Lee, L. A. Croen, K. H. Backstrand, et al., "Maternal and infant characteristics associated with perinatal arterial stroke in the infant," *The Journal of the American Medical Association*, vol. 293, no. 6, pp. 723–729, 2005.

[7] R. W. Hunt and T. E. Inder, "Perinatal and neonatal ischaemic stroke: a review," *Thrombosis Research*, vol. 118, no. 1, pp. 39–48, 2006.

[8] E. A. Chalmers, "Perinatal stroke—risk factors and management," *British Journal of Haematology*, vol. 130, no. 3, pp. 333–343, 2005.

[9] P. Monagle, E. Chalmers, A. Chan, et al., "Antithrombotic therapy in neonates and children: American College of Chest Physicians Evidence-Based Clinical Practice Guidelines (8th edition)," *Chest*, vol. 133, supplement 6, pp. 887S–968S, 2008.

[10] U. Nowak-Göttl, C. Duering, B. Kempf-Bielack, and R. Sträter, "Thromboembolic diseases in neonates and children," *Pathophysiology of Haemostasis and Thrombosis*, vol. 33, no. 5-6, pp. 269–274, 2003.

[11] M. J. Manco-Johnson, "How I treat venous thrombosis in children," *Blood*, vol. 107, no. 1, pp. 21–29, 2006.

[12] C. R. Burak, M. D. Bowen, and T. F. Barron, "The use of enoxaparin in children with acute, nonhemorrhagic ischemic stroke," *Pediatric Neurology*, vol. 29, no. 4, pp. 295–298, 2003.

[13] R. C. Punzalan, C. A. Hillery, R. R. Montgomery, J. P. Scott, and J. C. Gill, "Low-molecular-weight heparin in thrombotic disease in children and adolescents," *Journal of Pediatric Hematology/Oncology*, vol. 22, no. 2, pp. 137–142, 2000.

[14] D. Dix, M. Andrew, V. Marzinotto, et al., "The use of low molecular weight heparin in pediatric patients: a prospective cohort study," *Journal of Pediatrics*, vol. 136, no. 4, pp. 439–445, 2000.

[15] W. Streif, G. Goebel, A. K. C. Chan, and M. P. Massicotte, "Use of low molecular mass heparin (enoxaparin) in newborn infants: a prospective cohort study of 62 patients," *Archives of Disease in Childhood Fetal and Neonatal Edition*, vol. 88, no. 5, pp. F365–F370, 2003.

[16] L. A. Michaels, M. Gurian, T. Hegyi, and R. A. Drachtman, "Low molecular weight heparin in the treatment of venous and arterial thromboses in the premature infant," *Pediatrics*, vol. 114, no. 3, pp. 703–707, 2004.

2

Minor Trauma Causing Stroke in a Young Athlete

Vineet Gupta,[1] Naveen Dhawan,[2] and Jaya Bahl[3]

[1]*Department of Medicine, University of California San Diego (UCSD), San Diego, CA 92103, USA*
[2]*Nova Southeastern University, 3301 College Avenue, Fort Lauderdale, FL 33314, USA*
[3]*Florida International University (FIU), 11200 SW 8th Street, Miami, FL 33174, USA*

Correspondence should be addressed to Vineet Gupta; vineetgsvm@gmail.com

Academic Editor: Chin-Chang Huang

A 17-year-old Caucasian male presented with sudden dizziness, ataxia, vertigo, and clumsiness lasting for a couple of hours. He had a subtle trauma during a wrestling match 2 days prior to the presentation. A CT Angiogram (CTA) and MRI showed left vertebral artery dissection (VAD). The patient was treated with anticoagulation with heparin drip in the ICU. The patient was discharged home on the third day on Lovenox-warfarin bridging. This case underscores the importance of considering VAD as a differential diagnosis in patients with sports-related symptoms especially in activities entailing hyperextension or hyperrotation of neck. Due to a varied latent period, often minor underlying trauma, and subtle presentation, a low index of suspicion is warranted in timely diagnosis and treatment of VAD. Considering recent evidence in treatment modality, either antiplatelet therapy or anticoagulation may be used for treatment of VAD.

1. Background

Vertebral artery dissection (VAD) is an underrecognized cause of stroke in patients younger than 45 years [1]. VAD is marked by several causes. It can be due to hyperextension of the neck by a variety of sports-related activities or cervical manipulation [2]. VAD is much less common than carotid artery dissection, but it can be a potentially life-threatening episode. The mortality rate of VAD in the acute phase is about 10% [1]. We present an interesting case of young male with subtle clinical manifestations who was later diagnosed with VAD.

2. Case Presentation

A 17-year-old Caucasian male backyard wrestler with no significant past medical history presented with acute onset of transient dizziness, ataxia, vertigo, and clumsiness lasting for a couple of hours while watching a baseball game. The patient complained of the onset of symptoms while turning his head to left. The patient was asymptomatic on presentation; the physical examination was unremarkable for any focal neurological deficits or constitutional symptoms.

During a thorough history-taking, it was revealed that the patient hyperextended his neck during a mock wrestling match 2 days prior to presentation. The patient did not develop any headache, loss of consciousness, or focal neurologic deficits at that time. The patient remained asymptomatic during the intervening days.

3. Investigations

A CT scan head was unremarkable for any intracranial bleed. CT Angiogram (CTA) and MRI were notable for the dissection of almost the entire length of the left vertebral artery (extracranially) not involving the basilar artery (Figure 1). Dissection was further characterized by filling defect and mural thickening (Figures 2 and 3).

4. Differential Diagnosis

The differential diagnosis for the presenting symptoms of ataxia, vertigo, and dizziness includes stroke (hemorrhagic and ischemic), cervical spine fracture, cervical strain, subarachnoid hemorrhage, and atherothrombotic disease of the vertebrobasilar region and tension headache [1]. Migraine

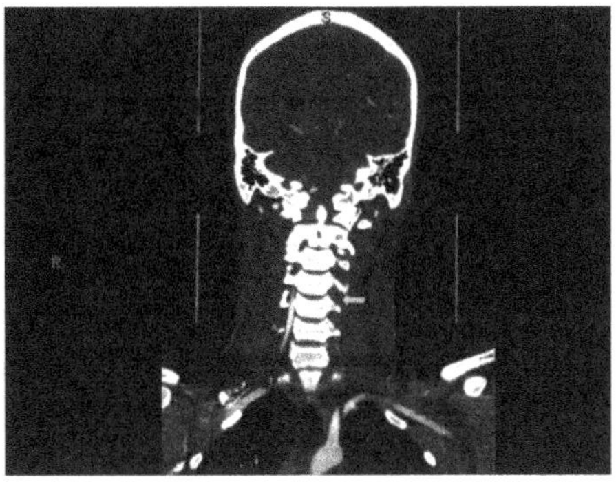

FIGURE 1: CT Angiogram shows attenuated filling of left vertebral artery (extracranial) almost in its entire length secondary to dissection (marked by solid arrow).

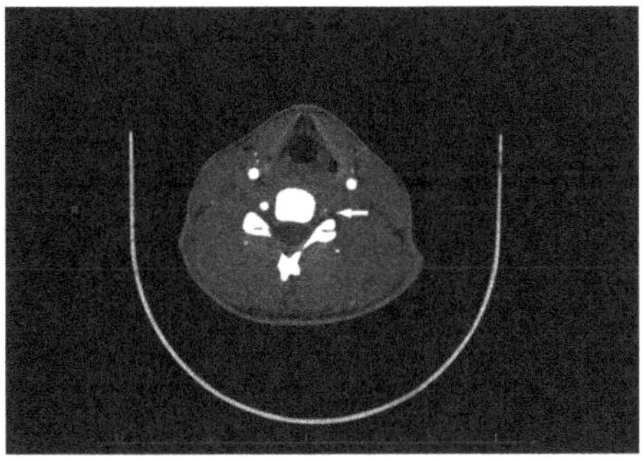

FIGURE 2: CT Angiogram showing the filling defect in left vertebral artery (marked by white solid arrow).

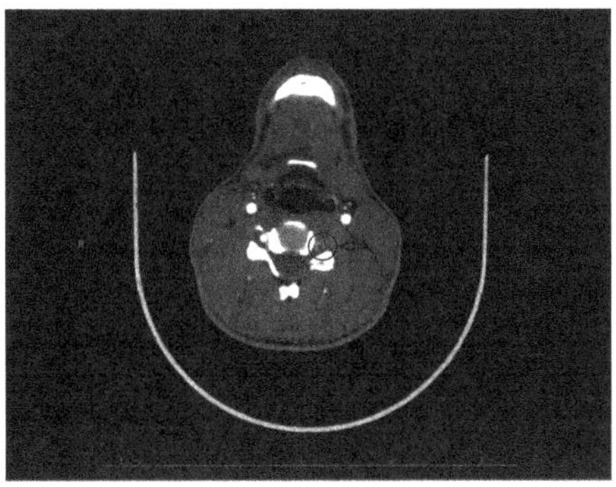

FIGURE 3: CT Angiogram showing hyperattenuating crescent shaped mural thickening of left vertebral artery (marked by black circle and arrow).

headaches must also be excluded as a cause [3]. VAD is associated with collagen disorders such as Ehlers-Danlos syndrome, Marfan's syndrome, and osteogenesis imperfecta which render the vertebral arteries more prone to dissection [4]. Additionally, hyperhomocysteinemia and MTHFR mutations may also lead to VAD [5].

5. Treatment

Given the absence of intracranial bleed on CT scan brain and primarily extracranial involvement of vertebral artery, the patient was started on a heparin drip for anticoagulation and admitted to the intensive care unit (ICU) for closer observation. The patient had unremarkable ICU course for any neurological changes. The patient was discharged home on the third day on Lovenox-warfarin bridging with follow-up CT Angiogram in 3 months.

6. Outcome and Follow-Up

When last contacted, the patient had been neurologically stable. He has not engaged in any wrestling activities and has not experienced any trauma.

7. Discussion

The underlying lesion in VAD is an expanding intramural hematoma, secondary to hemorrhage of the vasa vasorum within the media of vertebral artery, arising either spontaneously or after minor trauma [1]. Intimal disruption and decreased flow states predispose to a thrombogenic milieu that can lead to emboli formation and propagation.

It is estimated that VAD occurs at an incidence of about 1–1.5 per 100,000 [6]. Females are generally three times as likely to experience VAD as compared to males. The disease is usually seen in young patients (less than 45 years of age). The mortality rate in the acute phase is about 10% due to extensive intracranial dissection, brainstem infarction, or subarachnoid hemorrhage.

Causes of VAD include activities that entail hyperrotation or hyperextension of the neck, ranging from trivial activities to sports [7]. Trivial trauma may include spinal manipulation, nose blowing, yoga, and ceiling painting. Sports-related injuries that have been previously described include golf, judo, Kung Fu, and swimming [8–11]. Hyperextension of neck was noted to be the cause in our patient.

Unique anatomical attributes of vertebral arteries render them more prone to dissection than the carotid arteries. The vertebral arteries are particularly vulnerable to spinal compression, particularly at the level of the C1 and C2 vertebrae, where the rotation of the head takes place [12]. In contrast to the carotid artery, which is positioned in a less taut manner within the neck's soft tissue, the vertebral arteries traverse around the C1 vertebrae, making them more prone to injury caused by hyperextension or hyperrotation of the neck [7, 13].

Typical presentation of VAD includes severe occipital headache and posterior nuchal pain following a recent, relatively minor, head or neck injury involving some degree of cervical distortion [5]. Patients most commonly report neurological symptoms attributable to lateral medullary dysfunction as noted in our patient. The occipital and nuchal pain associated with VAD mimics musculoskeletal pain and often is attributed to the mechanical strain that precipitated the dissection. Thus, the symptoms are often mistaken for musculoskeletal prior to the development of neurological symptoms [5]. Focal neurological signs attributable to brainstem and cerebellum ischemia (typically signs of lateral medullary dysfunction) eventually develop in up to 85% of the patients. The latent period between trauma and neurological symptoms may be variable, ranging from days to weeks and even years [1].

CT Angiogram or MRA/MRI is the investigation of choice. MRI shows vertebral arteries that are enlarged with a rim of hyperintense signal around a hypointense signal (lumen) [5].

Treatment for VAD lacks consensus with the option of using either anticoagulation or antiplatelet therapy for stroke prevention [14]. Rationale for anticoagulation is to prevent thrombogenic or embolic occlusion in the intimal flap that results from the separation of the intima from the vascular wall [11]. It is typically instituted for 3–6 months after ruling out subarachnoid hemorrhage or intracranial VAD [11]. Antiplatelet therapy offers a less risky alternative for bleeding complications. Adding to the pool of evidence, the maiden randomized trial CADISS found no difference in efficacy of antiplatelet and anticoagulant therapy in preventing stroke and death in patients with symptomatic carotid and vertebral artery dissection [14, 15]. Currently, the VAD therapy is tailored on a case-by-case basis and is often influenced by the experience and preference of the treating physician.

In a young individual less than 45 years of age presenting with stroke-related symptoms, a diagnosis of VAD can be easily mistaken for other more common causes of stroke. This case underscores the importance of considering VAD on the list of differentials when evaluating symptoms related to sports activities. In particular, a thorough history is essential and one must consider hyperextension or hyperrotation of the neck as part of the patient's activity that may have caused VAD.

8. Learning Points

(i) VAD is an underrecognized cause of stroke especially in younger age groups (less than 45 years of age).

(ii) VAD should be considered in symptomatic cases of hyperextension or hyperrotation of the neck during sports-related activities.

(iii) Due to a varied latent period, minor underlying trauma, and subtle presentation, a thorough history and strong index of suspicion are necessary for its timely diagnosis and treatment.

(iv) Antiplatelet therapy and anticoagulation are equally efficacious for the prevention of stroke in VAD.

Conflict of Interests

The authors declare that there is no conflict of interests.

References

[1] E. S. Lang, *Vertebral Artery Dissection*, 2014, http://emedicine.medscape.com/article/761451-overview.

[2] F. C. Albuquerque, Y. C. Hu, S. R. Dashti et al., "Craniocervical arterial dissections as sequelae of chiropractic manipulation: patterns of injury and management," *Journal of Neurosurgery*, vol. 115, no. 6, pp. 1197–1205, 2011.

[3] A. Pezzini, F. Granella, M. Grassi et al., "History of migraine and the risk of spontaneous cervical artery dissection," *Cephalalgia*, vol. 25, no. 8, pp. 575–580, 2005.

[4] C. Grond-Ginsbach and S. Debette, "The association of connective tissue disorders with cervical artery dissections," *Current Molecular Medicine*, vol. 9, no. 2, pp. 210–214, 2009.

[5] S. Debette and D. Leys, "Cervical-artery dissections: predisposing factors, diagnosis, and outcome," *The Lancet Neurology*, vol. 8, no. 7, pp. 668–678, 2009.

[6] G. J. Redekop, "Extracranial carotid and vertebral artery dissection: a review," *Canadian Journal of Neurological Sciences*, vol. 35, no. 2, pp. 146–152, 2008.

[7] R. Dziewas, C. Konrad, B. Dräger et al., "Cervical artery dissection—clinical features, risk factors, therapy and outcome in 126 patients," *Journal of Neurology*, vol. 250, no. 10, pp. 1179–1184, 2003.

[8] J. C. Maroon, P. Gardner, A. A. Abla, H. El-Kadi, and J. Bost, "'Golfer's stroke': golf-induced stroke from vertebral artery dissection," *Surgical Neurology*, vol. 67, no. 2, pp. 163–168, 2007.

[9] A. Lannuzel, T. Moulin, D. Amsallem, J. Galmiche, and L. Rumbach, "Vertebral-artery dissection following a judo session: a case report," *Neuropediatrics*, vol. 25, no. 2, pp. 106–108, 1994.

[10] F. Pacei, L. Valvassori, and L. Bet, "Vertebral artery dissection during Kung-Fu training," *Neurological Sciences*, vol. 35, no. 2, pp. 331–332, 2014.

[11] M. Ning and R. G. Gonzalez, "Case 34-2013—a 69-year-old man with dizziness and vomiting," *The New England Journal of Medicine*, vol. 369, no. 18, pp. 1736–1748, 2013.

[12] F. M. Amin, V. A. Larsen, and P. Tfelt-Hansen, "Vertebral artery dissection associated with generalized convulsive seizures: a case report," *Case Reports in Neurology*, vol. 5, no. 2, pp. 125–129, 2013.

[13] R. K. Menon and J. W. Norris, "Cervical arterial dissection. Current concepts," *Annals of the New York Academy of Sciences*, vol. 1142, pp. 200–217, 2008.

[14] S. E. Kasner, "CADISS: a feasibility trial that answered its question," *The Lancet Neurology*, vol. 14, no. 4, pp. 342–343, 2015.

[15] The CADISS trial investigators, "Antiplatelet treatment compared with anticoagulation treatment for cervical artery dissection (CADISS): a randomised trial," *The Lancet Neurology*, vol. 14, no. 4, pp. 361–367, 2015.

3

Case Series of Post-Thrombolysis Patients Undergoing Hemicraniectomy for Malignant Anterior Circulation Ischaemic Stroke

A. Williams,[1] M. Sittampalam,[2] N. Barua,[3] and A. Mohd Nor[2]

[1] *Department of Neurosurgery, Derriford Hospital, Plymouth, PL6 8DH, UK*
[2] *Department of Neurology, Derriford Hospital, Plymouth, PL6 8DH, UK*
[3] *Department of Neurosurgery, Frenchay Hospital, Bristol, BS16 1LE, UK*

Correspondence should be addressed to A. Williams, apwilliams13@gmail.com

Academic Editor: Gjumrakch Aliev

While ischaemic stroke remains a leading cause of death and disability, there have been recent advancements in treatment modalities including thrombolysis and decompressive hemicraniectomy. A retrospective review of patients treated in our NHS teaching hospital, in Plymouth (UK), over a 2 year period identified 17 thrombolysed patients, of whom two had undergone subsequent decompressive hemicraniectomy. These were non-dominant hemisphere strokes in young patients, aged 51 and 57. Initial NIHSS scores were 16 and 17, and they received thrombolysis at 2 hrs 42 min and 5 hrs 10 min post onset of symptoms respectively. CT imaging demonstrated cerebral swelling with significant midline shift in both cases, and decompressive hemicraniectomy was undertaken at 29 hrs 8 min and 27 hrs 30 min post-thrombolysis. We found no significant intra-operative complications attributable to prior use of thrombolytics. Both patients have had acceptable psychological and physical outcomes, with Barthel Index scores of 40 and 25, and MMSE scores of 29/30 and 27/30. We conclude that the use of thrombolytic therapy does not contra-indicate subsequent decompressive hemicraniectomy in well selected patients with non-dominant hemisphere strokes. More research in this field is required to elucidate factors which would facilitate recognition of stroke patients who will benefit most from aggressive medical and neurosurgical intervention.

1. Introduction

The acute treatment for ischaemic stroke, a leading cause of death and permanent disability in the Western world, underwent profound changes after the randomised double-blind NINDS study of intravenous thrombolysis in 1995 [1]. Despite its benefits, thrombolysis has remained an underused intervention perhaps due to its short window of efficacy, although this is being reconsidered [2], and delayed presentations to hospital are being addressed with multiple public health campaigns. Its benefits are, however, clearly documented. ECASS II [3], a multicentred European trial of 800 patients, using Alteplase (0.9 mg/kg) intravenously (IV), combined with strict CT and blood pressure inclusion criteria, supported the use of Alteplase within 3 hours of symptom onset. The potential benefits were counterbalanced by a 2- to 5-times increase in symptomatic intracranial haemorrhage. The NINDS study [1] suggested that intracerebral haemorrhage occurred in 5.8% of patients receiving tPA, which was associated with a 45% fatality rate.

In parallel with recent studies of thrombolysis, there has been an increase in interest in decompressive hemicraniectomy for anterior circulation ischaemic strokes since its initial description in 1935 [4]. Large cerebral infarcts are often associated with significant cerebral oedema, which may be significant enough to cause herniation and death. Hemicraniectomy was devised to counteract this postinfarction complication. This is most commonly a phenomenon of the second to fifth days after ictus [5], and half of deaths within the first month of young patients with ischaemic stroke can be attributed to space-occupying malignant infarction [6]. Again, this treatment is not without its controversies, the most predominant of which being that while it prevents death, it may promote life but with complete dependence.

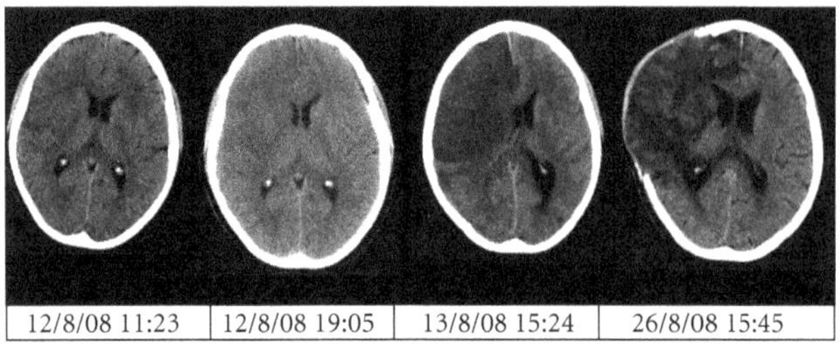

Figure 1

Recently, pooled data from three European multicentered, randomised, controlled trials (DECIMAL, DESTINY, and HAMLET) has suggested mortality and poor functional outcome can be improved by undertaking decompressive hemicraniectomy without increasing the numbers of completely dependent patients [7].

Combining these two interventions offers further opportunities to improve patient outcomes, but also raises further questions. Most predominant is the fear that precedent use of thrombolysis could predispose patients to excess risk of both intraoperative and postoperative haemorrhage. We sought to investigate this possibility in this retrospective analysis.

2. Methods

We examined clinical and surgical outcomes when decompressive hemicraniectomy was undertaken following intravenous thrombolysis in the same patients, and specifically when hemicraniectomy was undertaken for space-occupying cerebral oedema rather than post-thrombolysis haemorrhage. We analysed data from a cohort of patients treated in Derriford Hospital over a 30-month period from 13/05/2006 to 29/01/2009. Patients were identified by searching the hospital clinical coding database, using procedure codes for thrombolysis. The patients excluded either were thrombolysed for other reasons (e.g., myocardial infarction) or did not subsequently undergo hemicraniectomy. A total of 17 patients received intravenous thrombolysis between these dates, and two of these patients subsequently underwent decompressive hemicraniectomy. We undertook a detailed case notes study with interest focused on intraoperative and perioperative issues regarding the recent use of thrombolysis and patients' long-term outcome.

Case 1 (SK (Figure 1)). A 51-year-old right-handed female presented to the emergency department at 10:25 on 12/08/08, with a sudden onset left hemiplegia, occurring at 09:18, and involving the upper motor neurone of the VIIth cranial nerve and her upper and lower limbs, and a left-sided hemineglect. On admission her GCS was 15. Her past medical history included Hepatitis A in 1967. She had no medical allergies, and, aside from the oral contraceptive pill, she was on no medications. There was no contributory family history, and she was a life-long nonsmoker.

A noncontrast CT brain scan at 11:23 demonstrated characteristic grey and white matter changes in the right middle cerebral artery (MCA) territory and density within the right MCA, indicating acute infarct. There was no evidence of acute haemorrhage or hydrocephalus. Her admission blood profile was unremarkable (Hb 14.4, PLT 235, PT 12.8, APTT 23.2).

She was diagnosed with a right MCA ischaemic stroke, and, following appropriate consent, recombinant tissue plasminogen activator (rTPA), Alteplase was administered at 12:00. She was given a 5.4 mg bolus over 2 min, and then an infusion of 48.6 mg over the subsequent hour. A total of 54 mg rTPA was administered intravenously. Her blood pressure remained stable throughout.

Her neurological status remained unchanged until 13/08/08 when her GCS dropped to 9 (E3V1M5), and a CT brain scan (at 15:24) demonstrated an extensive right anterior cerebral artery (ACA) and MCA territory infarction. The associated mass effect resulted in 10 mm of midline shift to the left. There was radiological evidence of right uncal herniation. No intracranial haemorrhage was demonstrable.

After failed medical control of ICP, she underwent an emergency decompressive hemicraniectomy at 18:15 on 13/08/08. A standard operative protocol was used: a trauma flap was fashioned and frontotemporoparietal craniotomy was performed, and the dura was incised in a stellate pattern. The dura was left open, and an artificial dural patch (DuraGuard, Synovis, St. Paul, USA) was laid over the defect. No subgaleal drain was sited. Routine bipolar diathermy was sufficient for haemostasis. This was an uncomplicated procedure. Her postoperative haemoglobin was 11.7 (preoperative was 14.4). No intraoperative blood component transfusions were administered, though, one day later, she received a 2-unit packed red cell transfusion.

Thereafter, she was managed on the intensive therapy unit (ITU) for medical optimisation of her intracranial pressure (ICP). Clexane 40 mg s/c, Aspirin 75 mg, and Clopidogrel 75 mg were commenced within a week. A routine postoperative scan on 26/08/08 was satisfactory. The evolution of radiological changes on CT scanning are shown in Figure 1.

She was transferred for physical and neurological rehabilitation three weeks after surgery. At her most recent outpatient review (6 months after surgery), her MMSE was 29/30. She was able to move from lying to sitting independently, to transfer from bed to chair and chair to car with the assistance of one, to stand with supervision of one, and to walk 20 metres with hand-rail assistance. She lives in a nursing home, with no difficulties with swallowing or meeting her nutritional needs, and she is continent. She had required antidepressant medication during rehabilitation, though this is no longer the case. She has a Barthel Index Score of 40.

Case 2 (DH (Figure 2)). A 57-year-old right-handed male presented with sudden onset left hemiplegia at 13:30 on the 09/01/09 involving the upper motor neurone of the VIIth cranial nerve, and his left upper and lower limbs, but with a GCS of 15. His past medical history included right-sided sciatica and a childhood hypospadias repair. He had no medical allergies, nor used regular medications. He was a nonsmoker with an unremarkable family history.

A noncontrast CT brain scan at 17:03 demonstrated clear evidence of an acute, nonhaemorrhagic infarct in the right MCA territory, occupying greater than 50% of the usual MCA territory. Thrombus was seen in the right MCA. Routine investigations of blood parameters were unremarkable (Hb 14.9 PLT 242 PT 14.0 APTT 28.4).

He was consented for off-licence thrombolysis with Alteplase. This was commenced at 18:40 with a bolus of 6.3 mg over 2 minutes, followed by a 56.7 mg infusion over the subsequent hour. Thus, a total of 63 mg was prescribed intravenously. Blood pressure was monitored throughout the infusion, and there were no hypertensive episodes during administration.

The infusion was stopped early, after 53 mg total dose, as the patient developed a generalised tonic-clonic seizure. A repeat CT brain scan at 20:10 demonstrated evolving MCA territory malignant infarction with no evidence of acute haemorrhage, and the patient was subsequently intubated and ventilated on ITU.

Evolution of a fixed right mydriatic pupil was noted on the 10/01/09, and a repeat CT brain scan at 16:43 demonstrated that the cerebral oedema associated with the MCA infarct had significantly progressed with 12 mm shift in midline structures to the left. A left-sided intraparenchymal ICP bolt was inserted at 17:30, and ICP readings remained at 18–20 cm H20 despite optimal medical intervention.

On 10/01/09, a decision was made to proceed with decompressive hemicraniectomy due to refractory ICPs. A similar procedure was undertaken: the dura was opened, and an artificial dural patch (Dura-Guard) was laid over the defect. A subgaleal drain was sited for 48 hours. Bipolar diathermy was sufficient for haemostasis. There was a 220 mL blood loss intraoperatively. Postoperative Hb was 11.2 (14.3 preoperatively), and no intraoperative or postoperative blood component transfusions were required.

A routine postoperative scan demonstrated a maturing infarct involving the whole of the right MCA territory, but no intracranial haemorrhage. The shift of the midline structures had resolved, and the basal cisterns were patent. He was later discharged to intensive physical and neurological rehabilitation. Serial CT scan findings are shown in Figure 2.

On review nine months after stroke, his level of function allowed transfer from bed to chair with the assistance of one, and standing with two for short periods. He is independently mobile in a wheelchair. He is able to write independently, and his cognition is intact with only mild memory deficit (MMSE 27/30). There is no deficit in swallow safety, and no requirement for nutritional support. The cranial vault defect has been repaired with a titanium cranioplasty. He does, however, lack some insight into his physical condition and potential, and has required antidepressant medication. Due to impaired mobility, he has suffered with double incontinence. His Barthel Index Score is 25.

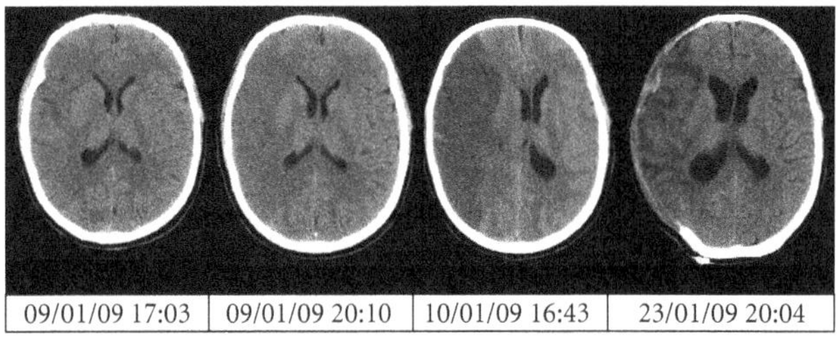

Figure 2

3. Discussion

Tissue plasminogen activator (t-PA) is an exogenous stimulator of the fibrinolytic system which degrades fibrin clots through activation of plasminogen to plasmin [8]. Plasmin not only lyses the fibrin component of a blood clot but also contributes to tissue remodelling by degrading extracellular matrix proteins, either directly or via the activation of matrix metalloproteinases [9].

In nonsurgically managed patients, serious complications of t-PA include systemic bleeding and anaphylaxis, but the most worrisome adverse reaction is intracerebral haemorrhage (ICH). Studies demonstrate symptomatic ICH occurs within 36 hours of treatment in 6.4% of patients treated with t-PA compared with 0.6% of patients treated with placebo. Despite this increased haemorrhage rate, mortality was similar in both groups with a trend toward increased mortality in the placebo group (21%) compared with the treatment group (17%) [1].

Moreover, there is a further concern that if neurosurgery is undertaken after intravenous thrombolysis, there may be an increased risk of perioperative haemorrhage, with significant risk of mortality. However, t-PA is rapidly cleared from the plasma at 550–680 mL/min, giving an initial distribution phase half-life of under 5 minutes, and a terminal elimination phase of approximately 40 minutes. Thus, 50% of t-PA is cleared from the plasma within 5 minutes after discontinuation of an IV infusion, and approximately 80% is cleared within 10 minutes.

Malignant infarction and resultant space-occupying cerebral oedema is most common between the second and fifth days postictus [5], and, given the short serum half-life of t-PA, it is likely that any excess haemorrhage risk has returned to baseline at the time when neurosurgical intervention is being considered. However, there is little experimental or anecdotal evidence to confirm this hypothesis at present, and the evidence will need to be examined in greater detail before definitive conclusions on the safety of major neurosurgical intervention following thrombolysis can be reached.

This study has identified two cases in which both thrombolysis and decompressive hemicraniectomy have been undertaken in the same patients. In both cases, the patients rapidly underwent thrombolysis, and subsequently underwent emergency neurosurgery, and both patients survived with the avoidance of a vegetative state (Table 1). Furthermore, neither patient suffered any haemorrhagic complication of undergoing both interventions.

A recently published study [10] of mortality following stroke reported 17 patients who underwent hemicraniectomy following initial thrombolysis. It was demonstrated that thrombolysis prior to hemicraniectomy had no effect on inpatient hospital mortality (odds ratio 1.21, 95% confidence interval 0.43, 3.39). In support of this finding, our case reports may point the way for further studies into the

Table 1

	Patient 1	Patient 2
Age	51	57
Time from onset of symptoms to arrival to hospital	1 hr 7 min	2 hrs 8 min
NIHSS scores on admission	16	17
Time from onset of symptoms to thrombolysis	2 hrs 42 min	5 hrs 10 min
Time from onset of symptoms to operation	32 hrs 57 min	32 hrs 40 min
Time between thrombolysis and operation	29 hrs 8 min	27 hrs 30 min
Barthel index scores	40	25
Mini-mental state examination	29/30	27/30

role of neurosurgical intervention following intravenous thrombolysis. While it is impossible to make any definitive conclusions from a case series of two patients, we found no evidence that hemicraniectomy is associated with excess haemorrhage risk in patients receiving prior thrombolysis. More research into these treatments is needed to further elucidate the potential for both modalities to be used in appropriate patients.

Despite these successful cases, our findings clearly have caveats. These are both young patients, and selection for such aggressive interventions is appropriately biased in favour of the younger patient in whom the outcomes after stroke are demonstrably better. Both were nondominant hemisphere stokes, and clearly remained significantly disabled. Therefore, it would be unwise to extrapolate any findings to dominant hemisphere strokes.

4. Conclusions

Intracerebral haemorrhage is a potentially fatal complication of intravenous thrombolysis. However, there is very little evidence to support or refute the hypothesis that prior thrombolysis results in excess haemorrhage risk for patients who suffer space-occupying cerebral oedema and are selected for subsequent decompressive hemicraniectomy. Decompressive hemicraniectomy following thrombolysis represents an aggressive treatment paradigm, and the decision to proceed with such intervention requires a multidisciplinary team approach and a frank and open discussion with patients and/or their relatives. Whilst decompressive hemicraniectomy may preserve both life and function in well-selected patients, the potential risks of surgery, including life-threatening haemorrhage, must be discussed with patients and/or relatives in order to obtain a fully informed consent. This case series supports the hypothesis that decompressive hemicraniectomy following intravenous thrombolysis is not associated with excess haemorrhage risk. However, definitive guidelines must be based on larger prospective clinical studies.

References

[1] J. R. Marler, "Tissue plasminogen activator for acute ischemic stroke," *The New England Journal of Medicine*, vol. 333, no. 24, pp. 1581–1587, 1995.

[2] A. Stemer and P. Lyden, "Evolution of the thrombolytic treatment window for acute ischemic stroke," *Current Neurology and Neuroscience Reports*, vol. 10, no. 1, pp. 29–33, 2010.

[3] D. Jenkinson, "ECASS-II: intravenous alteplase in acute ischaemic stroke. European Co-operative Acute Stroke Study-II," *The Lancet*, vol. 353, no. 9146, pp. 67–68, 1999.

[4] T. Greco, "Post-traumatic thrombosis of the carotid artery," *Archivio Italiano di Chirurgia*, vol. 29, pp. 757–784, 1935.

[5] J. I. Frank, "Large hemispheric infarction, deterioration, and intracranial pressure," *Neurology*, vol. 45, no. 7, pp. 1286–1290, 1995.

[6] J. Biller, H. P. Adams, A. Bruno, B. B. Love, and E. E. Marsh, "Mortality in acute cerebral infarction in young adults—a ten-year experience," *Angiology*, vol. 42, no. 3, pp. 224–230, 1991.

[7] K. Vahedi, J. Hofmeijer, E. Juettler et al., "Early decompressive surgery in malignant infarction of the middle cerebral artery: a pooled analysis of three randomised controlled trials," *The Lancet Neurology*, vol. 6, no. 3, pp. 215–222, 2007.

[8] H. R. Lijnen and D. Collen, "Tissue-type plasminogen activator," *Annales de Biologie Clinique*, vol. 45, no. 2, pp. 198–201, 1987.

[9] H. R. Lijnen, "Plasmin and matrix metalloproteinases in vascular remodeling," *Thrombosis and Haemostasis*, vol. 86, no. 1, pp. 324–333, 2001.

[10] A. Alshekhlee, C. Horn, R. Jung, A. Alawi, and S. Cruz-Flores, "In-hospital mortality in acute ischemic stroke treated with hemicraniectomy in US hospitals," *Journal of Stroke and Cerebrovascular Diseases*. In press.

4

Ischemic Stroke of the Artery of Percheron with Normal Initial MRI

Guillaume Cassourret,[1] Bertrand Prunet,[1] Fabrice Sbardella,[2] Julien Bordes,[1] Olga Maurin,[1] and Henry Boret[1]

[1] *Intensive Care Unit, Sainte-Anne Hospital, Boulevard Sainte Anne, 83000 Toulon, France*
[2] *Department of Radiology, Sainte-Anne Hospital, 83000 Toulon, France*

Correspondence should be addressed to Bertrand Prunet, bertrand.prunet@orange.fr

Academic Editor: Huy M. Do

The artery of Percheron is a solitary trunk representing an uncommon anatomic variant that provides bilateral arterial supply to the paramedian thalami and the rostral midbrain. Occlusion of this artery results in bilateral thalamic and mesencephalic infarctions. The clinical diagnosis is difficult because the complex anatomy causes large clinical variability. We report a case of a comatose patient with normal early head-computed tomography and magnetic resonance imaging. A bilateral paramedian thalamic infarct due to an occlusion of the artery of Percheron was revealed two days later by a new head computed tomography. To our knowledge, this is the first report in the literature of a symptomatic patient presenting an acute Percheron stroke with normal early brain magnetic resonance imaging. Our case indicates that a normal initial magnetic resonance imaging cannot formally eliminate the diagnosis of acute stroke of the artery of Percheron. We discuss the causes of noncontributive brain magnetic resonance imaging at the onset of this acute Percheron stroke and the alternative diagnosis and therapy methods.

1. Introduction

Percheron described four normal variations of the neurovascular anatomy of the thalami and midbrain (Figure 1). The medial part of the thalami is supplied from the posterior circulation via the perforating thalamic arteries, also called paramedian arteries [1]. Variation I is the most common, where each perforating artery arises from each left and right posterior cerebral artery. In variation IIb, the bilateral perforating thalamic arteries arise from one central artery called the artery of Percheron, which arises from the P1 segment of one posterior cerebral artery. It supplies the paramedian thalami and the rostral midbrain [2–4]. Consequently, occlusion of the artery of Percheron causes a bilateral paramedian thalamic and mesencephalic infarction [2, 5]. Magnetic resonance imaging (MRI) normally allows visualization of the initial infarct in cases of acute cerebral ischemia and is usually used in stroke centers as the primary or early secondly imaging modality.

We report a case of a patient admitted for coma without evident cause and normal early imaging by head computed tomography (CT) and MRI. A new head CT two days later revealed a bilateral paramedian thalamic infarct at the origin of the initial symptoms.

2. Case Presentation

A 64-year-old right-handed Caucasian man presented with a sudden loss of consciousness at home, 5 minutes after feeling discomfort with dysarthria. His past medical history included dyslipidemia, diabetes, obesity, and chronic atrial fibrillation. He was treated with long-term oral anticoagulants (fluindione), but with poor therapeutic observance. He was found comatose by the prehospital team. On examination, the patient had the following initial vital signs: temperature 36.4°C, pulse 78 beats/min, respiratory rate 16 breaths/min, and blood pressure 148/87 mmHg. On

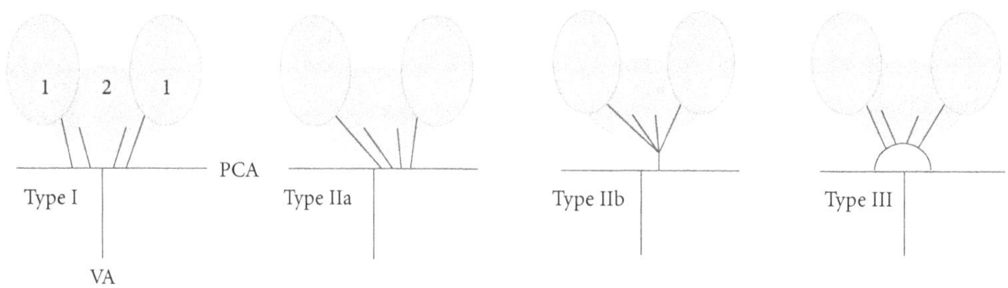

FIGURE 1: The four variations of the vascularization of the thalami and the midbrain described by Percheron (1: Thalami, 2: Midbrain, PCA: Posterior Cerebral Artery, VA: Vertebral Artery).

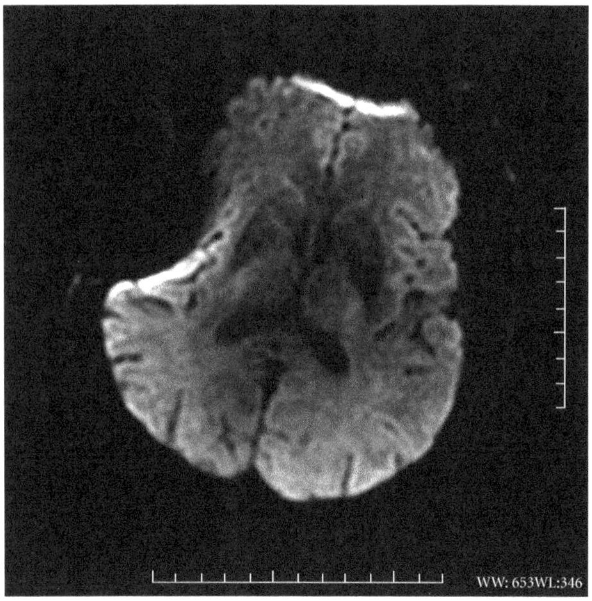

FIGURE 2: Axial cerebral DWI ($b = 1000\,s/mm^2$) performed 95 minutes after the onset symptoms show no ischemic lesion.

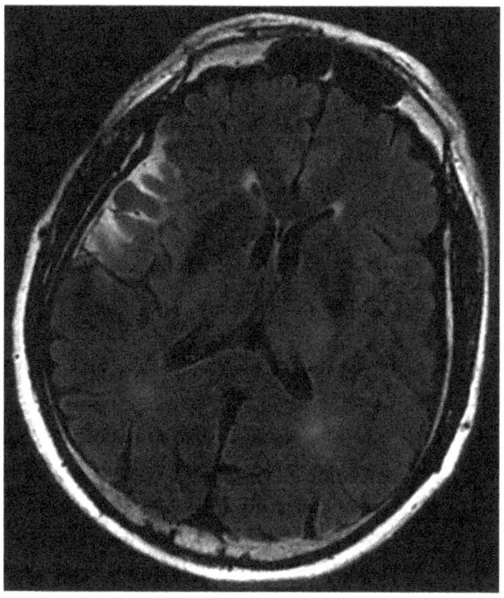

FIGURE 3: Axial cerebral FLAIR performed 95 minutes after the onset symptoms show no ischemic lesion.

neurological examination, the Glasgow coma-scale score was 7 with localizing pain being the best motor response and no opening of eyes or verbal response. Pupillary light reflex in the right eye was 4 mm nonreactive and that in the left eye was 3 mm reactive. The deep tendon reflexes were present and symmetric. Babinski sign was found on both feet. Capillary blood glucose was found to be 123 mg/dL. The electrocardiogram showed atrial fibrillation, with no abnormal repolarization. He was intubated and mechanically ventilated and then brought to the emergency department. The initial head CT, performed 65 minutes after loss of consciousness, showed no acute hemorrhage or other abnormality. To eliminate an acute ischemic infarction, a brain MRI was then performed 95 minutes after the onset symptoms. It did not reveal significant acute infarction signals: no lesion was found on diffusion-weighted (DW) images (Figure 2), on apparent diffusion coefficient images, or on T2-weighted fluid-attenuated inversion recovery (FLAIR) images (Figure 3). The T2* images confirmed the absence of hemorrhage. This MRI was of inferior quality because of right artifacts due to osteosynthesis material for a right zygomatic fracture a few years previously. Cerebral arteriography was not performed, and the patient was admitted to the intensive care unit. Ionogram and complete blood count were normal. No drugs were found in the blood. The anticoagulant therapy was inefficient with an index normalized ratio of 1.2. The cerebrospinal fluid analysis was normal. Electroencephalogram recording did not show epileptiform activity.

A new head CT was performed 48 hours later (Figure 4). It revealed a bilateral paramedian thalamic hypodensity corresponding to an obstruction of the artery of Percheron. A transesophageal echocardiography revealed a left atrial thrombus. The patient was anticoagulated with intravenous heparin. Sedation was stopped on day 3, and the patient was extubated on day 6. At first, neurologic examination showed altered levels of consciousness, eyes opening and vertical gaze palsy, and progressive response to simple orders. He was then gradually able to open his eyes normally, to speak, and to walk, but partial memory impairments were still present. After four weeks in a neurology department, the patient was discharged home in good condition with oral long-term anticoagulants.

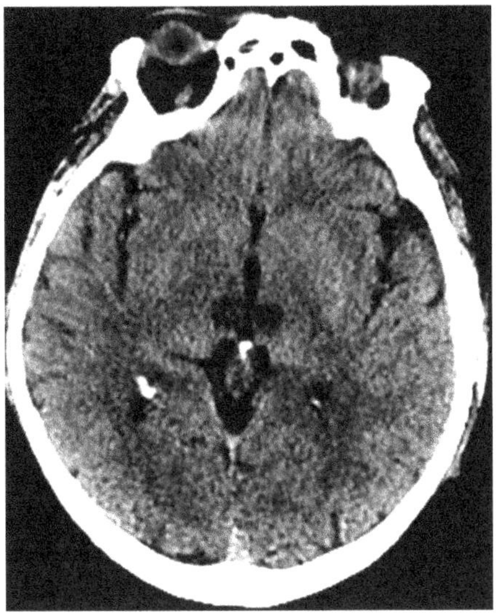

Figure 4: Head CT on day 2 showing bilateral symmetrical hypodensity of the medial part of the thalami corresponding to the occlusion of the artery of Percheron.

3. Discussion

Bithalamic paramedian infarcts are rare, and it is painful to suspect them because of the complex anatomy causing large clinical variability [5–7]. The four main symptoms found in the literature are vertical gaze palsy (65%), memory impairment (58%), confusion (53%), and coma (42%) [7]. The prognosis is fairly good, as in our observation [4, 7, 8]. It may be ameliorated with the treatment of acute stroke, the thrombolytic therapy. It can be performed if the diagnosis of an acute stroke is done [9]. In stroke centers, MRI is the reference exam to diagnose acute brain ischemia. The combination of pathologic diffusion-weighted images and normal findings on T2-weighted FLAIR images in the paramedian thalami and possibly the mesencephalic area suggests an acute stroke of the artery of Percheron [9]. With a brain MRI showing an acute stroke, intravenous thrombolysis can be performed, if the deadline for achieving it is not exceeded (4 hours and 30 minutes after the onset symptoms). Presence of a hypersignal in T2-weighted FLAIR images and blood supply study also affect the decision of thrombolytic therapy. In our case, the early MRI was inconclusive and did not allow thrombolytic therapy. To our knowledge, this is the first case describing an artery of Percheron acute stroke with early nonsignificant MRI.

Several reasons can explain the MRI results. The imaging was achieved with a head and neck antenna, which is probably less precise on this part of the brain compared with a head antenna. In addition, the brain MRI, performed 95 minutes after the onset of symptoms, was probably done earlier than in other reported cases. This demonstrates that modern neuroimaging is extremely valuable in making a positive diagnosis but normal imaging studies alone, however, do not exclude a vascular etiology. Small lesion size, brainstem lesions, small cortical lesions, and DW-imaging performed within a few hours after stroke onset are features associated with a particular risk of false-negative DW-images [10, 11]. In our case, there was no indication to perform a cerebral arteriography because of the negative MRI result. Furthermore, the efficiency and risks of such a therapy have not been evaluated. Moreover, such vessels are usually not visible on angiograms. Nevertheless, a case report describing successful artery of Percheron in situ thrombolysis in a patient similar to ours has been reported. However, the diagnosis suspicion was clinical with normal head CT, and MRI obtained after the arteriography [8].

4. Conclusion

In conclusion, our case indicates that a normal initial MRI cannot formally eliminate the diagnosis of acute stroke of the artery of Percheron, especially if performed very early or if the technical conditions are not optimal. These findings suggest the presentation of acute rostral brain stem stroke accompanied by a nonconclusive brain MRI should encourage to perform a new brain imaging by MRI within therapeutic times or should consider doing interventional explorations focused on the vertebrobasilar territory. On that basis, intravenous or in situ thrombolytic therapy should be performed. Interventional explorations focused on the vertebrobasilar territory have not been evaluated but may allow to confirm the diagnosis of Percheron artery lesion. However, only one successful case has been described. Anytime the initial imaging is normal, new brain imaging by MRI or CT scan should be performed within the first 48 hours.

References

[1] A. Cosson, L. Tatu, F. Vuillier, B. Parratte, M. Diop, and G. Monnier, "Arterial vascularization of the human thalamus: extra-parenchymal arterial groups," *Surgical and Radiologic Anatomy*, vol. 25, no. 5-6, pp. 408–415, 2003.

[2] G. Percheron, "The anatomy of the arterial supply of the human thalamus and its use for the interpretation of the thalamic vascular pathology," *Journal of Neurology*, vol. 205, no. 1, pp. 1–13, 1973.

[3] G. Percheron, "Arteries of the human thalamus. II. Arteries and paramedian thalamic territory of the communicating basilar artery," *Revue Neurologique*, vol. 132, no. 5, pp. 309–324, 1976 (French).

[4] G. Raphaeli, A. Liberman, J. M. Gomori, and I. Steiner, "Acute bilateral paramedian thalamic infarcts after occlusion of the artery of Percheron," *Neurology*, vol. 66, no. 1, p. E7, 2006.

[5] L. Ben Slamia, H. B. Jemaa, S. Benammou, and K. Tlili-Graiess, "Occlusion of the artery of percheron: clinical and neuroimaging correlation," *Journal of Neuroradiology*, vol. 35, no. 4, pp. 244–245, 2008.

[6] M. G. Matheus and M. Castillo, "Imaging of acute bilateral paramedian thalamic and mesencephalic infarcts," *American Journal of Neuroradiology*, vol. 24, no. 10, pp. 2005–2008, 2003.

[7] P. Monet, P.-Y. Garcia, G. Saliou, et al., "Bithalamic infarct: is there an evocative aspect? Radioclinical study," *Revue Neurologique*, vol. 165, no. 2, pp. 178–184, 2009 (French).

[8] V. Kostanian and S. C. Cramer, "Artery of Percheron thrombolysis," *American Journal of Neuroradiology*, vol. 28, no. 5, pp. 870–871, 2007.

[9] W. Krampla, B. Schmidbauer, and W. Hruby, "Ischaemic stroke of the artery of Percheron," *European Radiology*, vol. 18, no. 1, pp. 192–194, 2008.

[10] S. T. Engelter, S. G. Wetzel, L. H. Bonati, F. Fluri, and P. A. Lyrer, "The clinical significance of diffusion-weighted MR imaging in stroke and TIA patients," *Swiss Medical Weekly*, vol. 138, no. 49-50, pp. 729–740, 2008.

[11] P. N. Sylaja, S. B. Coutts, A. Krol, M. D. Hill, and A. M. Demchuk, "When to expect negative diffusion-weighted images in stroke and transient ischemic attack," *Stroke*, vol. 39, no. 6, pp. 1898–1900, 2008.

5

Hyperacute Therapies for Childhood Stroke: A Case Report and Review of the Literature

Jose Irazuzta[1] and Kevin J. Sullivan[1,2]

[1] *Division of Pediatric Critical Care Medicine, University of Florida Health Science Center at Jacksonville and The Wolfson Children's Hospital, 800 Prudential Drive, Jacksonville, FL 32207, USA*
[2] *Department of Anesthesia, Mayo Clinic Rochester, Rochester, MN 55905, USA*

Correspondence should be addressed to Jose Irazuzta, jose.irazuzta@jax.ufl.edu

Academic Editor: Guillaume Sebire

Objective. The optimal management of pediatric patients with arterial ischemic stroke (AIS) is not known. Despite this, goal-oriented, time-sensitive therapies geared to rapid reestablishment of arterial blood flow are occasionally applied with beneficial effects. The inconsistent approach to AIS is in part due to a lack of knowledge and preparedness. *Methods.* Case report of a 12-year-old male with right middle cerebral artery (MCA) occlusion resulting in dense left hemiplegia and mutism and review of the literature. *Intervention(s).* Mechanical thrombectomy, intra-arterial administration of rt-PA, vasodilators, and platelet inhibitors, and systemic anticoagulation and subsequent critical care support. *Results.* Restoration of right MCA blood flow and complete resolution of neurologic deficits. *Conclusion.* We report the gratifying outcome of treatment of a case of AIS in a pediatric patient treated with hyperacute therapies geared to arterial recanalization and subsequent neurologic critical care and review the pertinent literature. Guidelines for the emergency room management of pediatric AIS from prospective, randomized trials are needed.

1. Introduction

Arterial ischemic stroke (AIS) occurs more commonly in adults than children. In children the clinical presentation is often interpreted as other neurologic conditions or intoxications resulting in a delay in diagnosis due to the lack of awareness of pediatrician or that the symptoms do not systematically evoke a stroke. Adult AIS occurs in the setting of the principal risk factors of hypertension and atherosclerosis, while pediatric risk factors are heterogeneous and include focal intracranial arteriopathies, congenital cardiovascular diseases, and hemoglobinopathies [1, 2]. Recent advances in the management of AIS have emphasized the importance of timely diagnosis and restoration of arterial flow in the affected vascular territories. Adult victims have access to time-sensitive or hyperacute therapies due to an awareness of the severity of the disease, organization of delivery of medical care from the emergency room that includes designation of stroke centers, and protocol-driven preparedness for such emergencies [3–6]. Unfortunately, this is not the case for pediatric victims, because it is not known whether thrombolytic therapies are appropriate.

We describe the case of a 12-year-old male with AIS who presented to medical attention with a potentially devastating neurological injury. A resolute strategy utilizing hyperacute therapies aimed at restoring blood flow followed by neurointensive care support was provided. The patient had a very good outcome that may be related to this management but a complete causation cannot be ascribed to it as 1 out of 3 patients with lenticulostriate stroke may have a spontaneous favorable evolution. Herein we review the literature to date describing the challenges in analyzing and preparing for the application of time-sensitive therapies in the treatment of AIS.

2. Case Report

The institutional IRB was consulted and waved the need for approval of the publication of this case. The patient is a 12-year-old, right-handed, 52 kg African-American male

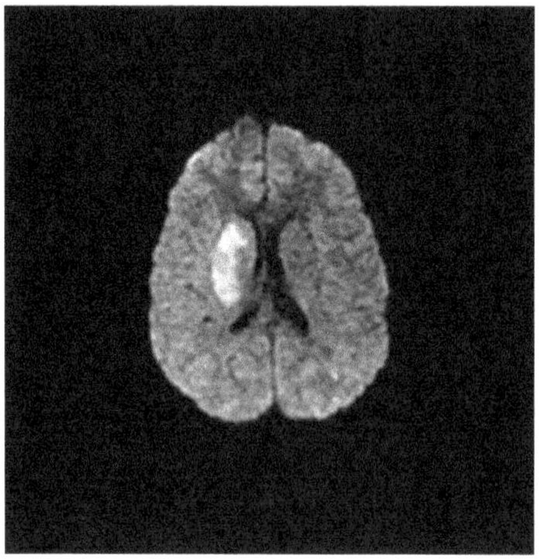

FIGURE 1: Diffusion weighted imaging (DWI) showing area of restricted diffusion.

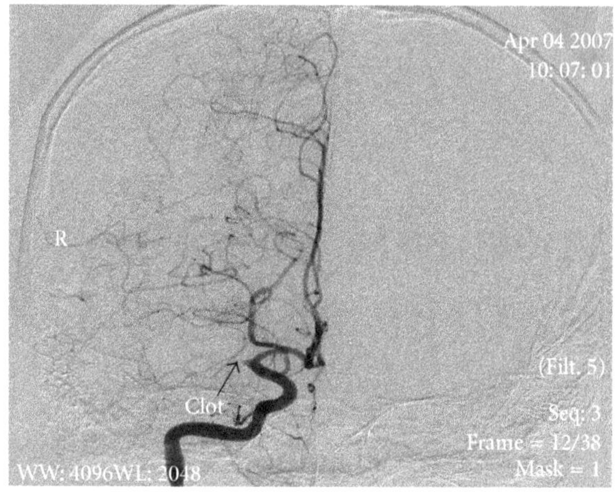

FIGURE 2: Coronal view of angiography arrow pointing to the area the Middle Cerebral Artery occlusion.

without any significant medical history other than nocturnal enuresis. His father woke him up at 04:00 on the morning of admission as was customary in their home to prevent bedwetting. While initially he responded appropriately, the child collapsed to the ground after standing and became unresponsive. He was transported to an outlying emergency department where he was noted to have aphasia and left dense hemiplegia. Computed tomography demonstrated signal attenuation and edema in the vascular distribution of the right middle cerebral artery. Right lateral ventricle compression and midline shift were noted.

The patient was transferred to our institution by helicopter and was briefly examined in the emergency room prior to transfer to the magnetic resonance (MR) imaging suite. He was awake, with stable airway, anxious and frustrated by inability to speak, but was cooperative and able to follow some commands. Heart rate was 50–60 beats per minute and blood pressure was 130–140/80–90 mm Hg. He demonstrated lack of language expression, flaccid paralysis of the left face, upper extremity, and lower extremity. His NIH stroke score was 16. MRI and MRA studies revealed occlusion of the right middle cerebral artery with restricted diffusion in the right basal ganglia and the posterior lateral aspect of the caudate head (Figure 1). There was mass effect on the right lateral ventricle and midline shift. Our information was that 6 h had elapsed since the onset of neurologic symptoms. Taking into account the possibility of a devastating clinical outcome and in conjunction with adult stroke and interventional radiologist specialist, the decision was made to attempt to restore arterial patency.

The patient was anesthetized, intubated, and cooled to 33–35°C (mild therapeutic hypothermia). A thrombus was located (Figures 2 and 3); endovascular mechanical embolectomy with a Merci retrieval device was attempted without success. Recombinant tissue plasminogen activator (rt-PA) was infused into the MCA in doses of 0.7, 2, and 4 mg with minimal improvement in blood flow. Abciximab and nitroglycerin (25 μg) were then infused with considerable improvement in blood flow (Figures 4 and 5).

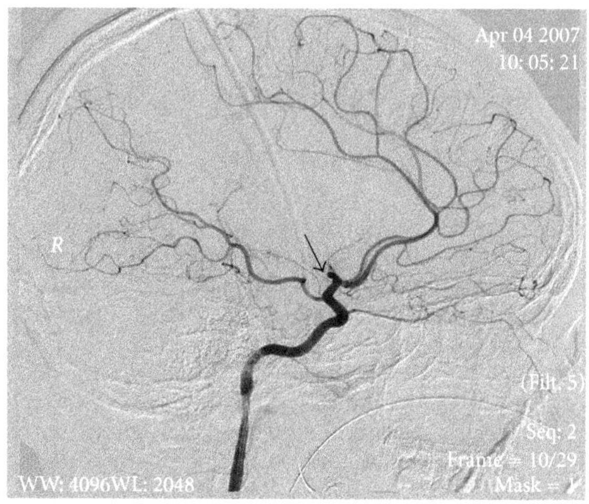

FIGURE 3: Sagittal view of angiography arrow pointing to the area the Middle Cerebral Artery occlusion.

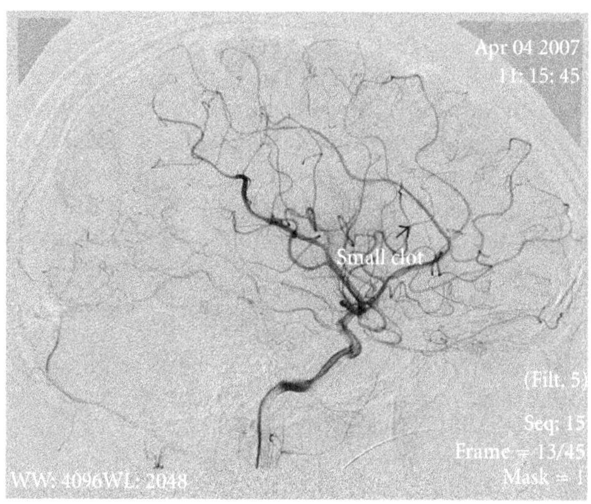

FIGURE 4: Sagittal view demonstrating a significant improvement in blood flow after rt-PA Abciximab and nitroglycerin were infused. Arrow points to a small residual occlusion.

The patient was transferred to the pediatric ICU and remained sedated and mechanically ventilated. Neurosurgical consultation was obtained for an intracranial pressure (ICP) monitoring, but this was not placed due to recent thrombolytic administration and the initiation of systemic anticoagulation. Heparin was administered for 7 days, Abciximab ($10\,\mu g$/min for the first 12 h), aspirin (325 mg/day), magnesium sulfate (2000 mg/24 hrs), 25% albumin (1 g/kg IV every 6 h for the first 5 days), and memantine HCL (10 mg nasogastric each day for 3 days). Mild therapeutic hypothermia was maintained for 4 days to decrease acute postischemic cerebral edema followed by passive rewarming over a 24-hour period. A CT scan obtained at 24 hrs showed a decrease in the midline shift.

The central venous pressure (CVP) was maintained at 8–10 cm H_2O and mean arterial pressure (MAP) at 75–80 mm Hg. A dual channel near infrared spectroscopy (NIRS) probe was applied to the scalp overlying both frontal lobes. Initially, there was a discrepancy between the two sides with the ischemic right side 10%–15% lower than the left side (40%–50% versus 65%–70%). Increasing CVP or MAP served only to augment the discrepancy. Subsequently, the partial pressure of arterial carbon dioxide was allowed to increase from 35–40 to 46–55 mm Hg with resolution of the discrepancy (both sides equal to 60%–65%).

MR studies on the 7th day revealed appropriate MCA blood flow and partial resolution of the ischemic changes in the basal ganglia. Mass effect and right lateral ventricle compression by the basal ganglia were improved. He was extubated on day 10 and was able to communicate verbally, written, and receptive but had a small degree of residual left hemiparesis. He was transferred to a rehabilitation facility on day 15 where he exhibited an almost complete recovery within the following two weeks and was discharged home. Subsequent followup by our pediatric neurology service over the next year has demonstrated complete recovery to baseline without deficits. One year later he is taking advanced placement classes in school, playing junior high school basketball and baseball, and having no demonstrable neurological deficits.

Cerebral angiography and serologic studies did not find the presence of dissection, vasculitis, or autoimmune disease; transthoracic echocardiography ruled out structural heart disease, intracardiac thrombus, and right to left intracardiac shunt, and hemoglobin electrophoresis, hypercoagulability studies, and lipid panels were all unremarkable. Doppler studies of the veins of the lower extremities and pelvis were all negative for deep venous thrombosis. An etiology for this patient AIS has not been found. An MRI performed 3 months after the events showed resolution of the edema and restricted diffusion with a residual hyperdense signal abnormally in the periventricular region (Figure 6).

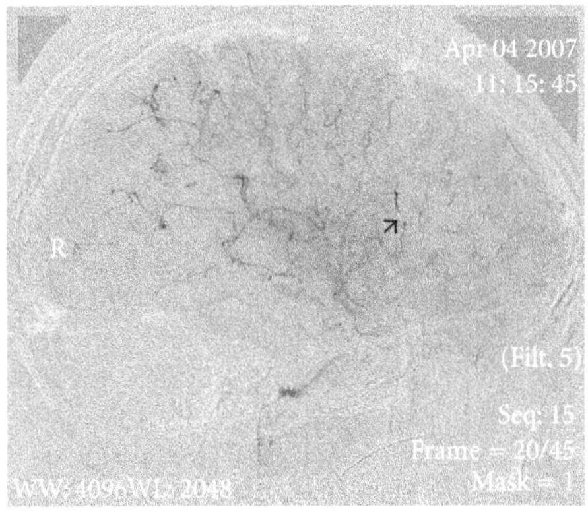

Figure 5: Sagittal view demonstrating a significant improvement in blood flow after rt-PA Abciximab and nitroglycerin were infused. Arrow points to a small residual occlusion.

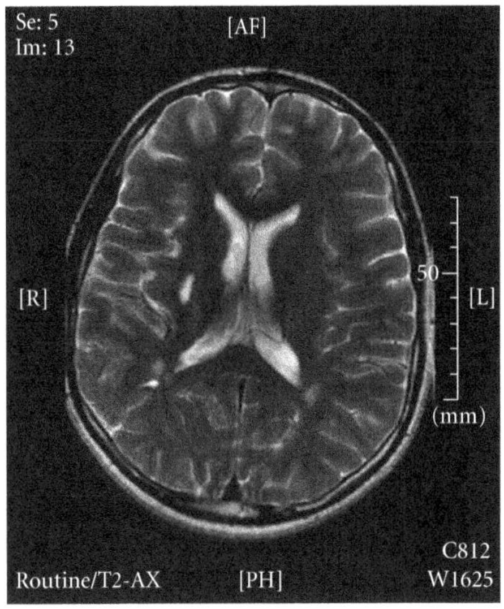

Figure 6: MRI 3 month after the initial insult showing a residual hyperdense signal abnormally in the periventricular region.

3. Discussion

Our case report differs from others in the literature in that intra-arterial thrombolysis was undertaken 6 h after the onset of symptoms than most other reports of anterior circulation occlusion and few other patients have made as complete a recovery. Several provocative issues relevant to AIS in children are raised by his management: (a) the use of hyperacute therapies, (b) the role of antiplatelet agents and anticoagulants in the management of AIS, and (c) the role of adjunctive pharmacological neuroprotective agents.

The growing recognition that AIS in adults is reversible if treated in a prompt manner has fostered a sense of urgency in clinicians who regard this condition as a "brain attack" and hospitals preparedness with designation of stroke centers for rapid triage and treatment. The resolve of the physician has a decisive effect on the timely implementation of therapies for stroke in adults [3].

By comparison, little sense of urgency to aggressively restore vascular patency exists for pediatric patients, and with the exception of AIS in the setting of sickle cell disease and Moyamoya disease, therapeutic approaches that embrace supportive care and rehabilitation are more common in pediatric hospitals. Development of a similar sense of determination and urgency is hampered by several obstacles. First, pediatric emergency room practitioners encounter AIS infrequently, and it is therefore not uncommon for considerable delay to occur in the diagnosis excluding the patient from the accepted time windows for hyperacute therapies. Second, the outcome of children with stroke is incorrectly thought to be better than that of adults. The outcome of AIS is mainly determined by size, location, and etiology of stroke. While the pediatric mortality is described to be between 5%–10% and is favorable when compared to adult patients, pediatric survivors of AIS are left with persistent neurologic and psychosocial deficit or seizure disorder for the rest of their lives [7, 8]. Third, the pathophysiology underlying the heterogeneous disorders of pediatric AIS makes it difficult to extrapolate the adult AIS literature to children, and many children's hospitals do not have preplanned algorithms for rapid diagnosis and treatment of AIS. Finally, many practitioners are uncomfortable administering thrombolytic medications in the absence of pediatric-specific data or clinical guidelines to support their use. Indeed, most recommendations for the treatment of AIS in children are derived from consensus and expert opinion, and neither the Royal College of Physicians (RCP) in the United Kingdom nor the American College of Chest Physicians (ACCP) in the United States recommends the administration of rt-PA to children with AIS [9, 10]. Despite this reluctance, several case reports to date have described their use in children [11–16], and a review of a national inpatient database registry indicates that a small minority of pediatric patients with AIS are receiving thrombolytic therapy [17, 18].

3.1. Thrombolysis/Embolectomy. The term "hyperacute therapies" has been coined to refer to therapies which must be initiated within an acceptable time interval in order to be effective, and they are designed to restore blood flow through obstructed vascular beds. Hyperacute therapies that are offered to adults include intravenous thrombolysis with rt-PA, intra-arterial thrombolysis with rt-PA, and mechanical embolectomy.

The use of intravenous thrombolysis is now well established in the literature and is recommended for the treatment of AIS in adults without contraindications who present to medical attention within 3 h of symptoms onset [4, 5]. Patients treated with 0.9 mg/kg rt-PA (10% as a bolus and the remainder infused over 1 hour) had better functional outcomes at 3 months when compared to patients who received placebo, and mortality rates were similar between the two groups. Symptomatic intracranial hemorrhage occurred in 6.4% of patients treated with rt-PA and 0.6% of controls. The time period from onset of stroke symptoms to beneficial treatment with thrombolytic medications remains a subject of continuous debate. The debate addresses the observation that as time from symptom onset increases the likelihood of outcome benefit from thrombolysis decreases while thrombolytic therapy is associated with a substantial increase in likelihood of intracranial hemorrhage. However, a recent publication demonstrated benefit while extending the administration up to 4.5 h after the onset of symptoms [6]. Furthermore, whether strict adherence to predefined time interval cutoffs should be used to determine whether thrombolytic therapy should be offered is unclear. Comparison of MRI diffusion-weighted imaging (DWI) and perfusion-weighted imaging (PWI) may allow the clinician to determine for each patient how much brain tissue is receiving inadequate blood flow (abnormal PWI) to still viable brain tissue (intact DWI). Such an examination might allow clinicians to determine for patients presenting after more prolonged time intervals from onset of neurologic symptoms whether thrombolytic therapy could still be beneficial to a given patient [10, 11, 18, 19].

Intra-arterial administration of thrombolytics (urokinase and rt-PA) is sometimes offered as a potential, viable alternative for the delivery of thrombolytic medications to obstructed cerebral vascular beds for patients who are not candidates for systemic intravenous thrombolysis or those who present to medical attention between 3 and 6 h after symptom onset. Intra-arterial administration of recombinant prourokinase and intravenous heparin within 6 h of onset of stroke symptoms resulted in improved functional outcomes when compared to intravenous heparin alone [20], but intra-arterial and intravenous thrombolyses have not been compared to each other.

Other options for recanalization of obstructed cerebral vasculature include the use of endovascular mechanical retrieval devices for clot removal. Intra-arterial and endovascular mechanical embolectomies have extended the time window for treatment up to 8 h for AIS in the anterior circulation, and even longer in cases involving the posterior circulation. While mechanical intra-arterial thrombectomy has demonstrated a high recanalization rate [21], randomized trials that describe functional outcome are lacking.

There is evidence that thrombolytic medications are being administered to 1.6% of the children with AIS, and this data suggests that children may have inferior clinical outcomes with respect to mortality [18]. However, it cannot be determined from this data whether inferior outcomes are related to AIS severity or the treatment itself. Pediatrics encompasses a wide range of ages with maturational differences. Optimal rt-PA dosing is likely to differ as there are age-dependent differences in hemostasis [22, 23], younger individuals demonstrating diminished specific indices of fibrinolysis and global, increased fibrinolytic capacity [22]. Case reports over the past eight years have described the administration of thrombolytic medications to pediatric patients with good result at widely different interval from onset of symptoms [13, 16, 24–29]. Location of the AIS and anticipated neurological deficits is a major consideration. Indeed, due to the dire outcome of vertebrobasilar thrombosis (VBT), case reports in the pediatric literature describe successful administration of thrombolytic therapy 17 h after the onset of symptoms [24, 25].

3.1.1. Anticoagulation and Antiplatelet Therapy. The role of anticoagulation in pediatric AIS patients is unclear. The RCP and ACCP guidelines provide recommendations for acute treatment and secondary prevention of AIS. Their recommendations differ with respect to the role of anticoagulation in the acute management of AIS in children. RCP guidelines for the management of acute AIS in children (not associated with intracranial hemorrhage or sickle cell disease) recommend the administration of aspirin (5 mg/kg/day) [10]. The ACCP guidelines for management of acute AIS in children have a Class II recommendation in regard to the initiation of unfractionated heparin or low-molecular weight heparin (LMWH) for 5–7 days or until cardioembolic stroke and vascular dissection have been excluded [2, 9, 10]. Heparin may be safe for the treatment of strokes secondary to sinovenous thrombosis even though studies in regard to efficacy are lacking. The ACCP points out that while LMWH may offer reproducible pharmacokinetics and fewer monitoring tests in comparison with unfractionated heparin the effects of LMWH cannot be rapidly reversed after its discontinuation [2]. Adult guidelines from the AHA recommend the administration of aspirin (325 mg/day) within 24–48 h of stroke onset [4, 5].

For secondary prevention of AIS recurrence the ACCP recommends initiation of aspirin therapy (2–5 mg/kg/day) after discontinuation of anticoagulation [9]. For children with vascular dissection or cardioembolic stroke the ACCP recommends continuation of anticoagulation with low-molecular weight heparin or vitamin K antagonists for 3–6 months [9]. The RCP recommends continuation of aspirin (1–3 mg/kg/day) for all children except those with Moyamoya disease, sickle cell disease, or arterial dissection [6]. The RCP recommends treatment with anticoagulation for prevention of secondary AIS in patients with arterial dissection or cardioembolic stroke [10].

While aspirin is the major antiplatelet agent in clinical use, the roles for other antiplatelet and anticoagulant medications are under investigation. Adjuvant medications such as thrombin inhibitors and inhibitors of platelet glycoprotein IIb/IIIa (GIIb/IIIa) are being evaluated as monotherapy and in combination with rt-PA for the treatment of acute ischemic stroke. Current studies also evaluate the use of argatroban (a thrombin inhibitor) [30], ancrod (a viper-derived enzyme that cleaves fibrinogen and promotes endogenous release of plasminogen activator) [31, 32], and desmoteplase (a bat saliva-derived protease similar in function to human plasminogen activator) [33, 34]. A recently completed phase III trial with an intravenous administration of a glycoprotein IIb/IIIa antagonists, Abciximab, did not demonstrate safety or efficacy with an increased incidence of intracranial hemorrhage [35].

3.1.2. Attempts to Prevent Secondary Neuronal Injury. The literature is not clear how to prevent secondary injury in AIS. Once blood flow through the MCA was restored, and measures were taken to protect the ongoing patency of the vessel, we next considered measures that attempted to minimize secondary neuronal injury during reperfusion of the ischemic regions of the brain. Included among these were (a) the maintenance of adequate cerebral blood flow, (b) the prevention of hyperglycemia, (c) the continuation of mild therapeutic hypothermia, and (d) administration of 25% albumin, magnesium salts, and N-methyl-D-aspartate receptor (NMDA) antagonists.

Maintenance of adequate cerebral perfusion pressure may be of importance in optimizing neurologic outcome after AIS if regional autoregulation is lost or in cases of severe increase in intracranial pressure. While verification of adequacy of cerebral perfusion pressure might have been optimized with the assistance of an ICP monitor, the risks of ICP monitor placement in this anticoagulated child were felt to be prohibitive. In the absence of ICP monitoring we assumed that our patient probably had at least moderately increased ICP. Accordingly, we allowed moderate permissive hypertension, maintained a high osmolarity with hypertonic saline and mild hypothermia. Fever should be aggressively treated [36] in AIS, and mild hypothermia has shown to decreases acute postischemic cerebral edema, a transient phenomenon that is maximal at 2–4 days postinfarct [37–39]. However it has been difficult to ascertain a positive impact in outcome with its use, and a large randomized study is needed [40]. A rebound in intracranial pressure can occur when rewarming a patient that was hypothermic.

As an indirect monitor of the adequacy of cerebral perfusion, near infrared spectroscopy (NIRS) monitoring was applied to both cerebral hemispheres. In the initial h, regional cerebral oxygen saturation (rSO_2) was significantly lower in the compromised hemisphere. The stepwise preload augmentation and addition of norepinephrine to augment mean arterial pressure only increased the differences as a "steal" phenomenon by the nonaffected area. The subsequent introduction of mild permissive hypercapnia produced an increase and equalization of rSO_2 in both hemispheres.

While these trends in rSO_2 could be interpreted to indicate the restoration of adequate oxygen supply/demand in the affected hemisphere, prior studies employing NIRS in the noninvasive monitoring of patients with middle cerebral artery infarction and cerebral edema suggest that disappearance of the rSO_2 difference between hemispheres may indicate worsening cerebral edema and herniation in the infarcted hemisphere [41]. Computed tomography of the brain on day 3 and reassuring neurologic examinations during improving rSO_2 values in the affected hemisphere assured us that the disappearance of the rSO_2 gradient between hemispheres was not due to an ominous process. The role of NIRS as a noninvasive monitor of cerebral circulation in pediatric stroke remains to be delineated.

3.1.3. Other Potentially Neuroprotective Pharmacologic Interventions. Our patient was treated with scheduled infusions of hypertonic albumin after returning from the angiography suite. The administration of hypertonic solutions of albumin is recommended for the treatment of adult ischemic stroke patients in our institution and is based on studies that demonstrate improved functional neurologic outcome in adult patients suffering from ischemic stroke [42, 43]. Preclinical and phase I and II trials of the administration of albumin in acute ischemic stroke suggest that the time to administration of albumin after ischemic stroke is critically important (within 4-5 h) [44] and that a synergistic effect may exist when rt-PA is also administered [42]. The physiologic benefit of albumin administration is believed to be related to its effect on the endothelium [45–49], blood viscosity and aggregation [50], interactions with nitric oxide [51], and inhibition of platelet aggregation [52, 53]. Studies of albumin administration in experimental models of central nervous system ischemia demonstrate that albumin administration rapidly improves blood flow in cerebral vessels with critically reduced flow and clears thrombotic material adherent to the endothelium in ischemic venules [53, 54]. While preliminary studies of high dose albumin administration to AIS patients have been encouraging, the results of the multicenter, randomized, placebo-controlled efficacy trial of albumin in acute ischemic stroke—ALIAS Phase III trial is underway and may provide definitive answers on the role of albumin therapy in adult AIS. Pediatric trials on the use of albumin in this setting are still lacking. Hypertonic albumin administration may induce pulmonary edema in adults; however it is frequently utilized in pediatric intensive care in patients with other conditions without deleterious effects. Decompressive craniotomy is an effective treatment to treat increased intracranial pressures in patients with extensive stroke [55].

We administered memantine HCl and magnesium sulfate on a scheduled basis. This is the routine practice of our adult stroke team, and their administration is predicated on several theoretical principles. The magnesium ion regulates cellular energy metabolism, vascular tone, and cell membrane ion transport [56]. Magnesium may regulate ATP concentrations and is a prerequisite for ATP regeneration after ischemia and reperfusion [57, 58]. The magnesium ion also blocks the ion channel of the N-methyl-D-aspartate (NMDA) receptor in a voltage-dependent fashion, and increasing extracellular magnesium concentrations in vitro cause noncompetitive NMDA blockade [59, 60]. In vitro and in vivo models of focal and global ischemia have demonstrated neuronal protection that in some instances is as great as that seen with noncompetitive NMDA antagonists. Magnesium protects both hippocampal neurons from glutamate-mediated necrosis and white matter tracts from prolonged ischemia [61]. Systemic $MgCl_2$ decreased cerebral infarct volume by 20% after permanent middle cerebral artery occlusion in the rat [62]. Memantine hydrochloride, another NMDA receptor antagonist, was also administered to attenuate reperfusion injury. While a neuroprotective role has been ascribed to magnesium sulfate and NMDA receptor antagonists, no data from human trials have shown conclusive benefit to adult patients with AIS, and data is therefore certainly lacking to make recommendations regarding use in pediatric AIS.

4. Conclusions

The case described is a paradigmatic observation of the possibility of using hyperacute therapies in children with strokes: early recognition of the event, probable thromboembolism mechanism, MCA distribution, and rapid consultation with multiple specialists were crucial factors influencing the decision process. Thrombolysis is probably less favorable when other types of vasculopathy, that most often affect young children (e.g., basal arterial stenosis), are present. There is a need to increase awareness of childhood stroke by pediatricians and emergency room physicians caring for children with the aim of reducing the time lag from symptoms to the correct diagnosis. It is imperative to have in place a preplanned diagnostic algorithm as well as therapeutic algorithm. Most of emergency departments do not receive regularly children with stroke. Except in very specific cases, it is thus not possible to build autonomic pediatric stroke centers. Nevertheless, as it is well documented in the present case report, collaboration between emergency room physicians, pediatric neurologists, and physicians working in adult stroke centers should be highly considered.

References

[1] W. J. Molofsky, "Managing stroke in children," *Pediatric Annals*, vol. 35, no. 5, pp. 379–384, 2006.

[2] E. S. Roach, M. R. Golomb, R. Adams et al., "Management of stroke in infants and children: a scientific statement from a special writing group of the american heart association stroke council and the council on cardiovascular disease in the young," *Stroke*, vol. 39, no. 9, pp. 2644–2691, 2008.

[3] J. F. Maestre-Moreno, M. D. Fernández-Pérez, C. Arnáiz-Urrutia, A. Mínguez, P. Navarrete-Navarro, and J. Martínez-Bosch, "Thrombolysis in stroke: inappropriate consideration of the 'window period' as the time available," *Revista de Neurologia*, vol. 40, no. 5, pp. 274–278, 2005.

[4] H. P. Adams Jr., G. del Zoppo, and M. J. Alberts, "Guidelines for the early management of adults with ischemic stroke: a guideline from the american heart association/american stroke association stroke council, clinical cardiology council, cardiovascular radiology and intervention council, and the atherosclerotic peripheral vascular disease and quality of care outcomes in research interdisciplinary working groups: the american academy of neurology affirms the value of this guideline as an educational tool for neurologists," *Circulation*, vol. 115, pp. e478–e534, 2007.

[5] R. L. Sacco, R. Adams, G. Albers et al., "Guidelines for prevention of stroke in patients with ischemic stroke or transient ischemic attack: a statement for healthcare professionals from the American Heart Association/American Stroke Association Council on Stroke—co-sponsored by the Council on Cardiovascular Radiology and Intervention. The American Academy of Neurology affirms the value of this guideline," *Circulation*, vol. 113, no. 10, pp. e409–e449, 2006.

[6] W. Hacke, M. Kaste, E. Bluhmki et al., "Thrombolysis with alteplase 3 to 4.5 hours after acute ischemic stroke," *The New England Journal of Medicine*, vol. 359, no. 13, pp. 1317–1329, 2008.

[7] S. Lanthier, L. Carmant, M. David, A. Larbrisseau, and G. de Veber, "Stroke in children: the coexistence of multiple risk factors predicts poor outcome," *Neurology*, vol. 54, no. 2, pp. 371–378, 2000.

[8] G. DeVeber, E. Steve Roach, A. R. Riela, and M. Wiznitzer, "Stroke in children: recognition, treatment, and future directions," *Seminars in Pediatric Neurology*, vol. 7, no. 4, pp. 309–317, 2000.

[9] P. Monagle, A. Chan, P. Massicotte, E. Chalmers, and A. D. Michelson, "Antithrombotic therapy in children: the seventh ACCP conference on antithrombotic and thrombolytic therapy," *Chest*, vol. 126, no. 3, pp. 645S–687S, 2004.

[10] Royal College of Physicians PSWG, "Stroke in childhood: clinical guidelines for diagnosis, management, and rehabilitation," 2004, http://www.rcplondon.ac.uk/pubs/books/childstroke/.

[11] G. A. Ortiz, S. Koch, D. M. Wallace, and R. Lopez-Alberola, "Successful intravenous thrombolysis for acute stroke in a child," *Journal of Child Neurology*, vol. 22, no. 6, pp. 749–752, 2007.

[12] S. L. Benedict, O. K. Ni, P. Schloesser, K. S. White, and J. F. Bale, "Intra-arterial thrombolysis in a 2-year-old with cardioembolic stroke," *Journal of Child Neurology*, vol. 22, no. 2, pp. 225–227, 2007.

[13] M. D. Carlson, S. Leber, J. Deveikis, and F. S. Silverstein, "Successful use of rt-PA in pediatric stroke," *Neurology*, vol. 57, no. 1, pp. 157–158, 2001.

[14] M. R. Golomb, M. Rafay, D. Armstrong et al., "Intra-arterial tissue plasminogen activator for thrombosis complicating cerebral angiography in a 17-year-old girl," *Journal of Child Neurology*, vol. 18, no. 6, pp. 420–423, 2003.

[15] E. A. Noser, R. A. Felberg, and A. V. Alexandrov, "Thrombolytic therapy in an adolescent ischemic stroke," *Journal of Child Neurology*, vol. 16, no. 4, pp. 286–288, 2001.

[16] B. C. Cannon, N. J. Kertesz, R. A. Friedman, and A. L. Fenrich, "Use of tissue plasminogen activator in a stroke after radiofrequency ablation of a left-sided accessory pathway," *Journal of Cardiovascular Electrophysiology*, vol. 12, no. 6, pp. 723–725, 2001.

[17] C. Amlie-Lefond, G. deVeber, A. K. Chan et al., "Use of alteplase in childhood arterial ischaemic stroke: a multicentre, observational, cohort study," *The Lancet Neurology*, vol. 8, no. 6, pp. 530–536, 2009.

[18] N. Janjua, A. Nasar, J. K. Lynch, and A. I. Qureshi, "Thrombolysis for ischemic stroke in children: data from the nationwide inpatient sample," *Stroke*, vol. 38, no. 6, pp. 1850–1854, 2007.

[19] G. Thomalla, C. Schwark, J. Sobesky et al., "Outcome and symptomatic bleeding complications of intravenous thrombolysis within 6 hours in MRI-selected stroke patients: comparison of a German multicenter study with the pooled data of ATLANTIS, ECASS, and NINDS tPA trials," *Stroke*, vol. 37, no. 3, pp. 852–858, 2006.

[20] A. Furlan, R. Higashida, L. Wechsler et al., "Intra-arterial prourokinase for acute ischemic stroke. The PROACT II study: a randomized controlled trial," *Journal of the American Medical Association*, vol. 282, no. 21, pp. 2003–2011, 1999.

[21] A. C. Flint, G. R. Duckwiler, R. F. Budzik, D. S. Liebeskind, and W. S. Smith, "Mechanical thrombectomy of intracranial internal carotid occlusion: pooled results of the MERCI and multi MERCI part I trials," *Stroke*, vol. 38, no. 4, pp. 1274–1280, 2007.

[22] N. A. Goldenberg, W. E. Hathaway, L. Jacobson, K. Mcfarland, and M. J. Manco-Johnson, "Influence of factor VIII on overall coagulability and fibrinolytic potential of haemophilic plasma as measured by global assay: monitoring in haemophilia A," *Haemophilia*, vol. 12, no. 6, pp. 605–614, 2006.

[23] A. A. Smith, L. J. Jacobson, B. I. Miller, W. E. Hathaway, and M. J. Manco-Johnson, "A new euglobulin clot lysis assay for global fibrinolysis," *Thrombosis Research*, vol. 112, no. 5-6, pp. 329–337, 2003.

[24] E. C. Bourekas, A. P. Slivka, and M. J. Casavant, "Intra-arterial thrombolysis of a distal internal carotid artery occlusion in an adolescent," *Neurocritical Care*, vol. 2, no. 2, pp. 179–182, 2005.

[25] A. Sungarian and J. A. Duncan III, "Vertebrobasilar thrombosis in children: report of two cases and recom-mendations for treatment," *Pediatric Neurosurgery*, vol. 38, no. 1, pp. 16–20, 2003.

[26] M. Arnold, M. Steinlin, A. Baumann et al., "Thrombolysis in childhood stroke report of 2 cases and review of the literature," *Stroke*, vol. 40, no. 3, pp. 801–807, 2009.

[27] M. I. Shuayto, J. I. Lopez, and F. Greiner, "Administration of intravenous tissue plasminogen activator in a pediatric patient with acute ischemic stroke," *Journal of Child Neurology*, vol. 21, no. 7, pp. 604–606, 2006.

[28] R. S. Prasad, L. A. Michaels, S. Roychowdhury, V. Craig, A. Sorrell, and S. Schonfeld, "Combined venous sinus angioplasty and low-dose thrombolytic therapy for treatment of hemorrhagic transverse sinus thrombosis in a pediatric patient," *Journal of Pediatric Hematology/Oncology*, vol. 28, no. 3, pp. 196–199, 2006.

[29] A. Kirton, J. H. Wong, J. Mah et al., "Successful endovascular therapy for acute basilar thrombosis in an adolescent," *Pediatrics*, vol. 112, no. 3, part 1, pp. e248–e251, 2003.

[30] R. M. Sugg, J. K. Pary, K. Uchino et al., "Argatroban tPA stroke study: study design and results in the first treated cohort," *Archives of Neurology*, vol. 63, no. 8, pp. 1057–1062, 2006.

[31] D. G. Sherman, R. P. Atkinson, T. Chippendale et al., "Intravenous ancrod for treatment of acute ischemic stroke. The STAT study: a randomized controlled trial," *Journal of the American Medical Association*, vol. 283, no. 18, pp. 2395–2403, 2000.

[32] The Ancrod Stroke Study Investigators, "Ancrod for the treatment of acute ischemic brain infarction," *Stroke*, vol. 25, no. 9, pp. 1755–1759, 1994.

[33] A. J. Furlan, D. Eyding, G. W. Albers et al., "Dose escalation of desmoteplase for acute ischemic stroke (DEDAS): evidence of safety and efficacy 3 to 9 hours after stroke onset," *Stroke*, vol. 37, no. 5, pp. 1227–1231, 2006.

[34] W. Hacke, G. Albers, Y. Al-Rawi et al., "The desmoteplase in acute ischemic stroke trial (DIAS): a phase II MRI-based 9-hour window acute stroke thrombolysis trial with intravenous desmoteplase," *Stroke*, vol. 36, no. 1, pp. 66–73, 2005.

[35] H. P. Adams Jr., M. B. Effron, J. Torner et al., "Emergency administration of abciximab for treatment of patients with acute ischemic stroke: results of an international phase III trial: abciximab in emergency treatment of stroke trial (AbESTT-II)," *Stroke*, vol. 39, no. 1, pp. 87–99, 2008.

[36] M. D. Ginsberg and R. Busto, "Combating hyperthermia in acute stroke: a significant clinical concern," *Stroke*, vol. 29, no. 2, pp. 529–534, 1998.

[37] S. E. Kasner, A. M. Demchuk, J. Berrouschot et al., "Predictors of fatal brain edema in massive hemispheric ischemic stroke," *Stroke*, vol. 32, no. 9, pp. 2117–2123, 2001.

[38] A. Terent, G. Ronquist, K. Bergstrom, R. Hallgren, and H. Aberg, "Ischemic edema in stroke. A parallel study with computed tomography and cerebrospinal fluid markers of disturbed brain cell metabolism," *Stroke*, vol. 12, no. 1, pp. 33–40, 1981.

[39] K. Z. Guluma, H. Oh, S.-W. Yu, B. C. Meyer, K. Rapp, and P. D. Lyden, "Effect of endovascular hypothermia on acute ischemic edema: morphometric analysis of the ICTuS trial," *Neurocritical Care*, vol. 8, no. 1, pp. 42–47, 2008.

[40] H. M. Den Hertog, H. B. van der Worp, M.-C. Tseng, and D. W. J. Dippel, "Cooling therapy for acute stroke," *Cochrane Database of Systematic Reviews*, no. 1, Article ID CD001247, 2009.

[41] M. S. Damian and R. Schlosser, "Bilateral near infrared spectroscopy in space-occupying middle cerebral artery stroke," *Neurocritical Care*, vol. 6, no. 3, pp. 165–173, 2007.

[42] Y. Y. Palesch, M. D. Hill, K. J. Ryckborst, D. Tamariz, and M. D. Ginsberg, "The ALIAS Pilot Trial. A dose-escalation and safety study of albumin therapy for acute ischemic stroke—II: neurologic outcome and efficacy analysis," *Stroke*, vol. 37, no. 8, pp. 2107–2114, 2006.

[43] M. D. Ginsberg, M. D. Hill, Y. Y. Palesch, K. J. Ryckborst, and D. Tamariz, "The ALIAS pilot trial. A dose-escalation and safety study of albumin therapy for acute ischemic stroke—I: physiological responses and safety results," *Stroke*, vol. 37, no. 8, pp. 2100–2106, 2006.

[44] L. Belayev, Y. Liu, W. Zhao, R. Busto, and M. D. Ginsberg, "Human albumin therapy of acute ischemic stroke: marked neuroprotective efficacy at moderate doses and with a broad therapeutic window," *Stroke*, vol. 32, no. 2, pp. 553–560, 2001.

[45] J. E. Schnitzer, A. Sung, R. Horvat, and J. Bravo, "Preferential interaction of albumin-binding proteins, gp30 and gp18, with conformationally modified albumins. Presence in many cells and tissues with a possible role in catabolism," *Journal of Biological Chemistry*, vol. 267, no. 34, pp. 24544–24553, 1992.

[46] P. He and F. E. Curry, "Albumin modulation of capillary permeability: role of endothelial cell [Ca^{2+}](i)," *American Journal of Physiology*, vol. 265, no. 1, pp. H74–H82, 1993.

[47] L. Ghitescu, A. Fixman, M. Simionescu, and N. Simionescu, "Specific binding sites for albumin restricted to plasmalemmal vesicles of continuous capillary endothelium: receptor-mediated transcytosis," *Journal of Cell Biology*, vol. 102, no. 4, pp. 1304–1311, 1986.

[48] J. E. Schnitzer, "Gp60 is an albumin-binding glycoprotein expressed by continuous endothelium involved in albumin transcytosis," *American Journal of Physiology*, vol. 262, no. 1, pp. H246–H254, 1992.

[49] J. E. Schnitzer and P. Oh, "Antibodies to SPARC inhibit albumin binding to SPARC, gp60, and microvascular endothelium," *American Journal of Physiology*, vol. 263, no. 6, pp. H1872–H1879, 1992.

[50] W. H. Reinhart and C. Nagy, "Albumin affects erythrocyte aggregation and sedimentation," *European Journal of Clinical Investigation*, vol. 25, no. 7, pp. 523–528, 1995.

[51] J. F. Keaney Jr., D. I. Simon, J. S. Stamler et al., "NO forms an adduct with serum albumin that has endothelium-derived relaxing factor-like properties," *Journal of Clinical Investigation*, vol. 91, no. 4, pp. 1582–1589, 1993.

[52] N. Maalej, R. Albrecht, J. Loscalzo, and J. D. Folts, "The potent platelet inhibitory effects of S-nitrosated albumin coating of artificial surfaces," *Journal of the American College of Cardiology*, vol. 33, no. 5, pp. 1408–1414, 1999.

[53] P. W. Huh, L. Belayev, W. Zhao, R. Busto, I. Saul, and M. D. Ginsberg, "The effect of high-dose albumin therapy on local cerebral perfusion after transient focal cerebral ischemia in rats," *Brain Research*, vol. 804, no. 1, pp. 105–113, 1998.

[54] L. Belayev, E. Pinard, H. Nallet et al., "Albumin therapy of transient focal cerebral ischemia: in vivo analysis of dynamic microvascular responses," *Stroke*, vol. 33, no. 4, pp. 1077–1084, 2002.

[55] V. Ramaswamy, V. Mehta, M. Bauman, L. Richer, P. Massicotte, and J. Y. Yager, "Decompressive hemicraniectomy in children with severe ischemic stroke and life-threatening cerebral edema," *Journal of Child Neurology*, vol. 23, no. 8, pp. 889–894, 2008.

[56] R. A. Reinhart, "Clinical correlates of the molecular and cellular actions of magnesium on the cardiovascular system," *American Heart Journal*, vol. 121, no. 5, pp. 1513–1521, 1991.

[57] F. A. X. Schanne, R. K. Gupta, and P. K. Stanton, "31P-NMR study of transient ischemia in rat hippocampal slices in vitro," *Biochimica et Biophysica Acta*, vol. 1158, no. 3, pp. 257–263, 1993.

[58] B. M. Altura, R. L. Barbour, T. L. Dowd, F. Wu, B. T. Altura, and R. K. Gupta, "Low extracellular magnesium induces intracellular free Mg deficits, ischemia, depletion of high-energy phosphates and cardiac failure in intact working rat hearts: a 31P-NMR study," *Biochimica et Biophysica Acta*, vol. 1182, no. 3, pp. 329–332, 1993.

[59] L. Nowak, P. Bregestovski, P. Ascher, A. Herbet, and A. Prochiantz, "Magnesium gates glutamate-activated channels in mouse central neurones," *Nature*, vol. 307, no. 5950, pp. 462–465, 1984.

[60] N. L. Harrison and M. A. Simmonds, "Quantitative studies on some antagonists of N-methyl D-aspartate in slices of rat cerebral cortex," *British Journal of Pharmacology*, vol. 84, no. 2, pp. 381–391, 1985.

[61] P. K. Stys, B. R. Ransom, and S. G. Waxman, "Effects of polyvalent cations and dihydropyridine calcium channel blockers on recovery of CNS white matter from anoxia," *Neuroscience Letters*, vol. 115, no. 2-3, pp. 293–299, 1990.

[62] Y. Izumi, S. Roussel, E. Pinard, and J. Seylaz, "Reduction of infarct volume by magnesium after middle cerebral artery occlusion in rats," *Journal of Cerebral Blood Flow and Metabolism*, vol. 11, no. 6, pp. 1025–1030, 1991.

6

HIV Infection and Acute Stroke: A Case Report and a Review of the Literature

Hussein Assallum, Mohammad Alkayem, and Nehad Shabarek

Department of Internal Medicine, Lincoln Medical and Mental Health Center, 234 E 149th Steet, Bronx, NY 10451, USA

Correspondence should be addressed to Hussein Assallum; hassallum@gmail.com

Academic Editor: Ingo W. Husstedt

Background. In the United States, ischemic stroke in HIV-infected patients has increased by 60%. However, unexpected cardiovascular events in relatively young patients have been observed. *Clinical Vignette.* A 31-year-old male who presented with a 5-hour history of sudden onset slurred speech and left hemiplegia. He has medical history of HIV infection for 2 years taking ARTs. On exam, a significant left hemiparesis was noticed. Brain MRI showed right anterior corona radiata and basal ganglia acute infarction. *Discussion.* Several mechanisms have been proposed for the relationship between HIV infection and cardiovascular risk. (i) HIV-associated dyslipidemia: HIV-infected patients tend to develop decrease in HDL-c and LDL-c levels. ART was associated with an increase in LDL-c but little change in HDL-c. (ii) Endothelial dysfunction: certain antiretroviral agents may independently contribute to endothelial damage. (iii) Hypertension: systolic blood pressure is higher in those using ART for greater than five years. (iv) Insulin resistance and diabetes have been noticed with ART. (v) Chronic inflammation. (vi) Hypercoagulability: decrease in proteins C and S was associated with HIV infection. *Conclusion.* Poorly controlled HIV infection and/or the introduction of ATR might be risk factors for cardiovascular events. More studies needed to address this medical dilemma.

1. Background

In the United States, stroke risk in human immunodeficiency virus- (HIV-) infected patients increased 60% over the decade from 1997 through 2006 [1]. Since the emergence of AIDS in 1981, substantial advances in our understanding of the acquired immune deficiency syndrome (AIDS) have been achieved.

In addition, therapy was dramatically altered with the introduction of antiretroviral drugs in 1987 and revolutionized by combination treatment, known as antiretroviral therapies (ARTs) in 1996 which dramatically decreased mortality and morbidity of HIV as EuroSIDA study had shown [2]. But soon after the introduction of protease inhibitors (PIs) and nonnucleoside reverse-transcriptase inhibitors (NNRTIs) for the management of HIV infection, clinicians observed unexpected cardiovascular events among patients receiving this new combination in patients who were relatively young. This concern was validated by several reports; the French Hospital Database on HIV found that patients who had been treated with protease inhibitor for 18 months or more had twice the risk of myocardial infarction that was seen among patients with less drug exposure [3]. A cross-sectional study carried out on HIV-infected patients had shown that stroke in patients with HIV/AIDS was not associated with opportunistic infections and tumors, and early assessment of the vascular status was recommended [4]. We are presenting the case of HIV-infected young patient with acute stroke to discuss the risk factors of cardiovascular events in patients with HIV infection on ART as stroke is a rising cause of disability in HIV and AIDS populations.

2. Epidemiology

In a cohort study comparing stroke incidence in HIV-infected patients versus non-HIV-infected patients, the incidence rate was 5.27 per 1000 person-years in HIV-infected patients compared with 3.75 in non-HIV-infected patients, with an unadjusted HR of 1.40 (95% confidence interval (CI): 1.17 to 1.69, $P < 0.001$) [5]. Another cohort study done by Vinikoor et al. in the University of North Carolina of a total of 2,515 HIV-infected adults contributed a median of 4.5 years of followup had shown that the ischemic stroke incidence was 2.26 per 1,000 person-years (95% CI: 1.53, 3.21), approximately 1.5 times the rate of a population-based cohort in North Carolina [6].

3. Clinical Vignette

Mr. H, a 31-year-old Hispanic male who was admitted to Lincoln Medical and Mental Health Center for acute right MCA territory stroke in view of 5-hour history of sudden onset slurred speech with left upper and lower extremities weakness. There were no history of loss of consciousness, seizures, fever, headache, nausea or vomiting. Review of systems was otherwise unremarkable.

The patient has medical history of HIV infection which was diagnosed 2 years prior to this admission and started on ARTs since then. Mr. H admits compliance to his ARTs but does not remember last CD4 cell count. On the day of admission, CD4 cell count was 32 cells/uL. He was taking Raltegravir 400 mg bid, emtricitabine/tenofovir 1 tablet PO daily, ritonavir 100 mg bid, and darunavir 600 mg bid as well as daily bactrim for pneumocystis (carinii) Jiroveci pneumonia (PCP) prophylaxis. The patient denies cigarettes smoking, alcohol, or substance abuse.

On examination, the patient was alert and oriented to person, place, and time; the pupils were equal and reactive to light and accommodation. The patient has significant left hemiplegia with strength of 1 : 5 in the left upper and lower extremities; left facial droop was also noted. Neurologic exam was otherwise unremarkable.

His labs showed normal lipid profile (LDL-c of 51 mg/dL and HDL-c of 62 mg/dL), negative Factor V Leiden and prothrombin mutation, normal serum levels of protein C function (222%, normal range: 70–140), protein S function (100%, normal range: 70–142), antithrombin III function (139%, normal range: 75–125), and Homocystein (8.24 umol/L, normal < 12.99). Urine toxicology was negative for cocaine. Serum ANA was negative. Routine CSF analysis was unremarkable and negative for VDRL, Toxoplasmosis Ig M/Ig G serology, and HSV PCR.

Brain imaging studies showed right anterior corona radiata and basal ganglia acute infarction (Figure 1) and more clearly shown on brain MRI with contrast (Figure 2). The patient was started on aspirin and statins as secondary prevention as he was not candidate for thrombolytic therapy. Bilateral vascular Doppler showed normal carotid arteries. Echocardiogram including bubble study was unremarkable. The patient was transferred to skilled nursing facility for rehabilitation.

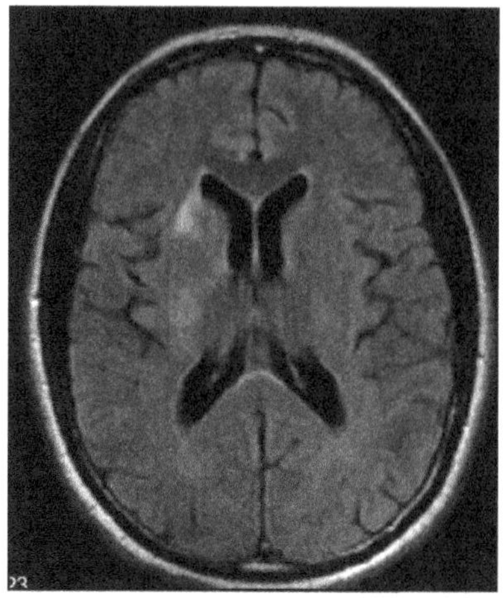

Figure 1: Brian MRI without gadolinium shows right anterior corona radiata and basal ganglia acute infarction.

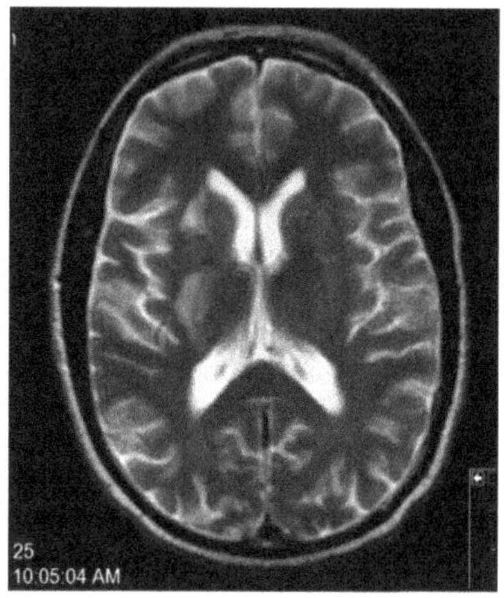

Figure 2: Brain MRI with gadolinium shows the infarct clearly.

4. Discussion

Before talking about the risk factors of atherosclerosis in HIV patients, we will talk in brief about the differential diagnosis of stroke-like symptoms in these particular patients. As a common concept, there are two main pathologies cross to our mind in any patient with HIV infection presented with focal neurologic deficits which are the following.

(1) Cerebral Toxoplasmosis. It typically presents with headache, confusion, and fever as well as focal neurological deficit in variant degrees. In one retrospective review of 115 cases, 55, 52, and 47% had headache, confusion, and fever, respectively, and 69% had focal neurologic deficits [7]. Cerebral toxoplasmosis usually affects HIV-infected patients with CD4 count of less than 200 cells per cubic millimeters and not taking toxoplasmosis prophylaxis.

(2) CNS Lymphomas. As the lifespan of HIV-infected patients has increased, malignancies have become a known cause of morbidity and mortality in this population. CNS lymphomas are more common in HIV-infected patients than in the non-HIV-infected patients (about 15 versus 1 percent of all lymphomas).

A rare culprit for stroke in HIV-infected patients is meningovascular syphilis. Syphilitic meningitis can cause an infectious arteritis that may affect any vessel in the subarachnoid space surrounding the brain or spinal cord and result in thrombosis, ischemia, and infarction. Many patients with meningovascular syphilis have prodromal symptoms, such as headache, dizziness, or personality changes, for days or weeks before the onset of ischemia or stroke. These symptoms are probably due to concomitant meningitis, but those patients may present with typical neurologic deficits leading to the diagnosis of stroke [8].

Several causative mechanisms have been proposed for the relationship between HIV infection and cardiovascular risk including HIV-associated dyslipidemia, endothelial dysfunction, inflammation, and hypercoagulability. Let us address these issues and review some of the related studies.

4.1. HIV-Associated Dyslipidemia. HIV-infected patients tend to develop decreases in high-density lipoprotein cholesterol (HDL-c) and low-density lipoprotein cholesterol (LDL-c) levels, followed by an increase in plasma triglyceride levels prior to developing AIDS and the degree of viremia may correlate with the amount of triglyceridemia [9].

A prospective study of 50 men from the Multicenter AIDS Cohort Study has shown significant declines in mean serum total cholesterol (TC), HDL-c, and LDL-c [10], and subsequent initiation of ARTs was associated with increases in TC and LDL-c but little change in HDL-c (it is noteworthy to mention that TC and LDL-C were observed after about 3 years of ARTs which possibly represent a return to pre-infection serum lipid levels after accounting for expected age-related changes).

A cross-sectional study done in India has shown that of the 306 patients taking ARTs for more than one year (126 controls, 30 on ZDV/3TC/NVP, and 150 on d4T/3TC/NVP), the prevalence of lipodystrophy was 46.1%, and lipoatrophy was significantly associated with d4T use [11]. However, discontinuation of ARTs may increase the risk of death by raising IL-6 and D-dimer levels [12].

4.2. Endothelial Dysfunction. An increased pulse wave velocity (which may be an early marker for atherosclerosis) has been noted in two small studies of HIV-infected patients taking ARTs compared to HIV-seronegative controls [13]. Endothelial function was assessed by brachial artery flow-mediated dilation (FMD) in treatment-naive patients initiating ARTs with either a PIs-based, NNRTIs-based, or nucleoside analog-sparing regimen [14]. Rapid and significant improvement in FMD was seen in all treatment arms compared to baseline, suggesting that suppression of HIV and not the specific drugs themselves led to improved endothelial function [14, 15].

However, antiretroviral medications may independently contribute to endothelial damage. In one study, plasma levels for markers of endothelial dysfunction (P-selectin and t-PA) were measured in 60 patients on ARTs and 60 treatment-naïve patients. Significantly higher levels of P-selectin and t-PA levels were found in those taking ARTs compared to the treatment-naïve group [16]. Certain antiretroviral agents may be more likely to disturb endothelial function than others like indinavir, [17] abacavir [18].

4.3. Hypertension. A Multicenter AIDS Cohort Study followed 5578 HIV-positive participants from 1984 to 2003 and observed a significantly higher systolic blood pressure in those using 8ARTs for greater than five years, [19] and there was no significant increase in systolic blood pressure in which ARTs were used for less than two years.

4.4. Insulin Resistance and Diabetes. ARTs are associated with an increased incidence of insulin resistance and diabetes. A multicenter AIDS cohort study done in Johns Hopkins University has shown that the incidence of DM in HIV-infected men with ARTs exposure was greater than 4 times that of HIV-seronegative men [20].

4.5. Chronic Inflammation. HIV infection per se may contribute to cardiovascular disease (CVD) risk via nonspecific inflammation. Uncontrolled HIV infection is associated with elevated markers of inflammation, including CRP; levels of these markers decline with treatment but not to normal levels, [21] and analysis from the FRAM study cohort has shown that fibrinogen and CRP are strong and independent predictors of mortality in HIV-infected adults even in those with relatively preserved CD4 counts >500 cells per microliter [22].

4.6. Hypercoagulability. Despite the endothelial damage and dysfunction discussed above, there is also evidence of an increased predisposition towards a hypercoagulable state. Researchers have described elevated plasma levels of endothelial cell products, including von Willebrand factor (vWF) and soluble thrombomodulin (sTM) in those living with HIV [23]. sTM was strongly raised in those patients with the lowest CD4+ cell count ($P < 0.001$), but levels of vWf increased at each incremental fall in CD4 cell count. A positive correlation has also been noted between HIV viral load and prothrombin fragment in 90 HIV-infected young individuals (mean age 38 ± 9 years, mean CD4 cell count 216 ± 198) not receiving ARTs suggesting that increasing levels of viremia may increase the risk of thrombosis [24].

In a study of 49 consecutive patients with acute opportunistic infections were screened for thrombophilic parameters, a followup investigation was performed after 10 ± 8 weeks in 26 patients. In acutely ill patients, the incidence of protein S deficiency was 67% (33/49) and of protein C deficiency 25% (12/49), while at the followup visit the incidences were 54% (14/26) and 8% (2/26), respectively, [25] which still above the national average of protein C and S deficiency.

By applying the aforementioned information to our case, this young patient without any of the classical risk factors for stroke and had negative thrombophilia workup found to have poorly controlled HIV infection despite being on ARTs for about 2 years. Although the acute thrombosis lowers the levels of protein C, protein S, and antithrombin as well as the initiation of Warfarin lowers the levels of protein C and protein S, normal values rule out those factors as risk factors for hypercoagulability in this patient. A negative VDRL in CSF and the lack of other symptoms of meningitis make the diagnosis of meningovascular syphilis very unlikely. By reviewing the literature, we found that the poorly controlled HIV infection and/or ARTs might be independent risk factors for stroke or acute cardiovascular event.

5. Conclusion

Despite the overall decrease in the number of stroke hospitalizations, data obtained from the Nationwide Inpatient Sample in the United States showed an increase in the number of stroke hospitalizations in the HIV-infected population.

The introduction of protease inhibitors and nonnucleoside reverse-transcriptase inhibitors for the management of human immunodeficiency virus (HIV) infection dramatically changed the prognosis and survivals, but unexpected cardiovascular events were observed. On the other hand, a poorly controlled HIV infection might be a independent risk factor.

More studies needed to address this medical dilemma in HIV-infected patients along with other classical risk factors modification which is a must.

References

[1] B. Ovbiagele and A. Nath, "Increasing incidence of ischemic stroke in patients with HIV infection," *Neurology*, vol. 76, no. 5, pp. 444–450, 2011.

[2] A. Mocroft, B. Ledergerber, C. Katlama et al., "Decline in the AIDS and death rates in the EuroSIDA study: an observational study," *The Lancet*, vol. 362, no. 9377, pp. 22–29, 2003.

[3] M. Mary-Krause, L. Cotte, A. Simon, M. Partisani, and D. Costagliola, "Increased risk of myocardial infarction with duration of protease inhibitor therapy in HIV-infected men," *AIDS*, vol. 17, no. 17, pp. 2479–2486, 2003.

[4] B. ILongo-Mbenza, M. Longokolo Mashi, M. Lelo Tshikwela et al., "Relationship between younger age, autoimmunity, cardiometabolic risk, oxidative stress, HAART, and ischemic stroke in Africans with HIV/AIDS," *ISRN Cardiology*, vol. 2011, Article ID 897908, 5 pages, 2011.

[5] F. C. Chow, S. Regan, S. Feske et al., "Comparison of ischemic stroke incidence in HIV-infected and non-HIV-infected patients in a US health care system," *Journal of Acquired Immune Deficiency Syndromes*, vol. 60, no. 4, pp. 351–358, 2012.

[6] M. J. Vinikoor, S. Napravnik, M. Floris-Moore et al., "Incidence and clinical features of cerebrovascular disease among HIV-infected adults in the Southeastern United States," *AIDS Research and Human Retroviruses*, vol. 29, no. 7, pp. 1068–1074, 2013.

[7] S. B. Porter and M. A. Sande, "Toxoplasmosis of the central nervous system in the acquired immunodeficiency syndrome," *The New England Journal of Medicine*, vol. 327, no. 23, pp. 1643–1648, 1992.

[8] S. Lachaud, L. Suissa, and M. H. Mahagne, "Stroke, HIV and meningovascular syphilis: study of three cases," *Revue Neurologique*, vol. 166, no. 1, pp. 76–82, 2010.

[9] C. Grunfeld, M. Pang, W. Doerrler et al., "Lipids, lipoproteins, triglyceride clearance, and cytokines in human immunodeficiency virus infection and the acquired immunodeficiency syndrome," *Journal of Clinical Endocrinology and Metabolism*, vol. 74, no. 5, pp. 1045–1052, 1992.

[10] S. A. Riddler, E. Smit, S. R. Cole et al., "Impact of HIV infection and HAART on serum lipids in men," *Journal of the American Medical Association*, vol. 289, no. 22, pp. 2978–2982, 2003.

[11] S. N. Pujari, A. Dravid, E. Naik et al., "Lipodystrophy and dyslipidemia among patients taking first-line, World Health Organization-recommended highly active antiretroviral therapy regimens in Western India," *Journal of Acquired Immune Deficiency Syndromes*, vol. 39, no. 2, pp. 199–202, 2005.

[12] L. H. Kuller, R. Tracy, W. Belloso et al., "Inflammatory and coagulation biomarkers and mortality in patients with HIV infection," *PLoS Medicine*, vol. 5, no. 10, article e203, 2008.

[13] G. Schillaci, G. V. L. de Socio, M. Pirro et al., "Impact of treatment with protease inhibitors on aortic stiffness in adult patients with human immunodeficiency virus infection," *Arteriosclerosis, Thrombosis, and Vascular Biology*, vol. 25, no. 11, pp. 2381–2385, 2005.

[14] F. J. Torriani, L. Komarow, R. A. Parker et al., "Endothelial function in human immunodeficiency virus-infected antiretroviral-naive subjects before and after starting potent antiretroviral therapy. The ACTG (AIDS Clinical Trials Group) Study 5152s," *Journal of the American College of Cardiology*, vol. 52, no. 7, pp. 569–576, 2008.

[15] R. Murphy and D. Costagliola, "Increased cardiovascular risk in HIV infection: drugs, virus and immunity," *AIDS*, vol. 22, no. 13, pp. 1625–1627, 2008.

[16] K. de Gaetano Donati, R. Rabagliati, M. Tumbarello et al., "Increased soluble markers of endothelial dysfunction in HIV-positive patients under highly active antiretroviral therapy," *AIDS*, vol. 17, no. 5, pp. 765–768, 2003.

[17] S. S. Shankar, M. P. Dubé, J. C. Gorski, J. E. Klaunig, and H. O. Steinberg, "Indinavir impairs endothelial function in healthy HIV-negative men," *American Heart Journal*, vol. 150, no. 5, pp. 933.e1–933.e7, 2005.

[18] F. J. Palella Jr., S. J. Gange, L. Benning et al., "Inflammatory biomarkers and abacavir use in the Women's Interagency HIV Study and the Multicenter AIDS Cohort Study," *AIDS*, vol. 24, no. 11, pp. 1657–1665, 2010.

[19] E. C. Seaberg, A. Muñoz, M. Lu et al., "Association between highly active antiretroviral therapy and hypertension in a large cohort of men followed from 1984 to 2003," *AIDS*, vol. 19, no. 9, pp. 953–960, 2005.

[20] T. T. Brown, S. R. Cole, X. Li et al., "Antiretroviral therapy and the prevalence and incidence of diabetes mellitus in the multicenter AIDS cohort study," *Archives of Internal Medicine*, vol. 165, no. 10, pp. 1179–1184, 2005.

[21] V. A. Triant, J. B. Meigs, and S. K. Grinspoon, "Association of C-reactive protein and HIV infection with acute myocardial infarction," *Journal of Acquired Immune Deficiency Syndromes*, vol. 51, no. 3, pp. 268–273, 2009.

[22] P. C. Tien, A. I. Choi, A. R. Zolopa et al., "Inflammation and mortality in HIV-infected adults: analysis of the FRAM study cohort," *Journal of Acquired Immune Deficiency Syndromes*, vol. 55, no. 3, pp. 316–322, 2010.

[23] A. D. Blann, M. Seigneur, J. Constans, J. L. Pellegrin, and C. Conri, "Soluble P-selectin, thrombocytopenia and von Willebrand factor in HIV infected patients," *Thrombosis and Haemostasis*, vol. 77, no. 6, pp. 1221–1222, 1997.

[24] M. Karmochkine, A. Ankri, V. Calvez, M. Bonmarchant, A. Coutellier, and S. Herson, "Plasma hypercoagulability is correlated to plasma HIV load," *Thrombosis and Haemostasis*, vol. 80, no. 1, pp. 208–209, 1998.

[25] M. Erbe, V. Rickerts, R. M. Bauersachs, and E. Lindhoff-Last, "Acquired protein C and protein S deficiency in HIV-infected patients," *Clinical and Applied Thrombosis/Hemostasis*, vol. 9, no. 4, pp. 325–331, 2003.

7

A Rare Case of Stroke Secondary to Iron Deficiency Anemia in a Young Female Patient

Kavitha Gopalratnam, Kevin Andrew Woodson, Jigarkumar Rangunwala, Kanaga Sena, and Manisha Gupta

Bridgeport Hospital-Yale New Haven Health, 267 Grant St, Bridgeport, CT 06610, USA

Correspondence should be addressed to Kevin Andrew Woodson; kevinwoodson@gmail.com

Academic Editor: Christos D. Lionis

Ischemic strokes occur when there is a sudden obstruction of an artery supplying blood flow to an area of the brain, leading to a focal neurological deficit. Strokes can be thrombotic or embolic in etiology and are associated with underlying conditions such as hypertension and atherosclerosis. Possible etiologies of strokes include cardioembolic disease, hematologic disorders, connective tissue disorders, and substance abuse or can be cryptogenic. Most stroke cases are seen in patients over 65 years of age. However, about one-fourth of strokes occur in young adults. Iron deficiency anemia (IDA) has been described as a known cause for strokes in children, but very few case reports describe this association in adults. We describe a 20-year-old female who presented with sudden onset left side weakness. Magnetic Resonance Imaging (MRI) of the brain demonstrated ischemic infarctions. Patient was also found to be severely anemic. Patient had a thorough work-up including Magnetic Resonance Angiography (MRA) of the brain, echocardiogram, and an extensive screen for thrombophilia disorders. This, however, did not demonstrate a clear etiology. As it has been suggested that IDA is a potential cause for stroke, it is possible the stroke in this young patient was attributable to severe IDA.

1. Introduction

Ischemic strokes are a common problem primarily in patients above 65 years of age [1]. In this case, we describe a young patient who suffered an ischemic stroke at 20 years of age. The patient's only comorbidity was severe IDA. This case is interesting as IDA is an etiology for stroke which is typically only seen in pediatric patients [2]. The case is significant as it suggests IDA as a possible etiology for stroke in young adults. IDA is not commonly associated with stroke in the minds of most clinicians. As IDA is a common condition in young adults, we suggest that prompt diagnosis and treatment of IDA should be a priority for young patients who present with stroke when all other more common etiologies are ruled out.

2. Case Presentation

A 20-year-old female presented to the hospital after being involved in a motor vehicle accident. The accident was preceded by a sensation of dizziness with blurring of vision and brief loss of consciousness. Her co-passengers, who witnessed the event, denied noticing any seizure-like activity. She regained consciousness within a few minutes, at which time she was alert and responding appropriately. Upon arrival to the hospital, she was noted to have some chest pain where the air bag had deployed but did not have any signs of significant trauma. She endorsed continued dizziness, blurring of vision, and photophobia. Also, she attested to some weakness in her left side involving her arms and legs. On physical exam, she demonstrated decreased motor strength in her left upper extremity but otherwise intact neurological exam. An initial head CT was negative for any ischemic changes. Laboratory tests revealed severe anemia with hemoglobin of 5.8 mg/dL and platelet count of 564, suggestive of reactive thrombocytosis. Patient also was found to have serum iron 20 μg/dL, TIBC 481 μg/dL, iron saturation 6%, and serum ferritin 39 ng/mL. MCV was 64 fL/cell and RDW was 18.2%. Other laboratory tests including white blood count, chemistry panel, lipid panel, urea, and creatinine were within normal limits. History revealed menorrhagia with multiple evaluations for near syncope and dizziness. However, she did not have active bleeding at the time of presentation. Her clinical course was further complicated by low grade fevers, confusion, lethargy, and changes in her mental status. She demonstrated significant neurological findings on physical exam with worsening left upper extremity strength, bilateral dysmetria, and a positive Romberg sign. A lumbar puncture did not reveal any infectious causes of her symptoms. MRI at the time revealed bilateral cerebellar and left occipital lobe nonhemorrhagic infarcts. An MRA of the brain ruled out arterial dissection or thrombus formation. She also had an echocardiogram, which did not show any signs of PFO or interatrial shunt with agitated saline study. A thorough work-up for underlying thrombophilia was unrevealing including protein S and C deficiency, lupus anticoagulant, anti-cardiolipin antibody, Factor V Leiden mutation, ANA positivity, antithrombin III deficiency, Vitamin B12 level, homocysteine level, hemoglobin electrophoresis, and rapid plasma reagin. The patient received multiple blood transfusions and showed good response with improvement in her hemoglobin. Additionally, patient received intravenous iron infusion and ferrous sulfate 325 mg TID was initiated to help correct the IDA. She showed improvement in neurological function over a period of two weeks with concurrent inpatient physical therapy. Patient was seen in the resident's continuity clinic in the following months with resultant improvement in iron saturation and serum ferritin. No additional neuroimaging was performed.

3. Discussion

IDA accounts for about 50% of all anemia cases worldwide. It has a prevalence of about 2–4% in nonpregnant women 12–49 years of age and about 2–5% prevalence in men and postmenopausal women [3, 4]. IDA can be caused by poor dietary intake, poor absorption of iron, or bleeding. Possible sources of blood loss include the gastrointestinal and genitourinary systems.

Strokes in adults over the age of 65 years constitute the majority of strokes. However, approximately 25% of strokes occur in patients under 65 years of age. Common causes of these strokes include hematologic disorders, connective tissue disease, substance abuse, trauma, and cardioembolic disease. About 30% of strokes in young adults have cryptogenic (undetermined) etiology [1].

Cerebrovascular disease associated with IDA has been attributed to three main mechanisms: venous sinus thrombosis from reactive thrombocytosis, arterial cerebral infarctions with possible thrombus formation, or severe hypoxia and severe anemia causing reversible neurologic deficits in the setting of atherosclerotic cardiovascular disease (ASCVD) [5, 6]. The association between IDA and stroke has been better defined in children than it has been in adults. Multiple case series have reported IDA to be associated with ischemic stroke or venous thrombosis in children (ages between 6 and 18 months) in the setting of acute viral illness as well [7]. However, very few case reports have been documented in young adults.

A 3-case report series by Akins et al. of women aged 20, 39, and 44 years described severe IDA secondary to menorrhagia associated with carotid artery thrombosis and a thrombus-induced stroke [8]. Transient ischemic attack (TIA) associated with carotid artery thromboembolism in severe iron deficiency was also described by a study conducted by Batur Caglayan et al., which hypothesized that IDA-induced microcytosis and thrombocytosis produce a hypercoagulable state [9]. It was theorized that increased blood flow to the brain causes endothelial injury, thereby leading to thrombus formation. Hypoxia from severe IDA is also hypothesized as one of the causes for stroke due to decreased oxygen-carrying capacity in the blood and, thereby, decreased delivery of oxygen to the brain [1].

Interestingly, it has been demonstrated by Huang et al. in a study that showed higher mortality within 3 years among patients with IDA at the time of admission during a first stroke from an atherosclerotic-related ischemic event [10]. This underscores the importance of identifying and correcting IDA in the setting of ischemic stroke, which can improve patient outcome.

The case of our patient who suffered an ischemic stroke at 20 years of age is intriguing because a thorough diagnostic work-up did not reveal any clear etiology apart from severe IDA. This adds to the small volume of case reports and case series that suggest IDA as a possible etiology for ischemic stroke in young adults. This is of interest as IDA is not a well-known cause of ischemic stroke in young adults. This highlights the importance of prompt diagnosis and treatment of IDA in young patients, especially after a thorough work-up has ruled out more widely recognized etiologies.

Competing Interests

The authors declare that they have no competing interests.

References

[1] P. J. Mehta, S. Chapman, A. Jayam-Trouth, and M. Kurukumbi, "Acute ischemic stroke secondary to iron deficiency anemia: a case report," *Case Reports in Neurological Medicine*, vol. 2012, Article ID 487080, 5 pages, 2012.

[2] J. L. Maguire, G. Deveber, and P. C. Parkin, "Association between iron-deficiency anemia and stroke in young children," *Pediatrics*, vol. 120, no. 5, pp. 1053–1057, 2007.

[3] Y.-L. Chang, S.-H. Hung, W. Ling, H.-C. Lin, H.-C. Li, and S.-D. Chung, "Association between ischemic stroke and iron-deficiency anemia: A Population-based Study," *PLOS ONE*, vol. 8, no. 12, Article ID e82952, 2013.

[4] S. Killip, J. M. Bennett, and M. D. Chambers, "Iron deficiency anemia," *American Family Physician*, vol. 75, no. 5, pp. 671–678, 2007.

[5] H. Knizley and W. D. Noyes, "Iron deficiency anemia, papilledema, thrombocytosis, and transient hemiparesis," *Archives of Internal Medicine*, vol. 129, no. 3, pp. 483–486, 1972.

[6] M. B. Alexander, "Iron deficiency anemia, thrombocytosis, and cerebrovascular accident," *Southern Medical Journal*, vol. 76, no. 5, pp. 662–663, 1983.

[7] D. S. Hartfield, N. J. Lowry, D. L. Keene, and J. Y. Yager, "Iron deficiency: a cause of stroke in infants and children," *Pediatric Neurology*, vol. 16, no. 1, pp. 50–53, 1997.

[8] P. T. Akins, S. Glenn, P. M. Nemeth, and C. P. Derdeyn, "Carotid artery thrombus associated with severe iron-deficiency anemia and thrombocytosis," *Stroke*, vol. 27, no. 5, pp. 1002–1005, 1996.

[9] H. Z. Batur Caglayan, B. Nazliel, C. Irkec, A. Dumlu, A. Filiz, and M. Panpalli Ates, "Iron-deficiency anemia leading to transient ischemic attacks due to intraluminal carotid artery thrombus," *Case Reports in Neurological Medicine*, vol. 2013, Article ID 813415, 3 pages, 2013.

[10] W.-Y. Huang, I.-C. Chen, L. Meng, W.-C. Weng, and T.-I. Peng, "The influence of anemia on clinical presentation and outcome of patients with first-ever atherosclerosis-related ischemic stroke," *Journal of Clinical Neuroscience*, vol. 16, no. 5, pp. 645–649, 2009.

8

Subacute Stroke in a Young Female: A Case of Moyamoya Syndrome Initially Anchoring with Anxiety

Saira Chaughtai, Zeeshan Chaughtai, Muhammad Shaheryar Haider, Hasnan M. Ijaz, Sarah Elmedani, Mohamed Bakr, Mohammad A. Hossain, and Arif Asif

Department of Medicine, Jersey Shore University Medical Center, Hackensack Meridian Health, Neptune, NJ 07753, USA

Correspondence should be addressed to Mohammad A. Hossain; mohammad.hossain@hackensackmeridian.org

Academic Editor: Mark E. Shaffrey

Moyamoya disease is an arterial disorder causing stroke in a young patient. This is a chronic condition causing progressive cerebrovascular disease due to bilateral stenosis and occlusion of the arteries around the circle of Willis, with prominent arterial collateral circulation. It was first described in Japan and subsequently reported in other Asian countries, but infrequently found in the Western world. Interestingly, there may be racial differences in the presentation and subsequent prognostication of treatment of moyamoya. It is diagnosed with classic angiographic findings of stenosis or occlusion of the circle of Willis vessels. Here, we describe a 28-year-old Caucasian female who was initially diagnosed with anxiety when she presented with symptoms of impaired concentration and fatigue. After the development of remitting slurred speech and facial droop, magnetic resonance imaging and cerebral angiogram yielded the discovery of high-grade stenosis of the origin of the left middle cerebral artery with associated thrombosis in that area. She did well after getting surgery and rehabilitation. This demonstrates a unique presentation of prominent psychiatric symptoms initially thought to be anxiety and culminated in the finding of ischemic stroke in an adult patient with moyamoya.

1. Introduction

Moyamoya disease (MMD) is an arterial disorder causing ischemic stroke in a young patient. This occurs primarily in the female sex in two age groups: the first decade of life and the fourth to fifth decades. Diagnosis relies on characteristic angiographic findings of bilateral stenoses of the arteries in the circle of Willis with collateral vessel formation [1]. This occlusion is located at the branching of the anterior cerebral artery and/or middle cerebral artery when they come off the internal carotid artery [1]. When it is only one-sided or associated with other medical conditions, it is termed moyamoya syndrome (MMS). These medical conditions include diseases such as Down's syndrome and sickle cell disease [1]. It is uncommon to have a case of moyamoya present with such prominent psychiatric symptoms. In this case summary, we discuss a case of a 28-year-old Caucasian woman who presented with prominent psychiatric symptoms. She was initially deemed to have anxiety, but subsequently developed remitting facial droop and slurred speech and found to have evidence of an ischemic stroke along with moyamoya syndrome on her cerebral imaging.

2. Case Summary

A 28-year-old Caucasian female, with a history of depression and breast fibroadenoma status postresection, presented to the hospital with a one-month history of fatigue, impaired concentration, and remitting slurred speech and right-sided facial droop. Three weeks prior to this admission, she came to the emergency department with the chief complaint of a "hard time processing thoughts" and had a normal neurologic examination. She was evaluated by computed tomography (CT) of the head and discharged home as the imaging study was unremarkable and symptoms were presumed to be anxiety related as they involved a strong psychiatric component. She subsequently developed slurred speech and facial droop. For further evaluation, magnetic resonance imaging (MRI) was ordered outpatient and showed a subacute infarct of her left middle cerebral artery, prompting her primary care physician to send her to the hospital for further evaluation and management. Family history includes a maternal grandfather who died of multiple strokes at age 45. On physical examination, her heart rate was 88/min, blood pressure was 139/93, respiratory rate was 15/min, temperature was 98 degrees Fahrenheit, and pulse oxygenation was 96% on room air. On mental status exam, she displayed anxiety regarding her condition. On neurological examination, she had word-finding difficulty and difficulty in repetition; however, her comprehension was intact. She also had a right-sided central facial droop of the upper motor neuron type. Her muscle strength was normal, and sensation was intact in all extremities. Magnetic resonance angiogram (MRA) of the head and neck demonstrated stenosis of the origin of the left middle and anterior cerebral arteries with thrombosis of the former (Figure 1). Cerebral angiogram (CTA) showed high-grade stenosis of the origin of the left middle cerebral artery with associated delayed filling in that territory. A neurologist was consulted, and he started her on aspirin, clopidegrol, and statin. She remained neurologically stable during the hospital course and was discharged with outpatient neurosurgery follow-up. She eventually underwent a direct and indirect bypass of the abnormal cerebral vasculature. She also had rehabilitation for her physical symptoms and had significant clinical improvement on follow-up.

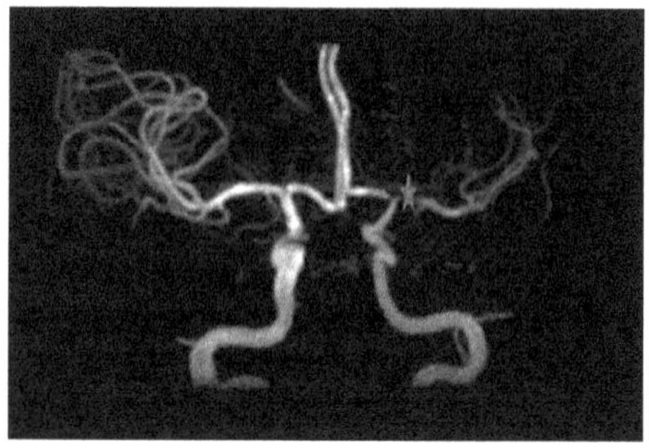

Figure 1: Our patient's magnetic resonance angiogram of the brain. The location of the red star shows the stenoses of the origin of the left anterior cerebral artery (A1 segment) and origin of the left middle cerebral artery (M1 segment), with associated thrombosis of the origin of the left middle cerebral artery.

3. Discussion

Moyamoya is a condition that involves progressive stenosis of the arteries of the brain with concomitant collateral vessel formation [2]. The term "moyamoya" is of Japanese origin meaning a "puff of smoke," which is the visual manifestation of the collateral circulation. Moyamoya disease is characterized by bilateral stenosis of the arteries of the circle of Willis; however, unilateral presentation is termed as moyamoya syndrome and bilateral disease eventually develops in many [2]. Moyamoya syndrome also applies to patients with certain associated conditions like Down's syndrome and sickle cell disease [2]. This condition is most commonly found in people of Asian heritage, but less so in North America [2]. Pathologic analysis shows that vessel occlusion results from a combination of hyperplasia of smooth-muscle cells and luminal thrombosis [2]. Genetic factors play a role as ten percent of Japanese cases have affected first-degree relatives. Some studies have identified mutations in proteins involved in extracellular-matrix remodeling and angiogenesis in the brain. Manifestations can be any signs of symptoms of a stroke and may cooccur with personality changes [2]. It predominantly occurs in two age groups: the first decade of life and the fourth to fifth decades of life [2]. The incidence in parts of the United States was found to be 0.086 per 100,000 [3]. Diagnosis is based upon characteristic angiogram findings involving stenosis of the distal internal carotid artery, with stenosis of the origins of the anterior and middle cerebral arteries [3]. The Suzuki grading system classifies the grade based on stenosis of the arteries with progressive collateral circulation development [3].

Treatment aims to reduce the risk of stroke and formation of collaterals by improving blood flow. However, there is no treatment that can reverse the disease [4]. Medical therapy includes antiplatelets, statins, and calcium channel blockers. However, surgery has better potential for improvement in symptoms and risk of recurrent stroke. Surgical options aim to revascularize the brain tissue and have been shown to be superior in improving the clinical course of patients with moyamoya [5]. These options include a direct and indirect approach. The indirect approach involves revascularizing the brain by placing connective tissue with vasculature on the cortical zone from which the vessels sprout [5]. The direct method involves a connection formed between a graft vessel and one of the cerebral vessels [5]. For example, the vasculature may be taken from the superficial temporal artery [5].

It is noteworthy that primarily psychiatric symptoms as the presentation of moyamoya is quite unique. Other case reports have described rare instances of patients initially presenting with anxiety, psychosis, prominent depression, and insomnia [6]. The significance of our case lies in the fact that our patient presented with prominent psychiatric symptoms of impaired concentration, anxiety, and fatigue. She was initially diagnosed as anxiety as her symptoms were associated with a prominent psychiatric component, and she was instructed to follow-up outpatient. She subsequently developed remitting facial droop and slurred speech and had an outpatient MRI done showing evidence of moyamoya. Her angiography confirmed findings, and she was able to get a direct and indirect bypass, along with rehabilitation, with ensuing improvement in symptoms. In a provider who is unaware of moyamoya, this may be labelled as a psychiatric case as her slurred speech and facial droop occurred after her initial presentation to the hospital. This highlights the importance of being aware of this diagnostic possibility in patients who we may label as having a psychiatric condition.

Since her facial droop and slurred speech were remitting, it is also easy for the provider to miss the fact that it was a stroke. Maheswari et al. mentioned in their case report that their patient had remitting symptoms of hemichorea and hemiparesis which was finally diagnosed after 3 months as being moyamoya [7]. So, it is important to know symptoms may remit and relapse.

Also, of note, most studies have involved the East Asian population; however, emerging evidence suggests that there may be a differing clinical presentation of moyamoya in other races [8]. It is noted that Asian patients are more likely to present with hemorrhage rather than ischemia [8]. Studies also suggest that non-Asian patients may have better outcomes after surgery [8]. Our Caucasian patient did have ischemia and did improve after surgery with no recurrence of stroke to date. Surgery has been noted to be an effective stroke-prophylaxis option for the ischemic type and maybe even for the hemorrhagic type [9].

4. Conclusion

Moyamoya disease is an unusual cause of stroke in a young adult. Early diagnosis of this rare disease can be complicated by psychiatric manifestation and anchoring bias, like in our case. The clinician should consider this rare condition while evaluating a young patient with stroke in appropriate clinical settings.

Consent

The patient described in the case report had given informed consent for the case report to be published.

Conflicts of Interest

The authors declare that they have no conflicts of interest.

Authors' Contributions

SC and MB contributed to the planning and case summary. ZC, MSH, and SE contributed to the discussion. MH and AA worked on the planning, manuscript revision, and final approval.

References

[1] R. Appireddy, M. Ranjan, B. A. Durafourt, J. Riva-Cambrin, W. J. Hader, and P. D. Adelson, "Surgery for Moyamoya disease in children," *Journal of Child Neurology*, vol. 34, no. 9, pp. 517–529, 2019.

[2] R. M. Scott and E. R. Smith, "Moyamoya disease and Moyamoya syndrome," *New England Journal of Medicine*, vol. 360, no. 12, pp. 1226–1237, 2009.

[3] N. C. Suwanwela, Moyamoya disease: etiology, clinical features, and diagnosis, 2017, https://www.uptodate.com/.

[4] S. Smith and C. Fox, Ischemic stroke in children and young adults: etiology and clinical features, 2017, https://www.uptodate.com/.

[5] S. U. Lee, C. W. Oh, O.-K. Kwon et al., "Surgical treatment of adult Moyamoya disease," *Current Treatment Options in Neurology*, vol. 20, no. 7, 2018.

[6] M. Richards, A. Grzenda, E. Nelson, and M. Gitlin, "Psychiatric comorbidity in Moyamoya disease and preliminary guidelines for treatment," *American Journal of Psychiatry*, vol. 176, no. 4, pp. 269–274, 2019.

[7] S. Maheshwari, A. Anthony, S. Kushwaha, S. Singh, R. Desai, and D. Madan, "Moyamoya disease presenting as alternating hemiparesis with relapsing remitting hemichorea: an unusual manifestation," *Journal of Pediatric Neurosciences*, vol. 13, no. 4, pp. 514–516, 2018.

[8] J. Feghali, R. Xu, W. Yang et al., "Differing surgical outcomes in a multi-ethnic cohort suggest racial phenotypes in Moyamoya disease," *World Neurosurgery*, vol. 128, pp. e865–e872, 2019.

[9] X. Deng, P. Ge, S. Wang et al., "Treatment of Moyamoya disease," *Neurosurgery*, vol. 65, no. CN_suppl_1, pp. 62–65, 2018.

9

Artery of Percheron Infarction: A Case Report of Bilateral Thalamic Stroke Presenting with Acute Encephalopathy

Charles Donohoe,[1] **Nooshin Kiani Nia**,[2] **Patricia Carey**,[3] **and Vamsi Vemulapalli**[3]

[1]*Department of Neurology Chair, Truman Medical Center, 2301 Holmes St, Kansas City, MO 64108, USA*
[2]*Department of Neurology, Truman Medical Center, 2301 Holmes St, Kansas City, MO 64108, USA*
[3]*University of Missouri-Kansas City School of Medicine, 2411 Holmes St, Kansas City, MO 64108, USA*

Correspondence should be addressed to Nooshin Kiani Nia; nkianinia@umkc.edu

Academic Editor: Dominic B. Fee

The artery of Percheron (AOP) is a relatively rare anatomic variant in which a solitary arterial trunk branches from the proximal segment of the posterior cerebral artery and provides arterial supply to the paramedian region of the thalami bilaterally and often to the rostral part of the midbrain. Occlusion of the artery of Percheron results in bilateral paramedian thalamic infarcts with and without midbrain involvement. Recognition of this condition as an acute stroke may be challenging due to various nonlocalized clinical presentations, given the wide range of neurological functions subserved by the thalamus. Prompt neuroimaging, preferably with magnetic resonance imaging (MRI), in conjunction with familiarity with this relatively rare vascular variation can facilitate initiation of appropriate time contingent thrombolytic treatment and improved long-term prognosis. We present a case of a 56-year-old African American female with a bilateral thalamic infarct secondary to the artery of Percheron thromboembolism. This patient presented unresponsive without focal neurologic findings but with an initial Glasgow Coma Score (GCS) of 7, and subsequent computed tomographic (CT) head revealed bilateral thalamic hypodensities. Confirmatory MRI exhibited bilateral subacute thalamic infarcts, which were thought to be embolic with the source from the left ventricular thrombus as the patient had at least three distinct clots. Unfortunately, the patient's mental status did not improve significantly, and she was discharged to a nursing facility for extended care. AOP infarction may be missed on vascular imaging utilizing CT, MRI, and even catheter angiography. Clinical recognition that the AOP is one of the only single artery occlusions that can affect bilateral structures and frequently present solely as altered mental status without focal neurologic deficits is crucial to the diagnosis.

1. Background

According to Gerald Percheron, who studied thalamic blood supply extensively in the twentieth century, the P1 segment of the posterior cerebral artery (PCA) supplies the paramedian thalamus through the paramedian arteries on each side [1, 2]. Paramedian arteries may sometimes arise from one common trunk from a P1 segment on either side: this common trunk is known as the artery of Percheron [2]. A bilateral paramedian thalamic infarct with or without the involvement of the rostral midbrain can result if the blood supply to the AOP is compromised [2]. Classic findings of this condition include impaired arousal, memory, or language impairment, and occasionally an ocular movement disorder [3, 4]. AOP infarctions are rarely associated with pyramidal symptoms, and initial noncontrast CT head imaging can be normal and misleading [5].

These varied clinical presentations without localizing findings and the rarity of this anatomic variant often cause significant delay in obtaining MR brain imaging and ultimately identifying an accurate diagnosis [5]. Figure 1 demonstrates four variations in the arterial supply of the thalamic circulation, and Table 1 provides a summarized description of each thalamic arterial supply variant. Variant I (tuberothalamic territory): this is the most common variant, where the perforating arteries on each side will arise

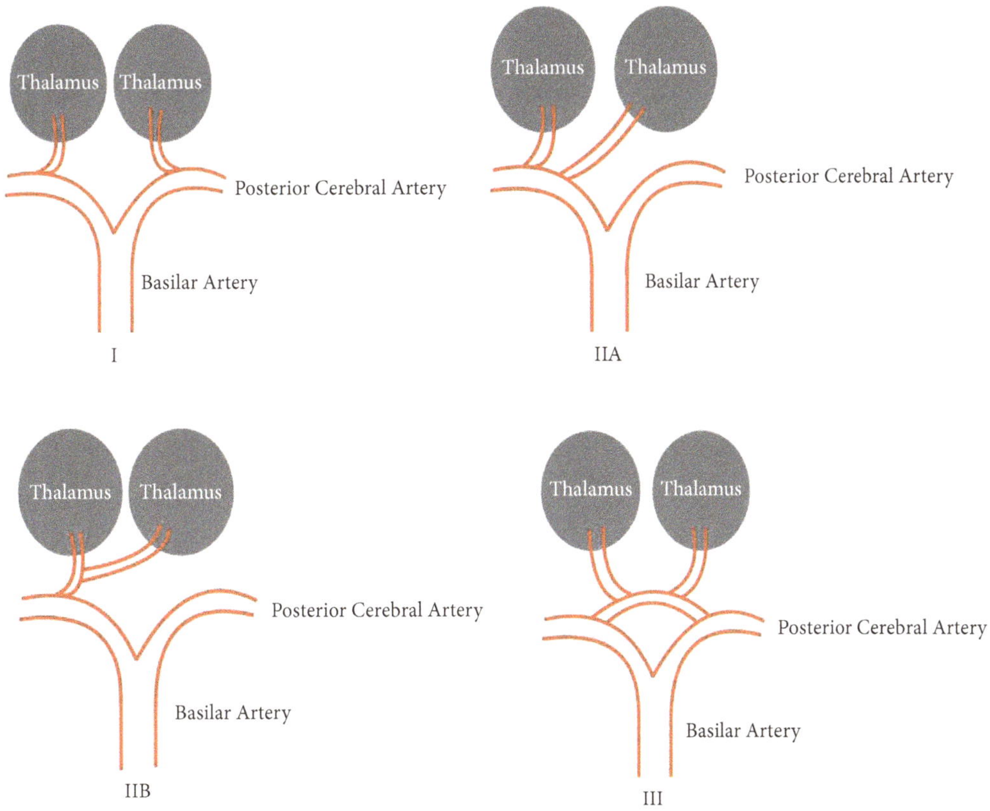

FIGURE 1: Anatomy of thalamic arterial supply variants.

TABLE 1: Description of thalamic arterial supply variants.

Type	Anatomical description
I	Normal paramedian artery anatomy: L and R PMAs arise from their respective PCA
IIA	Variant of paramedian artery anatomy: both PMAs arise from either L or R PCA
IIB	Artery of Percheron anatomy: one branch from either L or R PCA supplies both thalami
III	Variant of paramedian artery anatomy: both PMAs arise from an arterial branch connecting the L and R PCA

from each right and left posterior communicating artery (PCA). Vascular compromise leads to impaired orientation, arousal, memory, learning, personality, and executive dysfunction. Variant IIA (inferolateral territory): the proximal segment of one PCA gives rise to perforating arteries in an asymmetric pattern. The perforating arteries arise from the proximal segment of one PCA. Vascular compromise will lead to hemisensory loss, hemiparesis, hemi-ataxia of the contralateral side, and poststroke hyperalgesia, particularly with right-sided strokes. Variant IIB (posterior choroidal territory): bilateral perforating thalamic arteries arise from a single arterial trunk referred to as the artery of Percheron. Vascular compromise leads to sensory loss of the contralateral side, visual field defects, tremor, dystonia, weakness, and occasional language impairment. Variant III (paramedian territory): several small perforating branches arise from one arterial supply that bridges the P1 segments of both posterior communication arteries. Vascular compromise leads to hypersomnolence if the lesion is bilateral in addition to symptoms such as memory impairment, difficulty in learning, and language deficits [5].

2. Case Presentation

A 56-year-old African American female with a past medical history of nonischemic cardiomyopathy, hypertension, chronic obstructive pulmonary disease (COPD), hyperlipidemia, left ventricular thrombus on rivaroxaban, depression, anxiety, and polysubstance use disorder was found unresponsive at a house frequented by known drug abusers. She presented to the emergency room with acute encephalopathy of unknown cause. On admission, the patient had a GCS of 7, which improved with the administration of 2 milligrams of naloxone for concern of drug use as the cause of her encephalopathy. The patient did not have any focal neurologic findings, and no stroke alert protocol was initiated.

The patient then intermittently desaturated to 84% oxygen saturation levels with an episode of apnea and was subsequently placed on 3–4 liters of oxygen through a nasal cannula. As she was able to protect her airway, she was not intubated. In addition, the patient was hypertensive with a blood pressure of 152/100 mmHg on arrival.

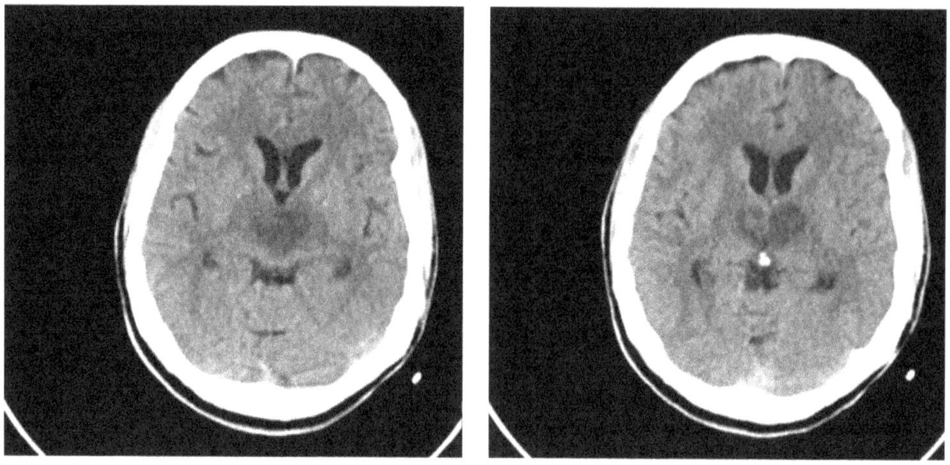

(a) (b)

Figure 2: Noncontrast CT brain demonstrating bilateral hypodensities in the medial thalami obtained at the time of admission.

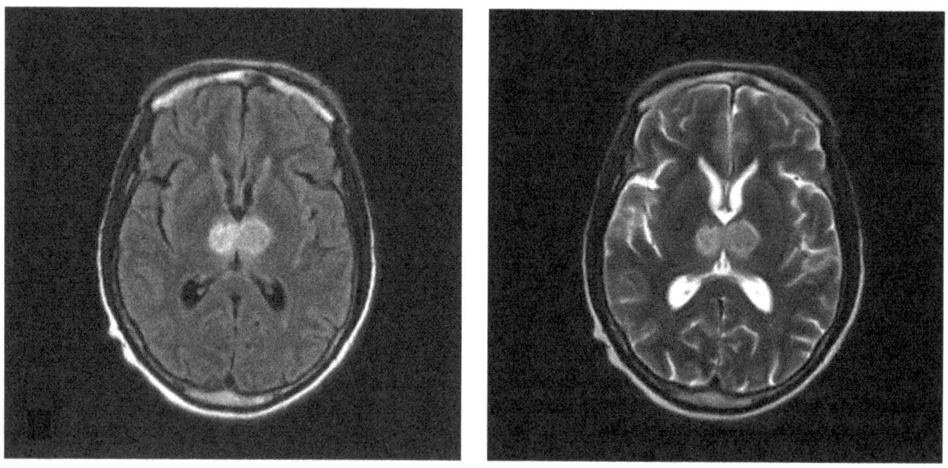

(a) (b)

Figure 3: Axial flair (a) and axial T2 (b) MR images obtained one week after the CT demonstrated increased signal bilaterally in the thalamic nuclei.

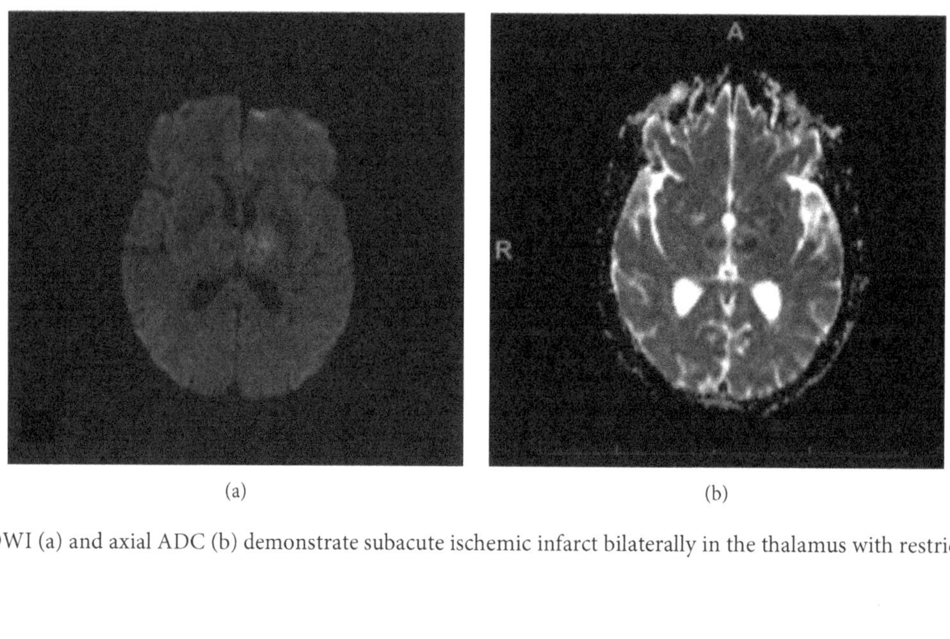

(a) (b)

Figure 4: Axial DWI (a) and axial ADC (b) demonstrate subacute ischemic infarct bilaterally in the thalamus with restricted diffusion and low ADC values.

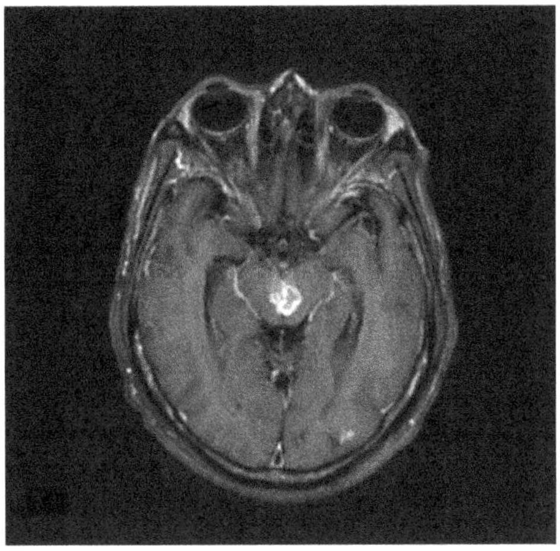

(a)

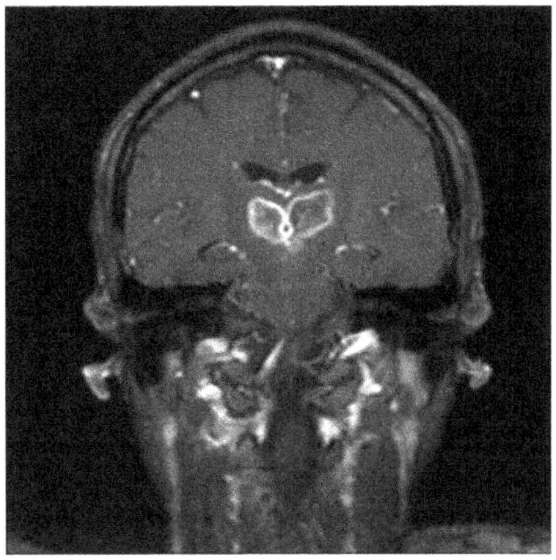

(b)

FIGURE 5: Postcontrast T1 MR images demonstrate vivid contrast enhancement involving the midbrain: (a) axial image and posterior thalami; (b) coronal image.

The initial basic metabolic panel in the emergency department was remarkable for hyponatremia at 133 mEq/L, but otherwise, the electrolytes were within normal limits. Further blood testing demonstrated an elevated creatinine kinase level of 1281 U/L and alcohol, salicylate, and acetaminophen levels within reference ranges. A urine drug screen was positive for amphetamines, cocaine, and cannabinoids.

CT head without contrast revealed hypodensity in both thalami, which prompted a teleneurology consult and they recommended that tissue plasminogen activator (TPA) not be administered because patient was taking rivaroxaban and the time last known well was unclear. CT angiogram (CTA) did not identify an isolated vessel occlusion. MRI brain confirmed bilateral thalamic infarcts. MR following gadolinium administration demonstrated vivid enhancement in both thalami and upper midbrain—characteristic of a subacute infarction (Figures 2–5). MR venogram (MRV) demonstrated a patent intracranial venous system (not shown).

An echocardiogram was then performed, which showed an ejection fraction of 20–25% and three distinct clots in the anterior, lateral, septal, and apical walls that were all more than 1 cm in size. On that basis, the thalamic infarcts were believed to be embolic, with the source as a left ventricular thrombus.

The patient's mental status failed to improve over her 48 days of hospital stay, and her Mini-Cog evaluation measured 0/5. She ultimately developed dysphagia requiring Percutaneous Endoscopic Gastrostomy (PEG) tube placement. Guardianship was instituted due to the patient's incapacity, and she was discharged to a skilled nursing facility for extended care.

3. Discussion

The AOP is the IIB variant of the thalamic circulation, where a single arterial trunk gives rise to bilateral perforating thalamic arteries [6]. Therefore, any compromise in the AOP will lead to compromised circulation to bilateral thalami with or without midbrain involvement [6]. The AOP can rarely be demonstrated on MRA, CTA, or conventional catheter angiography due to its small diameter, rendering it challenging to visualize. Therefore, confirmation by vascular imaging of the precise vessel occlusion is not a diagnostic requirement [7]. The AOP variant prevalence is estimated to occur in 4–30% of the general population and accounts for between 0.1% and 2% of ischemic strokes [1, 2, 8–11]. The bilateral and frequently symmetrical imaging abnormalities in the thalami and midbrain in conjunction with prominent mental status findings often initially point to a metabolic or toxic etiology, delaying the diagnosis of an uncommon stroke syndrome [3, 11].

The AOP infarction is an imaging diagnosis. MRI is the preferred modality approaching 100% sensitivity, while, unlike our patient, CT is frequently negative (50% sensitivity). Early diagnosis is best made with diffusion-weighted imaging (DWI) with apparent diffusion coefficient (ADC) sequences [11]. The AOP occlusion on CTA or MRA is an unlikely finding and not a diagnostic prerequisite [7, 12]. Thrombolysis is the treatment of choice when a diagnosis is made within the therapeutic window of 4.5 hours. Because of the nonlocalizing presentations associated with the change in mental status, many diagnoses are delayed and fall outside the therapeutic window. Prognosis can be favorable if the diagnosis is rapidly identified, and the patient receives appropriate treatment [7].

A series of 18 cases of paramedian infarction reported that 61% of them had favorable outcome and were able to perform activities of daily living without assistance [13]. There have been reported cases of bilateral thalamic strokes, who presented mainly with sudden onset of hypersomnia and fluctuating arousal as the thalamus plays an important role in sleep regulation and in maintaining arousal. Hypersomnolence can be due to the interruption of noradrenergic and dopaminergic pathways from the ascending reticular activating system to the thalamus [14–16].

One case report stated that there was significant improvement in the state of alertness after administering modafinil 100 mg twice a day [8]. In our case, we report a patient who was found unresponsive with a GCS of 7. Initial CT head without contrast showed abnormal hypodensity throughout the bilateral thalami consistent with an AOP infarction. MRI brain with and without contrast was performed and confirmed the earlier findings. MRV ruled out dural venous sinus thrombosis.

Unfortunately, this patient was outside the therapeutic window for thrombolysis. Her echocardiogram showed at least three distinct clots in the anterior, lateral, septal, and apical walls, all more than 1 cm in size. The thalamic infarcts were thought to be embolic from the source of a left ventricular thrombus, and she was started on warfarin. The role of multiple illicit substances including cocaine was considered a potential contributing factor. Due to the severity of the stroke and the corresponding clinical presentation, the prognosis of this patient was unfortunately poor, and she was supported throughout her hospital stay without significant clinical improvement.

4. Conclusion

Occlusion of the AOP can result in various clinical presentations, including acute encephalopathy, cognitive impairment, oculomotor defects, motor dysfunction, sensory symptoms, and behavioral abnormalities. In the setting of bilateral thalamic imaging abnormalities, a broad differential must be investigated, including cerebral venous thrombosis, basilar artery thrombosis, carbon monoxide toxicity, hypoxic ischemic encephalopathy, osmotic demyelination, Wernicke's encephalopathy, rabies, and flavivirus (Japanese) encephalitis. Demonstration of AOP occlusion by vascular imaging studies including MR angiography, CT angiography, and conventional angiography can be insensitive due to the small diameter of the AOP. Therefore, negative vascular imaging studies (MRA, CTA, and conventional catheter angiography) do not rule out the diagnosis. Timely diagnosis and treatment are facilitated by awareness of the diverse nonstroke-like clinical presentations and characteristic neuroimaging findings—improving the management of the infrequently encountered patient with an AOP infarction.

Abbreviations

AOP: Artery of Percheron
GCS: Glasgow Coma Score
CT: Computed tomography
CTA: Computed tomography angiography
MR: Magnetic resonance
MRI: Magnetic resonance imaging
MRA: Magnetic resonance angiography
CTA: Computed tomography angiography
PCA: Posterior cerebral artery
COPD: Chronic obstructive pulmonary disease
PEG: Percutaneous endoscopic gastrostomy
DWI: Diffusion weighted imaging
ADC: Apparent diffusion coefficient.

Conflicts of Interest

The authors declare that they have no conflicts of interest.

Acknowledgments

This study was funded by Department of Neurology, UMKC School Medicine, Clinical Research Division.

References

[1] G. Percheron, "Les artères du thalamus humain. II.--Artères et territoires thalamiques paramédians de l'artère basilaire communicante [Arteries of the human thalamus. II. Arteries and paramedian thalamic territory of the communicating basilar artery]," *Revue Neurologique*, vol. 132, no. 5, pp. 309–324, 1976.

[2] N. A. Lazzaro, B. Wright, M. Castillo et al., "Artery of percheron infarction: imaging patterns and clinical spectrum," *American Journal of Neuroradiology*, vol. 31, no. 7, pp. 1283–1289, 2010.

[3] P. E. Jiménez Caballero, "Bilateral paramedian thalamic artery infarcts: report of 10 cases," *Journal of Stroke and Cerebrovascular Diseases*, vol. 19, no. 4, pp. 283–289, 2010.

[4] A. Sandvig, S. Lundberg, and J. Neuwirth, "Artery of Percheron infarction: a case report," *Journal of Medical Case Reports*, vol. 11, no. 1, p. 221, 2017.

[5] K. M. I. U. Ranasinghe, H. M. M. T. B. Herath, D. Dissanayake, and M. Seneviratne, "Artery of Percheron infarction presenting as nuclear third nerve palsy and transient loss of consciousness: a case report," *BMC Neurology*, vol. 20, no. 1, p. 320, 2020.

[6] J. Musa, M. Rahman, A. Guy et al., "Artery of Percheron infarction: a case report and literature review," *Radiology Case Reports*, vol. 16, no. 6, pp. 1271–1275, 2021.

[7] G. Cassourret, B. Prunet, F. Sbardella, J. Bordes, O. Maurin, and H. Boret, "Ischemic stroke of the artery of percheron with normal initial MRI: a case report," *Case Reports in Medicine*, vol. 2010, Article ID 425734, 12 pages, 2010.

[8] R. López-Serna, P. González-Carmona, and M. López-Martínez, "Bilateral thalamic stroke due to occlusion of the artery of Percheron in a patient with patent foramen ovale: a case report," *Journal of Medical Case Reports*, vol. 3, no. 1, Article ID 7392, 2009.

[9] H. L. Teoh, A. Ahmad, L. L. L. Yeo, E. Hsu, B. P. L. Chan, and V. K. Sharma, "Bilateral thalamic infarctions due to occlusion of artery of Percheron," *Journal of the Neurological Sciences*, vol. 293, no. 1-2, pp. 110-111, 2010.

[10] J. Bogousslavsky, G. Van Melle, and F. Regli, "The Lausanne Stroke Registry: analysis of 1,000 consecutive patients with first stroke," *Stroke*, vol. 19, no. 9, pp. 1083–1092, 1988.

[11] Y. F. Shea, O. Y. Lin, R. S. Chang, and J. K. Luk, "Artery of percheron infarction," *Hong Kong Medical Journal*, vol. 18, no. 5, pp. 446–452, 2012.

[12] Y.-M. Chang and Y.-K. Fan, "Artery of percheron occlusion in an elderly male: a case report," *Journal of Clinical Medicine Research*, vol. 7, no. 2, pp. 126–128, 2015.
[13] Z. Xu, L. Sun, Y. Duan, J. Zhang, M. Zhang, and X. Cai, "Assessment of Percheron infarction in images and clinical findings," *Journal of the Neurological Sciences*, vol. 383, pp. 87–92, 2017.
[14] I. B. Saida, H. B. Saad, M. Zghidi, E. Ennouri, R. Ettoumi, and M. Boussarsar, "Artery of percheron stroke as an unusual cause of hypersomnia: a case series and a short literature review," *American Journal of Men's Health*, vol. 14, no. 4, Article ID 155798832093894, 2020.
[15] C. Bassetti, J. Marhis, M. Gugger, K. O. Lovblad, and C. W. Hess, "Hypersomnia following paramedian thalamic stroke: a report of 12 patients," *Annals of Neurology*, vol. 39, no. 4, pp. 471–480, 1996.
[16] O. A. M. Kheiralla, "Artery of Percheron infarction a rare anatomical variant and a diagnostic challenge: case report," *Radiology Case Reports*, vol. 16, no. 1, pp. 22–29, 2021.

10

A Case of Exertional Heat Stroke Complicated by Hypoxic Hepatitis

Bertram K. Woitok, Shawki Bahmad, and Gregor Lindner

Department of General Internal and Emergency Medicine, Buergerspital Solothurn, Solothurn, Switzerland

Correspondence should be addressed to Bertram K. Woitok; bertram.woitok@spital.so.ch

Academic Editor: Vasileios Papadopoulos

*Background.*Exertional heat stroke is a life-threatening condition often complicated by multiorgan failure. We hereby present a case of a 25-year-old male presenting with syncope after a 10 km run in 28°C outside temperature who developed acute liver failure. *Case Presentation.* Initial temperature was found to be 41.1°C, and cooling measures were rapidly applied. He suffered from acute renal failure and rhabdomyolysis and proceeded to acute liver failure (ASAT 6100 U/l and ALAT 6561 U/l) due to hypoxic hepatitis on day 3. He did not meet criteria for emergency liver transplantation and recovered on supportive care. *Conclusions.* Acute liver failure due to heat stroke is a life-threatening condition with often delayed onset, which nevertheless resolves on supportive care in the majority of cases; thus, a delayed referral to transplant seems to be reasonable.

1. Background

Exertional heat stroke is a life-threatening condition caused by excess heat generated from muscular exercise that exceeds the body's ability to dissipate it at the same rate. It is a form of hyperthermia associated with a systemic inflammatory response leading to a syndrome of multiorgan dysfunction in which encephalopathy predominates. Typical organ dysfunctions consists of liver failure due to hypoxic hepatitis, acute kidney injury, rhabdomyolysis, and disseminated intravascular coagulation [1, 2].

2. Case Presentation

We present case of severe heat stroke complicated by acute liver failure and rhabdomyolysis in a 25-year-old male after running 10 km in 28°C outside temperature presenting with syncope upon finishing the run. Paramedics on-site reported an initial GCS of 3, a body temperature of 41.1°C, and a blood glucose of 3.3 mmol/l. Cool packs were placed inguinal and 20 g parenteral glucose were administered.

The patient reported nausea and vomiting as well as a severe headache. His prior medical history was significant for an autism spectrum disorder, and otherwise unremarkable, he was taking no medication. The vital signs upon arrival showed GCS 15 with a tympanic temperature of 38.6°C, blood pressure was normal at 129/98 mmHg, and heart rate was 130 min^{-1}. The patient was hyperventilating at a respiratory rate of 45 min^{-1} and peripheral oxygen saturation was 98% breathing ambient air. The physical examination was otherwise unremarkable.

Laboratory findings are presented in Table 1. A urinalysis showed a leukocyturia and haematuria, and drug screen was negative. Leukocyte and erythrocyte casts as well as bacteria were present. An electrocardiogram and X-ray of the chest showed normal results.

After rehydrating with Ringers lactate solution, the body temperature stayed high between 38 and 39°C. He received symptomatic therapy with ondansetron. As leucocyte casts were present in urine, we treated a possible urinary tract infection with ceftriaxon, and to counteract possible concomitant fever, paracetamol and also metamizole were administered. The patient was admitted to the general medicine ward for further observation and rehydration.

On the third day after admission, the patient showed a slightly better general condition. Laboratory examinations revealed acute liver injury with ASAT 6100 U/l and ALAT 6561 U/l. The CK level elevated to a peak of 15969 U/l with a

Table 1: Blood test results, patient's evolution.

Test	Normal range	D1	D3	D4	D6
Hemoglobin (g/l)	137–165	182	156		154
WBC (10^9/l)	3.9–9.5	18.8	14.1		9.1
Platelet count (10^9/l)	140–360	90	97		132
INR		1.11			1.16
Sodium (mmol/l)	136–145	145	137	138	138
Potassium (mmol/l)	3.6–5.1	4.1	4.4	4.2	4.1
Calcium (mmol/l)	2.10–2.55	2.80		2.07	
Phosphorous (mmol/l)	0.74–1.52	0.22		0.61	
Creatinine (μmol/l)	64–104	195	127	103	103
Urea (mmol/l)	3.2–7.4	9.7		5.3	
CK (U/l)	30–200	842	15969	8743	2308
Total bilirubin (μmol/l)	<21	16	30	56	39
Aspartate aminotransferase (U/l)	5–35	48	6100	3062	411
Alanine aminotransferase (U/l)	<45	26	6561	5745	2811
Alkaline phosphatase (U/L)	40–150		72	82	86
Gamma-glutamyl transferase (U/L)	12–64	21	33	106	150
Lipase (U/l)	8–78	55			19
C-reactive protein (mg/l)	<5.1	0.3	2.4		1.1
Lactate (mmol/l)	0.5–2.2	4.7			

WBC: white blood cells; CK: creatinine phosphokinase; INR: international normalized ratio.

slightly improved kidney function (Table 1). The virus serology for hepatitis B, C, and E as well as HIV was negative.

As our patient did not meet the Kings College criteria for emergency liver transplantation, he was not referred to a tertiary centre for emergent transplant listing. Liver and kidney injury resolved with aggressive fluid resuscitation. The patient was discharged in good condition at the 8th day.

3. Discussion

Heat stroke is a form of hyperthermia associated with a systemic inflammatory response leading to a syndrome of multiorgan dysfunction in which encephalopathy predominates. Encephalopathy may be subtle, manifesting only as inappropriate behavior or impaired judgment. Heat stress leads to cutaneous vasodilation and splanchnic vasoconstriction, and also it triggers an acute phase response. The acute phase response plays a significant role in the development of hepatic injury, as is shown by an increase of interleukin-6 levels [1]. In addition, numerous animal models show that blockage of the release pathways for the cytokines IL-1β, IL-6, TNF-α, CD11b, CD68, IκBα, and NF-κB p65 and microRNA-155 [3–5].

Successful treatments with emergency liver transplantation [6–15], MARS [16], plasma exchange alone [17, 18], and hemofiltration [19] as well as cold dialysis and hemofiltration [20] have been published. There is growing evidence that conservative management seems to be sufficient for the management of most cases, and a delayed transplant strategy is reasonable [8, 12, 21–31], with cases reporting successful transplant after delaying transplantation in favour of spontaneous recovery [8, 12]. Most reported cases survived, but fatalities have been reported due to liver failure [8, 32–34] or transplant complications [35–37]. Nevertheless, early induction of cooling treatment, ideally reaching <38.9°C within 30 minutes, seems to be paramount [20, 38, 39]. Also, the administration of N-acetyl-cysteine was shown to improve transplant-free survival [40, 41] and has been reported in acute liver failure secondary to heat stroke [8, 21, 22]. It could also be shown that hypophosphatemia <0.5 mmol/l at admission, as was present in our patient, could predict the occurrence of acute liver failure [42], although it is unclear whether there is a causative connection. Predictors of an unfavorable outcome are core temperature >42°C, rapid multiorgan failure requiring artificial organ support and need of vasopressors [8].

4. Conclusions

We here present a case of heat stroke complicated by hypoxic hepatitis, acute renal failure, and rhabdomyolysis. A possible predisposing factor was urinary tract infection. Rapid cooling was achieved through convection cooling and transfer to air conditioned environment. Estimating the grade of encephalopathy was difficult due to autism spectrum disorder and mild hypoglycemia, but we interpreted the syncope as well as nausea and severe headache as manifestation of heat induced encephalopathy. Of note was the delayed onset of liver injury, presenting on day three after admission, which was also reported by the majority of published cases. After reviewing the literature, we decided to observe for spontaneous recovery and delay referral to a tertiary centre which was ultimately not necessary due to recovery.

The weakness of our case is that not all possible etiologies for acute liver injury were excluded as ceruloplasmin, iron studies, and an autoimmune panel were not obtained. In addition, there were no coagulation studies at the time of liver injury and the patient had received a single dose of paracetamol. We still decided to present the case due to the suggestive history and spontaneous resolve of the liver injury, which would neither be expected in metabolic or autoimmune liver injury or following a single dose of paracetamol, to raise awareness to this possible life-threatening complication of heat stroke.

Abbreviations

ASAT: Aspartate aminotransferase
ALAT: Alanine aminotransferase
CK: Creatinine phosphokinase.

Consent

The patient gave consent to publication of the case on 23.08.2019.

Conflicts of Interest

The authors declare that they have no conflicts of interest.

Authors' Contributions

Bertram K. Woitok was involved in collection of data and drafting of the manuscript. Shawki Bahmad and Gregor Lind were involved in the treatment of the patient, collection of data, and drafting of the manuscript.

References

[1] A. Bouchama and J. P. Knochel, "Heat stroke," *New England Journal of Medicine*, vol. 346, no. 25, pp. 1978–1988, 2002.

[2] J. L. Glazer, "Management of heatstroke and heat exhaustion," *American Family Physician*, vol. 71, no. 11, pp. 2133–2140, 2005.

[3] T. Kawasaki, K. Okamoto, C. Kawasaki, and T. Sata, "Thrombomodulin improved liver injury, coagulopathy, and mortality in an experimental heatstroke model in mice," *Anesthesia & Analgesia*, vol. 118, no. 5, pp. 956–963, 2014.

[4] P. Li, G. Wang, X. L. Zhang et al., "MicroRNA-155 promotes heat stress-induced inflammation via targeting liver X receptor alpha in microglia," *Frontiers in Cellular Neuroscience*, vol. 13, p. 12, 2019.

[5] H. Tong, Y. Tang, Y. Chen et al., "HMGB1 activity inhibition alleviating liver injury in heatstroke," *Journal of Trauma and Acute Care Surgery*, vol. 74, no. 3, pp. 801–807, 2013.

[6] B. Boni and C. A. Amann, "Exertional heat illness resulting in acute liver failure and liver transplantation," *Journal of Special Operations Medicine: A Peer Reviewed Journal for SOF Medical Professionals*, vol. 17, no. 17, pp. 15–17, 2017.

[7] S. Coenen, K. Tran, J. de Haan, and R. de Man, "Liver transplantation for non-exertional heat stroke-related acute liver failure," *BMJ Case Reports*, vol. 2017, 2017.

[8] B. C. Davis, H. Tillman, R. T. Chung et al., "Heat stroke leading to acute liver injury & failure: a case series from the Acute Liver Failure Study Group," *Liver International*, vol. 37, no. 4, pp. 509–513, 2017.

[9] F. Inayat and H. U. Virk, "Liver transplantation after exertional heatstroke-induced acute liver failure," *Cureus*, vol. 8, no. 8, p. e768, 2016.

[10] J. C. LaMattina, H. Akbar, S. Sultan et al., "Molecular adsorbent recirculating system support followed by liver transplantation for multiorgan failure from heatstroke," *Transplantation Proceedings*, vol. 50, no. 10, pp. 3516–3520, 2018.

[11] L. A. Martínez-Insfran, F. Alconchel, P. Ramírez et al., "Liver transplantation for fulminant hepatic failure due to heat stroke: a case report," *Transplantation Proceedings*, vol. 51, no. 1, pp. 87–89, 2019.

[12] P. N. Martins, I. M. A. Brüggenwirth, J. McDaid et al., "Heat stroke as a cause of liver failure and evaluation of liver transplant," *Experimental and Clinical Transplantation: Official Journal of the Middle East Society for Organ Transplantation*, 2018.

[13] M. Ramanathan, M. Pedersen, R. Ramsey, and A. Seetharam, "Diagnostic value of coagulation factor and intracranial pressure monitoring in acute liver failure from heat stroke: case report and review of the literature," *Transplantation Proceedings*, vol. 47, no. 3, pp. 817–819, 2015.

[14] R. S. Mateos, N. M. Hogan, D. Dorcaratto et al., "Total hepatectomy and liver transplantation as a two-stage procedure for fulminant hepatic failure: a safe procedure in exceptional circumstances," *World Journal of Hepatology*, vol. 8, no. 4, pp. 226–230, 2016.

[15] K.-I. Takahashi, K. Chin, K. Ogawa et al., "Living donor liver transplantation with noninvasive ventilation for exertional heat stroke and severe rhabdomyolysis," *Liver Transplantation*, vol. 11, no. 5, pp. 570–572, 2005.

[16] J. Sein Anand, Z. Chodorowski, and R. P. Korolkiewicz, "Heat stroke complicated by liver failure and hyperbilirubinaemia—a case report," *Przeglad Lekarski*, vol. 64, no. 64, pp. 344-345, 2007.

[17] K.-J. Chen, T.-H. Chen, Y.-M. Sue, T.-J. Chen, and C.-Y. Cheng, "High-volume plasma exchange in a patient with acute liver failure due to non-exertional heat stroke in a sauna," *Journal of Clinical Apheresis*, vol. 29, no. 5, pp. 281–283, 2014.

[18] V. M. S. Raj, A. Alladin, B. Pfeiffer et al., "Therapeutic plasma exchange in the treatment of exertional heat stroke and multiorgan failure," *Pediatric Nephrology*, vol. 28, no. 6, pp. 971–974, 2013.

[19] J. Jiao, F. Zhou, H. Kang, C. Liu, M. Yang, and J. Hu, "Unexpected extrapyramidal symptoms and pulmonary aspergillosis in exertional heatstroke with fulminant liver failure: a case report," *Journal of Medical Case Reports*, vol. 11, no. 1, 2017.

[20] S. Wakino, S. Hori, T. Mimura et al., "Heat stroke with multiple organ failure treated with cold hemodialysis and cold continuous hemodiafiltration: a case report," *Therapeutic Apheresis and Dialysis*, vol. 9, no. 5, pp. 423–428, 2005.

[21] A. Aquilina, T. Pirotta, and A. Aquilina, "Acute liver failure and hepatic encephalopathy in exertional heat stroke," *BMJ Case Reports*, vol. 2018, 2018.

[22] N. Azzopardi, S. Chetcuti, J. Sant, and J. Pocock, "Acute liver impairment in a young, healthy athlete: hypoxic hepatitis and rhabdomyolysis following heat stroke," *Case Reports in Gastroenterology*, vol. 6, no. 2, pp. 563–568, 2012.

[23] A. S. Carvalho, S. C. Rodeia, J. Silvestre, and P. Póvoa, "Exertional heat stroke and acute liver failure: a late dysfunction," *BMJ Case Reports*, vol. 2016, Article ID bcr2016214434, 2016.

[24] R. R. T. Castro, R. Costa Filho, and A. C. L. D. Nobrega, "Fulminant liver failure in a street runner: effects of heat stroke," *Revista da Associação Médica Brasileira*, vol. 64, no. 3, pp. 208–211, 2018.

[25] M. Deutsch, J. Koskinas, T. Emmanuel, D. Kountouras, and S. Hadziyannis, "Heat stroke and multi-organ failure with liver involvement in an asylum-seeking refugee," *The Journal of Emergency Medicine*, vol. 31, no. 3, pp. 255–257, 2006.

[26] T. Giercksky, K. M. Boberg, I. N. Farstad, S. Halvorsen, and E. Schrumpf, "Severe liver failure in exertional heat stroke," *Scandinavian Journal of Gastroenterology*, vol. 34, no. 34, pp. 824–827, 1999.

[27] E. Hadad, Z. Ben-Ari, Y. Heled, D. S. Moran, Y. Shani, and Y. Epstein, "Liver transplantation in exertional heat stroke: a medical dilemma," *Intensive Care Medicine*, vol. 30, pp. 1474–1478, 2004.

[28] Q. Jin, E. Chen, J. Jiang, and Y. Lu, "Acute hepatic failure as a leading manifestation in exertional heat stroke," *Case Reports in Critical Care*, vol. 2012, Article ID 295867, 4 pages, 2012.

[29] J. A. Kurowski, H. C. Lin, S. Mohammad, S. Krug, and E. M. Alonso, "Exertional heat stroke in a young athlete resulting in acute liver failure," *Journal of Pediatric Gastroenterology and Nutrition*, vol. 63, no. 4, pp. e75–e76, 2016.

[30] M. Wagner, P. Kaufmann, P. Fickert, M. Trauner, C. Lackner, and R. E. Stauber, "Successful conservative management of acute hepatic failure following exertional heatstroke," *European Journal of Gastroenterology & Hepatology*, vol. 15, no. 10, pp. 1135–1139, 2003.

[31] K. Weigand, C. Riediger, W. Stremmel, C. Flechtenmacher, and J. Encke, "Are heat stroke and physical exhaustion underestimated causes of acute hepatic failure?" *World Journal of Gastroenterology*, vol. 13, no. 2, pp. 306–309, 2007.

[32] E. Erarslan, í. Yüksel, and S. Haznedaroğ Lu, "Acute liver failure due to non-exertional heatstroke after sauna," *Annals of Hepatology*, vol. 11, no. 1, pp. 138–142, 2012.

[33] C. Ichai, J. Ciais, H. Hyvernat, Y. Labib, P. Fabiani, and D. Grimaud, "Insuffisance hépatique aiguë mortelle: une complication rare du coup de chaleur d'effort," *Annales Françaises d'Anesthésie et de Réanimation*, vol. 16, no. 1, pp. 64–67, 1997.

[34] S. Y. Kim, S. A. Sung, G. J. Ko et al., "A case of multiple organ failure due to heat stoke following a warm bath," *The Korean Journal of Internal Medicine*, vol. 21, no. 3, pp. 210–212, 2006.

[35] J. Berger, J. Hart, M. Millis, and A. L. Baker, "Fulminant hepatic failure from heat stroke requiring liver transplantation," *Journal of Clinical Gastroenterology*, vol. 30, no. 4, pp. 429–431, 2000.

[36] T. Hassanein, J. A. Perper, L. Tepperman, T. E. Starzl, and D. H. Van Thiel, "Liver failure occurring as a component of exertional heatstroke," *Gastroenterology*, vol. 100, no. 5, pp. 1442–1447, 1991.

[37] J. M. Saissy, L. Almanza, D. Samuel, and B. Pats, "Liver transplantation after exertion-induced heat stroke associated with fulminant liver failure," *La Presse Médicale*, vol. 25, pp. 977–979, 1996.

[38] D. J. Casa, L. E. Armstrong, G. P. Kenny, F. G. O'Connor, and R. A. Huggins, "Exertional heat stroke," *Current Sports Medicine Reports*, vol. 11, no. 3, pp. 115–123, 2012.

[39] T. P. Yeo, "Heat stroke," *AACN Clinical Issues: Advanced Practice in Acute and Critical Care*, vol. 15, no. 2, pp. 280–293, 2004.

[40] W. M. Lee, L. S. Hynan, L. Rossaro et al., "Intravenous N-acetylcysteine improves transplant-free survival in early stage non-acetaminophen acute liver failure," *Gastroenterology*, vol. 137, no. 3, pp. 856.e1–864e1, 2009.

[41] J. S. Will, C. J. Snyder, and K. L. Westerfield, "N-Acetylcysteine (NAC) for the prevention of liver failure in heat injury-mediated ischemic hepatitis," *Military Medicine*, vol. 184, no. 9-10, 2019.

[42] J. Garcin, J. Bronstein, S. Cremades, P. Courbin, and F. Cointet, "Acute liver failure is frequent during heat stroke," *World Journal of Gastroenterology*, vol. 14, no. 1, pp. 158-159, 2008.

11

Feasibility of Dual-Task Gait Training for Community-Dwelling Adults after Stroke: A Case Series

Prudence Plummer,[1] Raymond M. Villalobos,[2] Moira S. Vayda,[2] Myriam Moser,[2] and Erin Johnson[2]

[1] *Division of Physical Therapy, Department of Allied Health Sciences, The University of North Carolina at Chapel Hill, 3020 Bondurant Hall, Campus Box No. 7135, Chapel Hill, NC 27599, USA*
[2] *New England Rehabilitation Hospital, Woburn, MA 01801, USA*

Correspondence should be addressed to Prudence Plummer; pplummer@med.unc.edu

Academic Editor: Valery Feigin

This case series explored the feasibility and efficacy of cognitive-motor dual-task gait training in community-dwelling adults within 12 months of stroke. A secondary aim was to assess transfer of training to different dual-task combinations. Seven male participants within 12 months of stroke participated in 12 sessions of dual-task gait training. We examined single and dual-task performance in four different dual-task combinations at baseline, after 6 and 12 sessions, and if possible, at 1-month followup. Feasibility was assessed by asking participants to rate mental and physical fatigue, perceived difficulty, anxiety, and fear of falling at the end of each session. Five of the seven participants demonstrated reduced dual-task cost in gait speed in at least one of the dual-task combinations after the intervention. Analysis of the patterns of interference in the gait and cognitive tasks suggested that the way in which the participants allocated their attention between the simultaneous tasks differed across tasks and, in many participants, changed over time. Dual-task gait training is safe and feasible within the first 12 months after stroke, and may improve dual-task walking speed. Individuals with a combination of physical and cognitive impairments may not be appropriate for dual-task gait training.

1. Introduction

Cognitive-motor dual-task interference, defined as the decrement in performance that occurs when cognitive and motor tasks are performed simultaneously, has been well established in people after stroke [1–9]. This growing body of research has demonstrated significant dual-task decrements in gait speed [1, 5, 8], stride length [5, 8], cadence [6, 8], stride duration [2, 4, 8], and double limb support duration [1, 7]. In other words, compared to single-task walking, when individuals with stroke perform a cognitive task while walking they are less stable and take shorter, slower steps, resulting in a dramatic cost on gait speed. Gait-related dual-task deficits persist in community-dwelling stroke survivors many months after discharge from rehabilitation [3, 5, 8]. Since walking in the community is often performed concurrently with cognitive tasks, such as remembering directions or engaging in social interactions, a reduced capacity for dual-task walking may restrict the degree to which a person is able to physically function and participate in their life roles.

Conventional rehabilitation does not appear to adequately address gait-related dual-task interference. For example, in a longitudinal study of cognitive-motor interference, Cockburn and colleagues [2] found that 7 out of 10 patients showed a reduction in gait decrement associated with dual-task walking after usual rehabilitation; however, most patients continued to exhibit considerable dual-task interference during walking at discharge. Thus, even though single-task gait speed may recover to normal values after rehabilitation for stroke, dual-task capacity can remain considerably impaired.

There is promising evidence for dual-task training in older adults [10, 11] and individuals with Parkinson's disease [12, 13]. A recent study examined the effects of a cognitive-motor dual-task gait training intervention in people with neurological disorders [14], but only 2 of the 10 participants in the experimental group had experienced a stroke.

Table 1: Overview of gait activities for dual-task gait training.

	Predictable	Unpredictable
Stationary	Closed tasks (i) Walking in flat, wide space (ii) Walking over/around obstacles, all of the same height and equally spaced (iii) Walking with narrow BOS	Variable motionless tasks (i) Walking around obstacles with variable spacing (ii) Walking over obstacles of variable height (iii) Walking over changing floor surfaces
Moving	Consistent motion tasks (i) Walk toward/beside/behind a person moving at a consistent speed and direction (ii) Walk under different lighting conditions	Open tasks (i) Walking in a crowded corridor (ii) Walking outdoors in the car park (iii) Walking and negotiating a moving obstacle

To date, the only published dual-task training study in stroke is a dual-task exercise program involving patients with chronic stroke who walked while manipulating either one or two balls of various sizes (i.e., a motor-motor dual-task) [15]. Training was provided for 30 minutes, 3 times per week for 4 weeks. Compared to 12 patients who did not receive any intervention, the 13 patients who received dual-task training significantly improved their gait speed, cadence, stride duration, and stride length in single and dual-task (tray carrying) walking. Because this study focused on the coordination of simultaneous motor tasks and did not include any follow up, it is not known whether improvements transferred to other types of dual-tasks, such as cognitive-motor dual-tasks, or whether the improvements were maintained.

It is now well recognized that dual-task interference is influenced by the nature and difficulty of the cognitive tasks [9]. In a classic example, Maylor and Wing [16] found that age-related differences in postural stability were increased by cognitive tasks involving visuospatial cognition but not by counting tasks. Similar findings have been reported in gait-related dual-task interference in people with stroke [8]. Although these findings could be due to differences in task complexity, it is possible that the distinct cognitive processing demands of the tasks interfere differentially with postural control or gait, especially since gait is multifaceted with regard to its underlying cortical control mechanisms [17]. For this reason, it could be hypothesized that dual-task training in one type of task (e.g., executive function task) would not transfer to another type of cognitive task (e.g., visuospatial cognition task). Knowing whether the effects of dual-task training transfer to untrained dual-task combinations is essential for designing and planning rehabilitation interventions.

The purposes of this case series were to explore the feasibility and efficacy of a cognitive-motor dual-task training paradigm in community-dwelling adults within 12 months of stroke and to explore transfer of training to different dual-task combinations. To gain insight into whether dual-task gait training transfers across dual-task combinations, we examined the effects of the intervention on three different cognitive-motor dual-tasks and, where feasible, one motor-motor dual-task.

2. Case Descriptions

The case series included participants within 12 months of stroke who had completed conventional rehabilitation and were living in the community. Participants had to be able to walk at least 10 meters without the assistance of another person, follow a three-step command, and communicate verbally in English. Individuals were not eligible to participate if they had any pre-existing neurological disorders other than stroke, a previous stroke with residual deficits, uncorrected hearing impairment, severe visual impairment, severe dysarthria or aphasia, lower extremity amputation, any orthopedic problem affecting gait, concurrent participation in a trial of locomotor, or cognitive rehabilitation or were not living in the community prior to their stroke. Participants were screened for eligibility and approved for participation by a physician. Seven participants were recruited and provided written informed consent to participate.

3. Procedures

Study procedures were approved by the Institutional Review Board at Northeastern University (Boston, MA). Following baseline testing, participants completed 12 sessions of dual-task gait training (DTGT), 30 minutes each session, 3 times per week for 4 weeks. Maximum time to complete all sessions was 6 weeks. A midpoint assessment was conducted after 6 sessions. Posttraining assessments were completed within one week following the last session. If possible, a follow-up assessment 1 month later was also conducted. All training sessions and assessments took place in the outpatient therapy department at New England Rehabilitation Hospital (Woburn, MA). Licensed physical therapists were trained to provide the study intervention, and a trained research assistant conducted all of the outcome assessments.

4. Intervention

DTGT consisted of gait activities performed simultaneously with cognitive tasks. Gait training activities were based on Gentile's taxonomy of tasks [18]; the progressive sequence of gait training activities is presented in Table 1. Five categories of cognitive tasks with different levels of difficulty were used

Table 2: Summary of cognitive tasks for dual-task gait training.

Task	Description
Random number/letter generation	(i) Randomly naming numbers between 100 and 500 (without repetition or consecutively) (ii) Randomly naming odd (or even) numbers between 1 and 100 (without repetition or consecutively) (iii) Randomly naming consonants of the alphabet (without repetition or consecutively)
Word association	Easy: (i) naming as many words as possible in a category (e.g., animals, fruits) (ii) naming opposites of words Hard: (i) naming as many words as possible beginning with a particular letter (ii) naming as many words as possible in a category (e.g., European cities)
Working memory	Easy: (i) reciting a sequence of numbers (3 or 4 number sequences) (ii) reciting grocery list (3-4 items) Hard: (i) reciting a sequence of numbers (5 numbers per sequence) (ii) reciting grocery items (5 items)
Calculating a time	Easy: adding or subtracting minutes to a given time within the hour (e.g., 3:15 + 5 minutes; 1:30 − 15 minutes) Hard: adding or subtracting minutes to a given time into the next hour (e.g., 4:40 + 25 minutes; 1:15 − 30 minutes)
Backward recitation	(i) Reciting number sequences backward (ii) Months of the year (iii) Days of the week (iv) Backward spelling (4-5 letter words) (v) Counting backward (by 2, 3, 6, 7, and 8; starting between 75 and 100)

for the dual-task training (Table 2). The cognitive tasks used for DTGT were adapted from tasks used in previous dual-task training studies [10–12] and were selected to represent a range in level of difficulty. Tasks involving generation of spontaneous speech (e.g., telling a story) and visuospatial cognition (e.g., visualizing and reciting directions) were purposely excluded from the intervention regimen so that transfer of training to untrained tasks, such as these, could be assessed. The participants performed at least two different cognitive tasks in each training session.

Cognitive tasks were progressed according to individual abilities and progression occurred in concert with the progression of gait activities. The cognitive aspect of DTGT could be progressed in two ways: level of difficulty within the task (e.g., reciting a longer list of items from memory) or the category of task, recognizing that perceived task difficulty may vary between participants. For example, someone who is "good with numbers" might find the arithmetic-based tasks less difficult than someone who is not strong in arithmetic. Gait activities could be progressed by increasing speed, increasing the duration of continuous walking bouts, and changing the category/nature of the task (i.e., closed task versus open task). Therapists were instructed to ensure training activities were challenging, but not impossible, and were encouraged to try to progress training in both cognitive and gait domains within each session. However, several factors concerning the interaction between gait and cognitive tasks needed to be considered when progressing intervention activities. For example, walking speed may need to be decreased initially when a cognitive task is made more difficult; or an obstacle course activity may need to be made easier (e.g., closed task activity instead of variable activity) when a more difficult cognitive task is first attempted.

Therapists were provided with a comprehensive Manual of Procedures for the intervention and attended two 3-hour training sessions. The manual described each cognitive task and the progressive gait activities, as well as guidelines for progression of training. Therapists documented the duration, intensity, and type of treatment activities for each session on a standardized form. The importance of adhering strictly to the study protocol for the duration of the study was emphasized. The goal for all participants was to improve their ability to walk (increase speed, stride length, symmetry) while concurrently performing the cognitive tasks.

5. Outcome Measures

Gait and cognitive performances were assessed under single-task conditions and three different cognitive-motor dual-task conditions. Where feasible, we also assessed performance in a motor-motor dual-task. The three cognitive tasks were auditory Stroop, clock task, and spontaneous speech; the secondary motor task was a coin transfer task. The cognitive tasks were selected to represent different cognitive domains, one of which more closely resembled the cognitive activities used in training, while the others were considered "untrained" dual-task combinations (Table 3).

TABLE 3: Dual-task assessments.

Task	Description	Transfer
Stroop task	An executive function task representing the type of tasks trained during practice. Participants hear the words "high" and "low," spoken in either a high pitch or a low pitch; participants are instructed to report the pitch of the word (high/low), ignoring the actual word	Trained
Clock task	A visuospatial cognition task. Participants are instructed to generate a mental representation of a clock face and respond verbally (yes/no) based on where the hands of the clock would be for the given times	Untrained
Spontaneous speech	Spontaneous narrative in response to a stimulus question; highly relevant to everyday dual tasking	Untrained
Coin-transfer task	Participants wear a belt with pockets and transfer coins from one pocket to another	Untrained

In the auditory Stroop task [19] participants heard the words "high" and "low" spoken in either a high pitch (360 Hz) or a low pitch (180 Hz). The participants were instructed to indicate the pitch of the word they heard (ignoring the actual word presented) by responding "high" or "low" as quickly and as accurately as possible. In the clock task, the participants heard a time (e.g., ten-twenty-six) and were required to respond "yes" if the hands were in same half (left/right) and "no" if they were not. For the spontaneous speech task, speech samples were elicited using a set of questions designed to stimulate a verbal response lasting at least 30 seconds (e.g., tell me what you did on the weekend).

The coin transfer task, adapted from previous research [20, 21], involved participants transferring US 25-cent coins, one at a time using the dominant hand, from the dominant-side "pocket" to the nondominant side as quickly as possible. The pockets (16.5 × 14.5 cm) were attached to a belt worn around the participant's waist. In all dual-task conditions, the participants were not specifically instructed to prioritize either task because we were primarily interested in observing the spontaneous dual-task effects. Performance in both gait and nongait tasks was assessed in order to make inferences about attention prioritization and patterns of cognitive-motor interference during dual-task conditions [9].

Spatiotemporal metrics of gait were assessed using a 6-meter GAITRite walkway, with a 2-meter runoff at each end to allow deceleration and turning. Participants completed 4–6 continuous passes for each task. The average of all GAITRite passes for each condition was used for analysis. Order of the dual-tasks (Stroop, clock, speech, and coin transfer) was randomized for each participant, but each person completed the tasks in the same order on each testing occasion. In this report, we focus on gait speed as the primary measure of gait performance due to its functional importance [22] and to enable comparison of findings to previous dual-task studies.

Single-task performance on the Stroop, clock, speech, and coin transfer tasks was performed immediately prior to the respective dual-task condition. Single-task performance for the coin transfer task was assessed whilst standing; for the cognitive tasks, single-task performance was assessed while sitting. Average reaction times (in milliseconds) and overall accuracy (percent correct) on the auditory Stroop and clock tasks were measured using DirectRT software (Empirisoft, New York, NY). Discourse analysis of the speech transcripts was performed to evaluate dual-task effects on speech. We focused on two measures of speech discourse: clauses per utterance, a measure of sentence complexity, and pauses per utterance. This decision was based on our previous research, which demonstrated that individuals with stroke experienced a significant dual-task effect on pauses per utterance but not on clauses per utterance [8]. In the coin transfer task, the number of coins transferred (max. 12) was recorded, and the coin transfer rate (coins/min) was calculated. In the single-task condition of the coin-transfer task, the participants transferred as many coins as possible in 30 seconds.

To examine the effects of the intervention on the amount of dual-task interference, we calculated dual-task effects (DTE) on gait speed and each secondary-task measure (i.e., reaction time, accuracy, speech variables, and coin transfer rate). The DTE represents the relative change in performance in the dual-task condition compared to single-task performance and is calculated by dividing the difference in value (e.g., gait speed) between single and dual-task performance by the value of the single-task performance, expressed as percentage [23]. Negative DTE indicates that performance deteriorated in the dual-task condition relative to single-task performance (dual-task cost), while positive DTE represents improvement in performance (dual-task benefit). For the Stroop and clock tasks, we calculated a composite DTE for cognitive-task performance by summing the DTE for reaction time and accuracy, which accounts for speed-accuracy tradeoffs in the overall DTE [23]. We computed a composite DTE for the speech variables (clauses per utterance, pauses per utterance) in the same way.

Secondary outcome measures were the Timed Up and Go (TUG) test [24], the Activities-specific Balance Confidence (ABC) scale [25], and the Subjective Index of Physical and Social Outcome (SIPSO) [26]. The secondary outcome measures were assessed before and after intervention and at the one-month follow up assessment. These measures were collected immediately after the assessment of dual-task interference described above. The order of secondary outcome assessments was consistent across participants and timepoints (pre, post, follow-up). Additionally, at baseline, the participants were assessed on a range of measures to characterize severity of impairment in cognition (Montreal Cognitive Assessment [27]), executive function (Stroop color-word interference test [28]), language ability (Shipley

Vocabulary Test [29]), lower extremity motor function (Fugl Meyer et al. [30]), and depression (short form of the Geriatric Depression Scale [31]). The 6-minute walk test was conducted to provide a measure of walking endurance.

Feasibility of DTGT was assessed by measuring participants' perceptions of physical and mental fatigue as well as their perceptions of task difficulty, anxiety, and fear of falling on a 100-mm visual analogue scale [12], where 0 represented no fatigue/anxiety/difficulty/fear, and 100 represented maximum levels of the construct. Adherence to the 12-session training program was a further measure of feasibility. Safety of the intervention was assessed via monitoring of adverse events and falls. Overall patient acceptance of DTGT was measured using a feedback questionnaire regarding the participants' satisfaction with the intervention.

6. Outcomes

All seven participants completed 12 sessions of DTGT within 6 weeks (range: 3.7–5.4 weeks, mean: 4.3). One patient missed the midpoint assessment due to scheduling difficulties, and two participants were not available for the follow-up assessment. Only two participants were assessed on the motor-motor dual-task combination. The reasons for not assessing other participants on the coin transfer task included inability to perform the task due to upper extremity hemiparesis or use of assistive device in the unaffected hand and insufficient time/minimizing testing fatigue. The baseline characteristics and demographics of the participants are presented in Table 4.

6.1. Gait Speed. Table 5 presents single and dual-task gait speeds for each participant at each assessment. Dual-task changes are shown in both absolute (gait speed, m/s) and relative (dual-task effects, %) measures. Baseline single-task gait speeds ranged from 0.58 m/s to 1.07 m/s (mean: 0.84 m/s). After intervention, single-task gait speed was generally maintained in all participants (mean: 0.87 m/s, range: 0.66–1.10). Of the five participants with follow-up data, three had further improvements in single-task gait speed at 1-month follow up. As illustrated in Table 5, all participants had dual-task declines in gait speed in all of the dual-task combinations at baseline, except for Participant 2 who essentially maintained single-task walking speed during the speech dual-task (+0.01 m/s). After intervention, five of the seven participants demonstrated a reduced dual-task cost in gait speed in at least one of the dual-task combinations. Participant 3, who demonstrated an increase in single-task gait speed post intervention, only improved his dual-task walking speed in the speech dual-task. Participant 6 walked faster in all conditions after intervention, but continued to experience dual-task costs on gait speed in all three cognitive-motor dual-tasks.

The effects of the intervention on absolute and relative dual-task costs on gait speed appeared to be different across dual-task combinations (Table 5). The most consistent improvements were observed for the Stroop task. At baseline, absolute dual-task declines in gait speed for the Stroop task ranged from 0.03 to 0.38 m/s (mean: 0.13 m/s). After intervention, four participants (P1, P2, P4,and P5) had noticeably smaller dual-task declines in gait speed (range for all participants: −0.01–0.17 m/s, mean: 0.06 m/s). The improvements in gait-related dual-task performance were less consistent and, on average, of smaller magnitude for the clock and speech tasks. Baseline dual-task declines in gait speed during the clock task ranged from 0.05 to 0.22 m/s (mean: 0.11 m/s); after intervention the dual-task declines were 0.00–0.16 m/s (mean: 0.09 m/s). For the speech task, baseline dual-task declines in gait speed ranged from −0.01 to 0.23 m/s (mean: 0.11 m/s); after intervention the dual-task declines were 0.02–0.31 m/s (mean: 0.14 m/s). The two participants who performed the coin transfer task slowed their gait speed at baseline by 0.20 m/s (Participant 1) and 0.12 m/s (Participant 4); after intervention the dual-task declines were 0.19 m/s (Participant 1) and 0.00 m/s (Participant 4).

The magnitude of the absolute dual-task decline in gait speed at baseline meant that three of the four participants with usual gait speed ≥0.80 m/s (P4, P5, P7) walked <0.80 m/s in at least one of the dual-task conditions. This is important, since 0.8 m/s is the widely considered threshold for functional community ambulation [22, 32]. Thus, the dual-task decline in these participants is clinically significant; they were unable to maintain gait speed needed for functional community ambulation when walking while performing a cognitive task. After intervention, all three of these participants had dual-task gait speeds >0.80 m/s for the Stroop and clock tasks, and two (P5 and P6) also walked >0.80 m/s during the speech task. These represent clinically meaningful improvements, since dual-task walking speeds have crossed into the range needed for full community ambulation [22, 32]. Of the three participants with single-task gait speed <0.80 m/s at baseline (i.e., functionally limited community ambulators during single-task walking), two (P1 and P2) had improved dual-task gait speeds in all dual-task conditions at the 1-month follow up, but remained <0.70 m/s. Participant 3 was the only participant to walk slower than 0.60 m/s at baseline. Although his gait speed increased to 0.66 m/s after intervention, this was not retained at follow up. Despite improved dual-task walking speed in the speech dual-task after intervention, his relative dual-task costs after intervention were worse than at baseline (Table 5).

6.2. Pattern of Cognitive-Motor Interference. To examine changes in the pattern of cognitive-motor interference, we plotted the DTE on gait speed (DTEg) against the DTE on cognitive-task performance (DTEc) for each subject for the three cognitive-motor dual-task combinations before and after the intervention. Figure 1 explains the patterns of cognitive-motor interference, and Figure 2 presents the individual cognitive-motor interference patterns at baseline and postintervention assessments.

The data in Figure 2 indicate clearly the consistent negative DTE on gait speed (i.e., DTEg values consistently below the horizontal dotted line) and a range of positive and negative DTE in the cognitive task (i.e., DTEc values left

TABLE 4: Demographic and baseline characteristics of participants.

Participant	Age (years)	Gender	Time since stroke (months)	Side of hemiplegia	Fugl-Meyer	MoCA	Stroop test	Shipley	GDS	Education (years)	6 min walk (m)	Assistive device
1	72	M	12	L	24	27	39	32	3	16	243.2	None
2	74	M	11	R	25	25	49	31	3	16	230.9	Cane
3	86	M	4.5	L	26	23	NT	33	3	16	198.7	Cane
4	42	M	11	L	25	26	26	27	8	12	318.9	None
5	76	M	8.5	L	29	28	30	37	0	22	373.8	None
6	60	M	9.3	L	27	28	22	33	3	18	358.8	Cane
7	86	M	3	R	26	27	45	37	2	22	324.5	None
Mean	70.9		8.5		26.0	26.3	35.2	32.9	3.1	17.4	292.7	
SD	15.5		3.5		1.6	1.8	10.8	3.5	2.4	3.6	68.0	

Fugl-Meyer: Fugl-Meyer motor assessment for lower extremity (max. 34); MoCA: montreal cognitive assessment (maximum score 30); Stroop test: Stroop color-word interference score (color-word score minus color score); Shipley: Shipley vocabulary test (max. 40); GDS: geriatric depression scale (score > 5 indicates depression); NT: not tested.

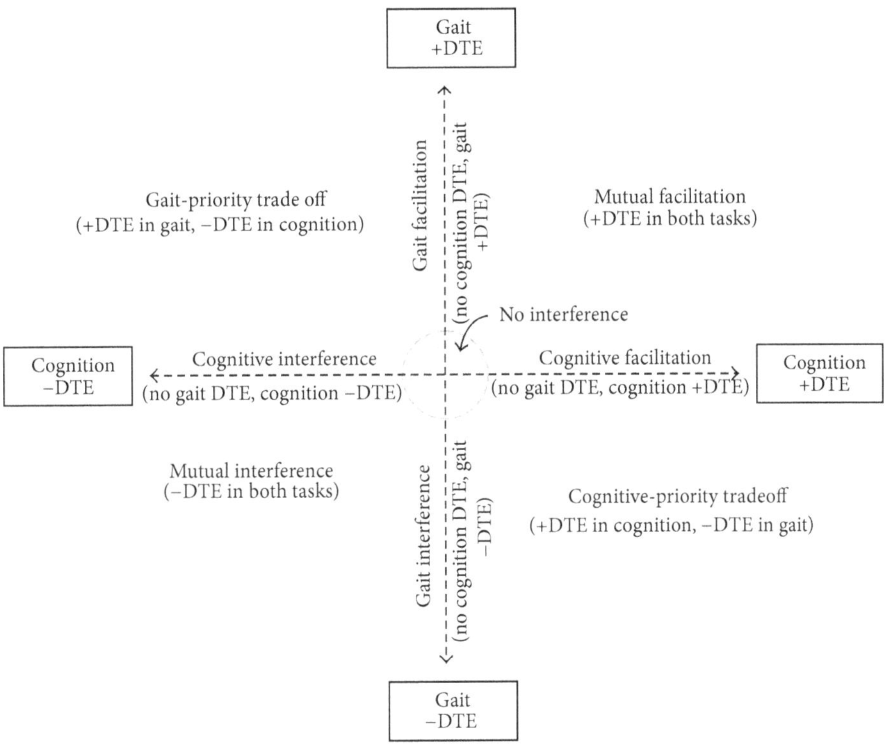

FIGURE 1: Patterns of cognitive-motor interference. Positive values for dual-task effects (DTE) indicate that performance improved in dual-task condition relative to single-task performance; negative values for DTE indicate that performance deteriorated in dual-task condition relative to single-task performance. Figure adapted from conceptual framework of Plummer et al. [9].

and right of the vertical dotted line). Indeed, the most common patterns of cognitive-motor interference were *mutual interference* (dual-task costs for both tasks), *gait interference* (dual-task costs on gait with little change in cognitive task performance), and *cognitive-priority trade-off* (dual-task costs on gait with concurrent dual-task improvements in cognition). Another noteworthy observation of the data in Figure 2 is the variability in dual-task interference across tasks and between participants. The variability suggests that the way in which the participants allocated their attention between the simultaneous tasks changed across tasks and, in some participants, changed over time.

For example, Participant 1 demonstrated *gait interference* in the Stroop and clock dual-tasks at baseline, but *mutual interference* after intervention in both the Stroop and clock dual-tasks (Figure 2). Specifically, after the intervention, there were smaller dual-task costs on gait speed in both tasks, but this came at a cost to cognitive-task performance. One

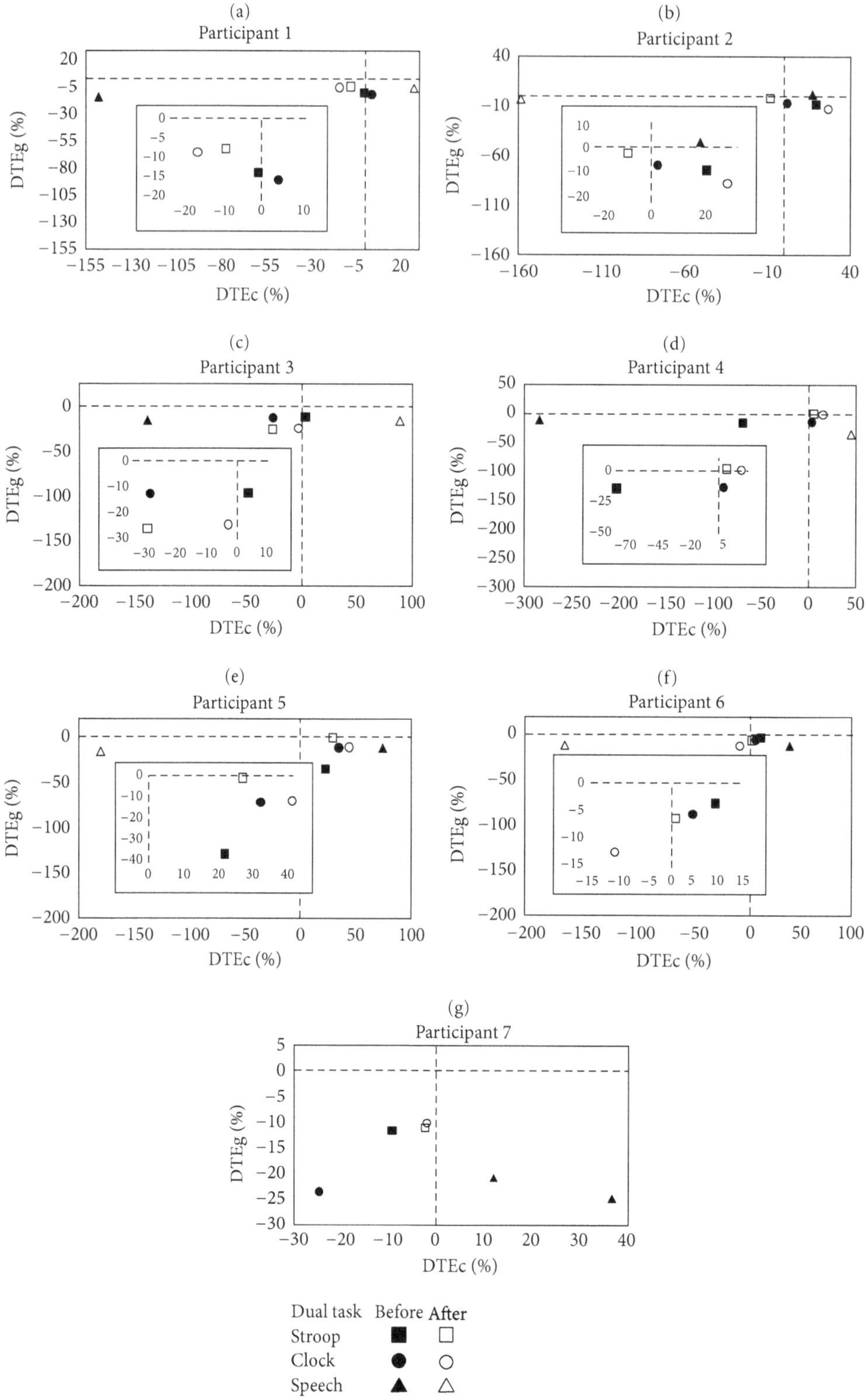

FIGURE 2: Plots showing patterns of cognitive-motor interference for each participant for each cognitive-motor dual-task combination before and after the intervention. Dual-task effects (DTE) represent percent change relative to single-task performance and are calculated by dividing the difference between single-task and dual-task values by the single-task value, expressed as a percentage. Positive values for DTE indicate that performance improved in the dual-task condition relative to single-task performance; negative values for DTE indicate that performance deteriorated in dual-task condition relative to single-task performance. DTEg is DTE on gait speed; DTEc is composite DTE for the three cognitive tasks (reaction time and accuracy for Stroop and clock tasks, clauses per utterance and pauses per utterance for spontaneous speech task).

TABLE 5: Absolute (gait speed, m/s) changes in gait speed for each participant at pre, mid, post intervention and 1-month follow up; and relative (dual-task effects, %) pre and post intervention. NT indicates not tested.

	Single task	Dual Stroop		Dual clock		Dual speech		Dual coin	
Participant 1									
Pre	0.77	0.67	(−13.7%)	0.66	(−14.8%)	0.64	(−17.0%)	0.57	(−26.1%)
Mid	0.74	0.69		0.72		0.66		0.65	
Post	0.75	0.69	(−7.3%)	0.69	(−8.1%)	0.68	(−8.8%)	0.58	(−22.6%)
Follow up	0.83	0.79		0.71		0.69		0.69	
Participant 2									
Pre	0.68	0.62	(−8.2%)	0.64	(−6.6%)	0.69	(+1.8%)	NT	
Mid	0.77	0.78		0.75		0.71			
Post	0.70	0.69	(−2.3%)	0.61	(−13.0%)	0.68	(−3.3%)		
Follow up	0.83	0.75		0.68		0.76			
Participant 3									
Pre	0.58	0.51	(−12.2%)	0.51	(−12.6%)	0.49	(−15.7%)	NT	
Mid	0.61	0.62		0.52		0.52			
Post	0.66	0.49	(−25.8%)	0.50	(−24.3%)	0.56	(−16.0%)		
Follow up	0.57	0.55		0.51		0.56			
Participant 4									
Pre	0.90	0.77	(−14.2%)	0.78	(−13.1%)	0.81	(−10.1%)	0.78	(−12.8%)
Mid	0.75	0.73		0.73		0.69		0.65	
Post	0.92	0.93	(+1.4%)	0.92	(0)	0.61	(−33.9%)	0.92	(0)
Follow up	1.03	1.04		0.96		0.76		0.98	
Participant 5									
Pre	1.07	0.68	(−36.0%)	0.94	(−12.1%)	0.94	(−12.3%)	NT	
Mid	0.99	0.86		0.91		0.84			
Post	1.02	1.01	(−1.0%)	0.90	(−11.4%)	0.86	(−16.1%)		
Follow up	NT	NT		NT		NT			
Participant 6									
Pre	0.97	0.93	(−3.5%)	0.91	(−5.5%)	0.85	(−12.2%)	NT	
Mid	1.03	0.94		0.90		0.87			
Post	1.11	1.05	(−6.2%)	0.98	(−12.2.%)	0.98	(−12.1%)		
Follow up	1.05	1.02		1.01		0.89			
Participant 7									
Pre	0.92	0.81	(−11.7%)	0.70	(−23.5%)	0.69	(−24.7%)	NT	
Mid	NT	NT		NT		NT			
Post	0.90	0.80	(−11.1%)	0.81	(−10.1%)	0.71	(−20.8%)		
Follow up	NT	NT		NT		NT			
Mean (SD)									
Pre	**0.84** (0.17)	**0.71** (0.14)	**−14.1%** (10.3)	**0.73** (0.15)	**−12.6%** (5.9)	**0.73** (0.15)	**−12.9%** (8.0)		
Post	**0.87** (0.17)	**0.81** (0.20)	**−7.5%** (9.1)	**0.77** (0.18)	**−11.3%** (7.3)	**0.72** (0.15)	**−15.8%** (9.8)		

interpretation is that, at baseline, the participant prioritized his attention during dual-task walking on the cognitive task (illustrated by the absent/minimal DTEc), but after training he was able to divide attention between both tasks. His cognitive-motor interference pattern was different for the speech dual-task; he had *mutual interference* at baseline (with greater dual-task costs on speech than gait), but demonstrated *cognitive-priority trade-off* after the intervention (Figure 2). Despite the apparent trade-off of attentional resources during the speech dual-task after training, gait dual-task costs were smaller, suggesting an overall improvement in dual-task capacity in this task.

Summarizing the data illustrated in Figure 2, Participants 2, 4, 5, and 7 demonstrated improved dual-task capacity in the Stroop dual-task after intervention; their dual-task interference "point" for the Stroop dual-task was closer to the *no interference* region after intervention. Only Participants 4 and 7 showed similar postintervention improvements in the clock dual-task: Participant 4 had only *gait interference* at baseline, and after intervention he had *no interference* on gait and some improvement in clock-task performance (positive DTEc, *cognitive facilitation*); Participant 7 had *mutual interference* during the clock dual-task at baseline, but less *gait interference* and *no interference*

Table 6: Secondary outcomes pre and, post training and, if possible, at one month follow up.

	Timed up and go (s)			ABC Scale (%)			SIPSO (max. 40)		
	Pre	Post	Follow up	Pre	Post	Follow up	Pre	Post	Follow up
Participant 1	14.4	13.8	14.6	88.6	92.5	94.4	33	27	32
Participant 2	13.5	14.3	13.5	60.6	73.8	83.1	25	30	33
Participant 3	15.0	19.3	20.1	48.8	53.1	34.4	22	23	22
Participant 4	11.3	9.0	10.2	66.9	71.9	85	14	19	25
Participant 5	11.5	11.5	NT	73.1	46.3	NT	26	32	NT
Participant 6	10.8	9.7	10.2	75	91.6	88.8	31	33	33
Participant 7	10.5	10.5	NT	81.9	81.9	NT	34	33	NT
Mean	12.4	12.5		70.7	73.0		26.4	28.1	
Median	11.5	11.5		73.1	73.8		26	30	

ABC: activities-specific balance confidence scale, SIPSO: subjective index of physical and social outcome, NT: not tested.

in cognition after intervention. Participants 2, 3, and 6 were similar to Participant 1 described above in that they demonstrated a change in pattern of interference for the clock dual-task, suggestive of a change in spontaneous prioritization of attention after intervention. However, the pattern change was not consistent (see Figure 2).

DTE on speech measures was typically much larger than those for the Stroop and clock task measures. The participants were also highly variable in whether they had negative or positive dual-task effects on measures of speech performance, and the pattern changed after intervention in most participants. For example, in Participants 1, 3, and 4, the pattern of dual-task interference in the speech dual-task changed from *mutual interference* to *cognitive-priority trade-off*; whereas in Participants 5 and 6, the patterns changed from *cognitive-priority trade-off* to *mutual interference* (in both cases, DTEg did not change but DTEc shifted from positive to negative).

6.3. Balance and Participation. Five of the seven participants had increased balance confidence (ABC scores) after intervention (Table 6), but only Participants 2 and 6 had increases that exceed the standard error of measurement (6.81 points) for the ABC in chronic stroke [33]. Compared to only two participants at baseline, four of the five participants tested 1 month after the intervention had ABC scores >80%, indicative of high physical functioning [34] and low likelihood of recurrent falls [35]. Participant 3 was low functioning at baseline (ABC < 50%); this improved slightly after intervention, but was worse than baseline at follow up. The reason why Participant 5 scored so low on the ABC scale after intervention is unclear. Three participants had increased SIPSO scores after intervention, suggestive of higher levels of social and physical reintegration, but the minimal clinically important difference values for this measure are not known. There were no meaningful changes in the TUG after intervention; the only participant whose pre-post change in TUG exceeded the minimal detectable change value for chronic stroke (2.9 seconds) [36] was Participant 3, whose baseline TUG indicated high fall risk [37]. He showed decline in functional mobility after training (4.3 seconds slower). Indeed, Participant 3 disclosed during the postintervention evaluation that he had experienced a fall (with associated vertigo) at home since the midpoint assessment.

6.4. Feasibility and Safety Outcomes. Most participants reported small increases in mental and physical fatigue in each session, with the ratings of physical fatigue typically greater than those of mental fatigue. The participants also reported low levels of difficulty, anxiety, and fear of falling. Participant 3 had the highest average ratings of perceived difficulty (mean: 55.3 mm, range: 34–68), anxiety (mean: 55.0 mm, range: 37–70), and fear of falling (mean: 47.5 mm, range: 28–72). None of the participants missed any session. Other than Participant 3 who reported a fall without injury at home during the second half of the intervention period, there were no adverse events reported. All participants indicated that they were "extremely satisfied" ($n = 4$) or "satisfied" ($n = 3$) with the treatment.

7. Discussion

This case series is the first study to examine cognitive-motor dual-task gait training in community-dwelling adults with stroke. The findings from this report provide evidence that cognitive-motor dual-task gait training is feasible in the first 12 months after stroke, and that cognitive-motor dual-task gait training can improve dual-task walking speed. The most consistent improvements were observed for the Stoop dual-task; improvements in dual-task walking speed during the clock and speech tasks were more variable. This may indicate low transfer of training to untrained cognitive-motor dual-tasks. The cognitive tasks used in the DTGT intervention largely involved executive functioning (which is a key function required for the Stroop task), thus it is possible that improvements in the Stroop dual-task were greater than the clock and speech dual-tasks because it resembled most closely the types of cognitive activities used during DTGT. Another possible explanation for the smaller and less consistent changes in dual-task performance in the clock and speech task, however, is that these tasks were relatively more difficult than the Stroop task. Previous research has shown significantly greater dual-task effects on gait in the clock [38] and speech tasks [8, 39] in people with stroke and healthy adults. Regardless of whether this finding can be attributed to poor transfer of training to untrained dual-task combinations, or differences in cognitive-task difficulty, the practical implication is that it may be important to include a wider range of cognitive tasks during DTGT to maximize transfer to different cognitive-motor dual-task combinations. Alternatively, therapists may choose to assess dual-task performance in a range of different dual-task combinations and then select dual-task activities for intervention that specifically target the person's greatest limitations.

An interesting finding from this case series is that most participants did not demonstrate remarkable improvements in single-task walking speed after the intervention. This may be due to the fact that there was no single-task practice during the DTGT sessions; the training focused exclusively on dual-task practice of gait. If gains in single-task walking speed are an important therapy goal, then it may be necessary to include both single and dual-task practice components in a dual-task gait training program. This may be a worthy consideration for future DTGT interventions, since single-task gait speed has been found to be correlated with dual-task costs on gait speed [39, 40]. Nevertheless, most of the participants in this case series showed improvements in dual-task walking in at least one of the dual-tasks.

Despite the improvements in the absolute and relative dual-task effects on gait speed by most of the participants in this study, our analysis of the patterns of cognitive-motor interference showed tremendous variability in dual-task performance and in the effects of the intervention on dual-task walking. While some participants showed evidence of improved dual-task capacity (e.g., decreased dual-task costs in both tasks), others demonstrated differences in the way they performed the task with no clear evidence of improvement in dual-task capacity. It is unclear whether a change in the pattern of cognitive-motor interference is indicative of a change in dual-task ability, and unfortunately this cannot be elucidated from the current data. However, our unique analysis highlights several important factors to be considered in future studies of dual-task gait training interventions. First, analysis of dual-task effects on gait may be inadequate to assess changes in dual-task performance. Performance on both gait and nongait tasks must be analyzed, and changes relative to each other should be considered when interpreting effects of treatment on dual-task performance. Second, reliability of dual-task performance needs to be established. To date, there have been no studies that have examined the reliability of dual-task performance: do individuals perform a particular dual-task the same way on multiple occasions? Until this is determined, it is not possible to conclude that changes in the pattern of interference are due to the intervention or just to a different strategy on a different day. This raises a third issue: the influence of instructions on dual-task performance. We did not provide any specific instruction about which task the individual should prioritize during the dual-task assessments. We were interested in examining the "default" performance of the participants. Lack of specific instruction about which task to prioritize means that each individual shall decide how to prioritize their attention in a given dual-task situation. While it is reasonable to assume that dual-task practice (i.e., dual-task intervention) may change the way a person chooses to spontaneously allocate their attention during dual-task walking, there are several other factors that may influence attention allocation in a particular dual-task situation, such as the perceived difficulty or importance of one task over another. Does dual-task training change a person's preferred attention allocation strategy or improve the efficiency and/or capacity for attention shifting, or simply improve gait automaticity such that attention can now be more easily allocated to other tasks?

Recent research has suggested that the ability to flexibly allocate attention between the two tasks during dual-task walking may be an important factor influencing dual-task interference [41]. It is not yet known whether individuals with stroke have the ability to voluntarily adapt their attentional focus during dual-task walking. While our results demonstrate variability within and between individuals in the way attention may be prioritized in different dual-tasks, determining the influence of dynamic attentional prioritization on dual-task performance will be important in order to establish the optimal instructions to use in dual-task assessment and training after stroke.

A potentially important clinical implication of the observations from this case series concerns the appropriateness of DTGT for individuals with more severe balance and gait deficits and/or limitations in cognitive ability. Participant 3 was the slowest walker and was at high risk for falls, with a baseline TUG greater than 15 seconds [37], and he had the lowest score on the MoCA. Relative to baseline, this participant had greater dual-task costs on gait speed in all three cognitive-motor dual-tasks after intervention, as well as clinically significant decline in the TUG. Furthermore, he perceived the intervention to be relatively difficult with some associated anxiety and fear of falling. It is possible that for individuals with considerable gait and balance impairments, improvements in walking and balance in undistracted conditions are needed before DTGT can be effectively implemented; or it may be that DTGT is not appropriate for individuals with a combination of physical and cognitive impairments. The findings from this case series have informed the selection criteria in the follow-up randomized controlled trial of dual-task gait training versus single-task gait training in community-dwelling stroke survivors within one year after stroke [42].

A limitation of this case series is that we did not include any postintervention assessments of cognition. In future, it would be of interest to determine whether DTGT has any effect on cognitive domains, such as executive function. The nature of the case series also limits the generalizability of the findings to other individuals with stroke. An unexpected scenario was that all of the participants in this case series were male. This is important because gender differences in gait-related dual-task interference have been reported among healthy adults [43, 44]. In general, there were only small changes in the self-reported measure of participation used in this study. Examination of spontaneous physical activity using activity monitoring devices may yield more accurate information about whether improvements in dual-task walking are translated to increased community ambulation. One of the participants (P5) in this case series for whom we captured physical activity data using the PAMSys (Biosensics, Cambridge, MA; data not shown) demonstrated notable increases in walking and standing activity, number of episodes of walking per day, and number of steps per day after the intervention [45].

8. Conclusion

The findings of this case series demonstrate the feasibility of DTGT in community-dwelling stroke survivors within one year of stroke. Our observations suggest that the potential benefits of DTGT may be limited in individuals with poor balance, slow usual walking speed, and/or impaired cognitive ability. The type and variety of cognitive tasks used during DTGT may influence transfer to untrained dual-task combinations. Importantly, even though dual-task costs on gait speed may improve with DTGT, the pattern of DTE suggests that changes in overall dual-task performance with intervention are highly variable.

Conflict of Interests

The authors declare that there is no conflict of interests regarding the publication of this paper.

Acknowledgments

The authors gratefully acknowledge the assistance of Keith Poulin, Gillian Shea, Colleen Dowd, Jacqueline Reinschmidt, Joy Huebner, Laura Hennessey, and Celina Cerf. This research was supported by the Kenerson Faculty Scholarship (P. Plummer).

References

[1] A. Bowen, R. Wenman, J. Mickelborough, J. Foster, E. Hill, and R. Tallis, "Dual-task effects of talking while walking on velocity and balance following a stroke," *Age and Ageing*, vol. 30, no. 4, pp. 319–323, 2001.

[2] J. Cockburn, P. Haggard, J. Cock, and C. Fordham, "Changing patterns of cognitive-motor interference (CMI) over time during recovery from stroke," *Clinical Rehabilitation*, vol. 17, no. 2, pp. 167–173, 2003.

[3] A. Dennis, H. Dawes, C. Elsworth et al., "Fast walking under cognitive-motor interference conditions in chronic stroke," *Brain Research*, vol. 1287, pp. 104–110, 2009.

[4] P. Haggard, J. Cockburn, J. Cock, C. Fordham, and D. Wade, "Interference between gait and cognitive tasks in a rehabilitating neurological population," *Journal of Neurology Neurosurgery and Psychiatry*, vol. 69, no. 4, pp. 479–486, 2000.

[5] D. Hyndman, A. Ashburn, L. Yardley, and E. Stack, "Interference between balance, gait and cognitive task performance among people with stroke living in the community," *Disability and Rehabilitation*, vol. 28, no. 13-14, pp. 849–856, 2006.

[6] S. Kemper, J. McDowd, P. Pohl, R. Herman, and S. Jackson, "Revealing language deficits following stroke: the cost of doing two things at once," *Aging, Neuropsychology, and Cognition*, vol. 13, no. 1, pp. 115–139, 2006.

[7] P. Plummer-D'Amato, L. J. P. Altmann, A. L. Behrman, and M. Marsiske, "Interference between cognition, double-limb support, and swing during gait in community-dwelling individuals poststroke," *Neurorehabilitation and Neural Repair*, vol. 24, no. 6, pp. 542–549, 2010.

[8] P. Plummer-D'Amato, L. J. P. Altmann, D. Saracino, E. Fox, A. L. Behrman, and M. Marsiske, "Interactions between cognitive tasks and gait after stroke: a dual task study," *Gait and Posture*, vol. 27, no. 4, pp. 683–688, 2008.

[9] P. Plummer, G. Eskes, S. Wallace et al., "Cognitive-motor interference during functional mobility after stroke: state of the science and implications for future research," *Archives of Physical Medicine and Rehabilitation*, vol. 94, pp. 2565–2574, 2013.

[10] P. Silsupadol, A. Shumway-Cook, V. Lugade et al., "Effects of single-task versus dual-task training on balance performance in older adults: a double-blind, randomized controlled trial," *Archives of Physical Medicine and Rehabilitation*, vol. 90, no. 3, pp. 381–387, 2009.

[11] P. Silsupadol, K.-C. Siu, A. Shumway-Cook, and M. H. Woollacott, "Training of balance under single- and dual-task conditions in older adults with balance impairment," *Physical Therapy*, vol. 86, no. 2, pp. 269–281, 2006.

[12] C. G. Canning, L. Ada, and E. Woodhouse, "Multiple-task walking training in people with mild to moderate Parkinson's disease: a pilot study," *Clinical Rehabilitation*, vol. 22, no. 3, pp. 226–233, 2008.

[13] S. G. Brauer and M. E. Morris, "Can people with Parkinson's disease improve dual tasking when walking?" *Gait and Posture*, vol. 31, no. 2, pp. 229–233, 2010.

[14] J. J. Evans, E. Greenfield, B. A. Wilson, and A. Bateman, "Walking and talking therapy: improving cognitive-motor dual-tasking in neurological illness," *Journal of the International Neuropsychological Society*, vol. 15, no. 1, pp. 112–120, 2009.

[15] Y.-R. Yang, Y.-C. Chen, C.-S. Lee, S.-J. Cheng, and R.-Y. Wang, "Dual-task-related gait changes in individuals with stroke," *Gait and Posture*, vol. 25, no. 2, pp. 185–190, 2007.

[16] E. A. Maylor and A. M. Wing, "Age differences in postural stability are increased by additional cognitive demands," *Journals of Gerontology B Psychological Sciences and Social Sciences*, vol. 51, no. 3, pp. P143–P154, 1996.

[17] R. Holtzer, J. Verghese, X. Xue, and R. B. Lipton, "Cognitive processes related to gait velocity: results from the Einstein aging study," *Neuropsychology*, vol. 20, no. 2, pp. 215–223, 2006.

[18] A. M. Gentile, "Skill acquisition: action, movement, and neuromotor processes," in *Movement Science: Foundations For Physical Therapy Rehabilitation*, J. Carr and R. Shepherd, Eds., Aspen Publishers, Gaithersburg, Md, USA, 2000.

[19] K.-C. Siu, R. D. Catena, L.-S. Chou, P. van Donkelaar, and M. H. Woollacott, "Effects of a secondary task on obstacle avoidance in healthy young adults," *Experimental Brain Research*, vol. 184, no. 1, pp. 115–120, 2008.

[20] N. Shkuratova, M. E. Morris, and F. Huxham, "Effects of age on balance control during walking," *Archives of Physical Medicine and Rehabilitation*, vol. 85, no. 4, pp. 582–588, 2004.

[21] S. O'Shea, M. E. Morris, and R. Iansek, "Dual task interference during gait in people with Parkinson disease: effects of motor versus cognitive secondary tasks," *Physical Therapy*, vol. 82, no. 9, pp. 888–897, 2002.

[22] J. Perry, M. Garrett, J. K. Gronley, and S. J. Mulroy, "Classification of walking handicap in the stroke population," *Stroke*, vol. 26, no. 6, pp. 982–989, 1995.

[23] V. E. Kelly, A. A. Janke, and A. Shumway-Cook, "Effects of instructed focus and task difficulty on concurrent walking and cognitive task performance in healthy young adults," *Experimental Brain Research*, vol. 207, no. 1-2, pp. 65–73, 2010.

[24] D. Podsiadlo and S. Richardson, "The timed "Up and Go": a test of basic functional mobility for frail elderly persons," *Journal of the American Geriatrics Society*, vol. 39, no. 2, pp. 142–148, 1991.

[25] L. E. Powell and A. M. Myers, "The Activities-specific Balance Confidence (ABC) scale," *Journals of Gerontology A Biological Sciences and Medical Sciences*, vol. 50, no. 1, pp. M28–M34, 1995.

[26] R. Trigg and V. A. Wood, "The Subjective Index of Physical and Social Outcome (SIPSO): a new measure for use with stroke patients," *Clinical Rehabilitation*, vol. 14, no. 3, pp. 288–299, 2000.

[27] Z. S. Nasreddine, N. A. Phillips, V. Bédirian et al., "The Montreal Cognitive Assessment, MoCA: a brief screening tool for mild cognitive impairment," *Journal of the American Geriatrics Society*, vol. 53, no. 4, pp. 695–699, 2005.

[28] J. R. Stroop, "Studies of interference in serial verbal reactions," *Journal of Experimental Psychology*, vol. 18, no. 6, pp. 643–662, 1935.

[29] W. C. Shipley, "A self-administering scale for measuring intellectual impairment and deterioration," *The Journal of Psychology*, vol. 9, no. 2, pp. 371–377, 1940.

[30] A. R. Fugl Meyer, L. Jaasko, and I. Leyman, "The post stroke hemiplegic patient. I. A method for evaluation of physical performance," *Scandinavian Journal of Rehabilitation Medicine*, vol. 7, no. 1, pp. 13–31, 1975.

[31] J. A. Yesavage, T. L. Brink, and T. L. Rose, "Development and validation of a geriatric depression screening scale: a preliminary report," *Journal of Psychiatric Research*, vol. 17, no. 1, pp. 37–49, 1982.

[32] A. Schmid, P. W. Duncan, S. Studenski et al., "Improvements in speed-based gait classifications are meaningful," *Stroke*, vol. 38, no. 7, pp. 2096–2100, 2007.

[33] E. M. Botner, W. C. Miller, and J. J. Eng, "Measurement properties of the activitites-specific balance confidence scale among individuals with stroke," *Disability and Rehabilitation*, vol. 27, no. 4, pp. 156–163, 2005.

[34] A. M. Myers, P. C. Fletcher, A. H. Myers, and W. Sherk, "Discriminative and evaluative properties of the activities-specific balance confidence (ABC) scale," *Journals of Gerontology A Biological Sciences and Medical Sciences*, vol. 53, no. 4, pp. M287–M294, 1998.

[35] M. Beninato, L. G. Portney, and P. E. Sullivan, "Using the international classification of functioning, disability and health as a framework to examine the association between falls and clinical assessment tools in people with stroke," *Physical Therapy*, vol. 89, no. 8, pp. 816–825, 2009.

[36] U.-B. Flansbjer, A. M. Holmbäck, D. Downham, C. Patten, and J. Lexell, "Reliability of gait performance tests in men and women with hemiparesis after stroke," *Journal of Rehabilitation Medicine*, vol. 37, no. 2, pp. 75–82, 2005.

[37] E. Nordin, N. Lindelöf, E. Rosendahl, J. Jensen, and L. Lundin-Olsson, "Prognostic validity of the Timed Up-and-Go test, a modified Get-Up-and-Go test, staff's global judgement and fall history in evaluating fall risk in residential care facilities," *Age and Ageing*, vol. 37, no. 4, pp. 442–448, 2008.

[38] P. Plummer-D'Amato, B. Brancato, M. Dantowitz, S. Birken, C. Bonke, and E. Furey, "Effects of gait and cognitive task difficulty on cognitive-motor interference in aging," *Journal of Aging Research*, vol. 2012, Article ID 583894, 8 pages, 2012.

[39] P. Plummer-D'Amato, L. J. P. Altmann, and K. Reilly, "Dual-task effects of spontaneous speech and executive function on gait in aging: exaggerated effects in slow walkers," *Gait and Posture*, vol. 33, no. 2, pp. 233–237, 2011.

[40] P. Plummer-D'Amato and L. J. P. Altmann, "Relationships between motor function and gait-related dual-task interference after stroke: a pilot study," *Gait and Posture*, vol. 35, no. 1, pp. 170–172, 2012.

[41] K.-C. Siu, L.-S. Chou, U. Mayr, P. van Donkelaar, and M. H. Woollacott, "Does inability to allocate attention contribute to balance constraints during gait in older adults?" *Journals of Gerontology A Biological Sciences and Medical Sciences*, vol. 63, no. 12, pp. 1364–1369, 2008.

[42] P. Plummer-D'Amato, A. Kyvelidou, D. Sternad, B. Najafi, R. M. Villalobos, and D. Zurakowski, "Training dual-task walking in community-dwelling adults within 1 year of stroke: a protocol for a single-blind randomized controlled trial," *BMC Neurology*, vol. 12, p. 129, 2012.

[43] G. Yogev-Seligmann, Y. Rotem-Galili, A. Mirelman, R. Dickstein, N. Giladi, and J. M. Hausdorff, "How does explicit prioritization alter walking during dual-task performance? Effects of age and sex on gait speed and variability," *Physical Therapy*, vol. 90, no. 2, pp. 177–186, 2010.

[44] J. H. Hollman, J. W. Youdas, and D. J. Lanzino, "Gender differences in dual task gait performance in older adults," *American Journal of Men's Health*, vol. 5, no. 1, pp. 11–17, 2011.

[45] P. Plummer-D'Amato, R. Villalobos, M. Vayda et al., "Feasibility of training dual task walking after stroke," *Archives of Physical Medicine and Rehabilitation*, vol. 92, no. 10, pp. 1717–1718, 2011.

12

Late Onset Postpartum Eclampsia: It is Really Never too Late—A Case of Eclampsia 8 Weeks after Delivery

Jens Minnerup,[1] Ilka Kleffner,[1] Heike Wersching,[1] Julian Zimmermann,[1] Wolf-Rüdiger Schäbitz,[1] Thomas Niederstadt,[2] and Rainer Dziewas[1]

[1] *Department of Neurology, University of Münster, Albert-Schweitzer Straße 33, 48149 Münster, Germany*
[2] *Department of Clinical Radiology, University of Münster, Albert-Schweitzer Straße 33, 48149 Münster, Germany*

Correspondence should be addressed to Jens Minnerup, minnerup@uni-muenster.de

Academic Editor: Marc Fisher

Introduction. Eclampsia is the combination of preeclampsia and seizures. Approximately one-half of all cases of eclampsia occur postpartum. Thereby late onset postpartum eclampsia is defined by its onset more than 48 hours after delivery. *Summary of Case.* We report a postpartum eclampsia occurring 8 weeks after delivery, which is the latest onset ever described. The course was complicated by an intracerebral hemorrhage (ICH). *Conclusion.* A late onset postpartum eclampsia even several weeks after delivery should be considered as possible diagnosis, since early treatment initiation with magnesium sulphate and antihypertensive medication prevents severe complications and reduces mortality.

1. Introduction

Preeclampsia is defined as the new onset of hypertension and proteinuria after 20 weeks of gestation in a previously normotensive woman [1]. The occurrence of generalized convulsions in a woman with preeclampsia without an alternative identifiable cause is referred to eclampsia. Approximately one-half of all cases of eclampsia occur postpartum [2, 3]. For a long time eclampsia was thought to not occur later than 48 hours after delivery [4]. This opinion was modified due to the onset of postpartum eclampsia occurring more than 48 hours after the onset of the postpartum period in some patients [5, 6]. Therefore late postpartum eclampsia (LPE) can be distinguished from early onset postpartum eclampsia by an onset later than 48 hours after term [5]. The latest onset of a LPE that has been reported in the literature so far was observed 23 days postpartum [5]. Characteristic findings on brain MRI include reversible white matter hyperintensities in T2-weighted images along with normal diffusion weighted imaging (DWI), thus representing a vasogenic edema [7, 8]. Usually, affected areas observed in the MRI are the parieto-occipital lobes, and less frequently other areas such as the frontal and the temporal lobe or the basal ganglia [9]. Here we report a postpartum eclampsia with the latest onset ever described, occurring 8 weeks after delivery. This case was complicated by an ICH due to the initially false diagnosis of an ischemic stroke and the consequently tolerated high blood pressure.

2. Case Report

A 30-year-old woman (gravida five, para five) having a migraine with aura in her medical history delivered a healthy girl in pregnancy week 38 by caesarean section. During her antenatal period, she developed edema of the legs and gestational diabetes. She was normotensive and had no proteinuria throughout pregnancy and during the postpartum course. On postpartum day 53, she complained of a rapidly developing severe headache and a transient visual loss in her left visual field. She was admitted to a local hospital. Her neurological examination there was normal except for a left-sided hemianopsia. The blood pressure was 180/90 mmHg. A CT scan of the head was performed immediately after admission and revealed hypodensities in the cerebellum. An MRI scan of the brain showed areas of hyperintense signal on T2-weighted images in the right rather than in the left cerebellar hemisphere (Figure 1). A lumbar puncture and a transesophageal echocardiogram were normal. The diagnosis

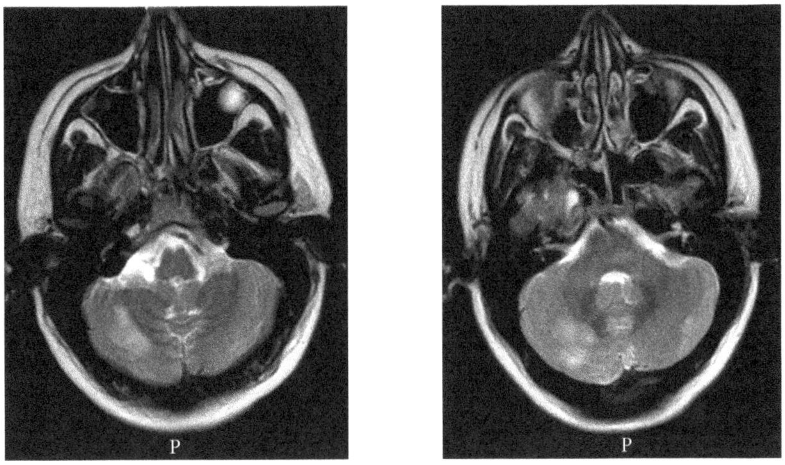

(a) (b)

Figure 1: Axial T2-weighted MRI shows areas of hyperintense signal in both the right and left cerebellar hemispheres. Findings in this MRI had led to the initial false diagnosis of an ischemic stroke in the posterior circulation.

of an ischemic stroke in the posterior circulation was made. Three days after admission, the patient experienced two generalized tonic-clonic seizures. A CT scan showed an ICH in the right frontal lobe. The patient was transferred to our neurological intensive care unit for further treatment of the ICH. On admission here, neurological examination revealed a somnolent state, a bilaterally reduced vision, and a left-sided moderate hemiparesis. Brain MRI and magnetic resonance arteriography/venography (MRA/MRV) showed an ICH (Figure 2(a)) of the right frontal lobe, hyperintensities on FLAIR sequences (Figure 2(b)) of the right frontal lobe rostral of the ICH and in the right occipital lobe, whereas DWI (Figure 2(c)) revealed no abnormalities, thus suggesting a vasogenic edema in these areas. There was no evidence for an intracranial sinus thrombosis on MRV. Urinanalysis indicated a proteinuria. A diagnosis of LPE was made. Treatment with intravenous magnesium was started and supplemented with valproic acid (VPA), which was subsequently changed to levetiracetam. No further seizures occurred. As her blood pressure was still increased, she was treated with urapidil. During her hospital stay, pulsoxymetry detected decreased oxygen saturation without symptoms of respiratory distress. The CT pulmonary angiography revealed subsegmental pulmonary embolism. A laboratory screening for thrombophilia was performed and a positive lupus anticoagulant test could be found. The patient was discharged four weeks after admission without any sequelae. A subsequent repeat MRI (Figure 3) of the brain three months after initial admission showed, apart from residues of the ICH, a complete resolution of the previous abnormalities.

3. Discussion

Important differential diagnoses of cerebellar lesions include multiple sclerosis and other inflammatory-demyelinating diseases, ischemic stroke, and neoplastic diseases [10]. Before referral to our hospital, the hyperintense lesions on the T2-weighted images in the posterior circulation were interpreted as stroke. However, no diffusion-weighted studies were done to corroborate the diagnosis. Furthermore, the arrangement of lesions was not consistent with an arterial supply. An eclampsia was initially not considered due to the long time interval between delivery and first symptoms even though the rapidly developing severe headache and the cortical visual deficit are typical symptoms [11]. In our department, the diagnosis of eclampsia was based on the clinical course, the detection of a vasogenic edema in absence of any cytotoxic edema on the MRI scan, and the combination of increased blood pressure with proteinuria and a recent childbirth in the patient's medical history. Frequent diseases causing seizures in puerperal period were ruled out. Particularly, there were no signs of a venous sinus thrombosis in the MRV. Other conditions causing seizures, such as meningitis and encephalitis, space-occupying lesions, and electrolyte or endocrine disturbances were also excluded. In addition, MRA, laboratory tests, and cerebrospinal fluid examination revealed no evidence for a vasculitis. Our patient had a pulmonary embolism and a positive lupus anticoagulant test, which is of interest, since thrombophilia and antiphospholipid antibodies have been found to be significantly associated with preeclampsia [12].

Complications in eclampsia are common and include acute renal failure, acute liver failure, and respiratory complications, such as aspiration pneumonia and acute pulmonary edema [13]. Mortality in eclampsia is mostly related to ICH [14]. Because of the severe complications, the appropriate therapy of eclampsia should be initiated as early as possible. For preventing and treating seizures in eclamptic patients magnesium sulphate is the drug of choice, as it is associated with a significant reduction of recurrent seizures, the risk for pneumonia, and admission to an intensive care unit [15, 16]. Mortality rates were also found to be substantially lowered compared to diazepam and tended to be reduced compared to phenytoin treatment [15, 16]. This is quite remarkable, since neurologists have a tendency toward using these classic anticonvulsants in patients with seizures that are due to

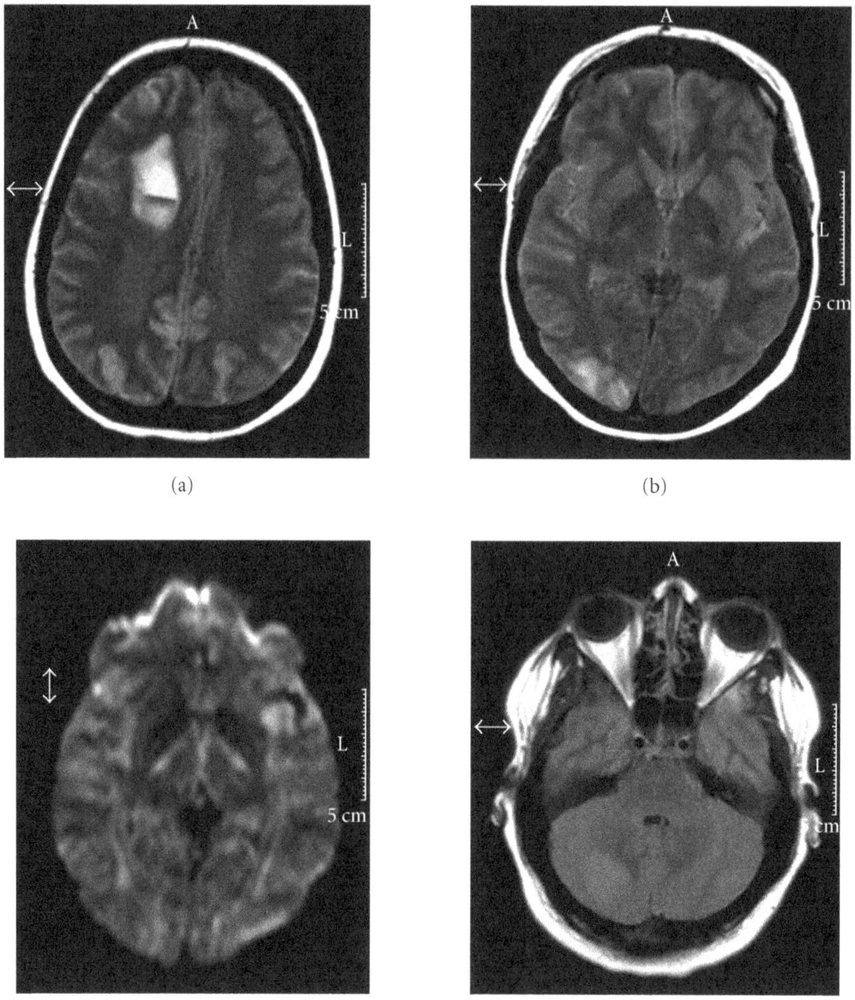

Figure 2: Axial FLAIR sequences show an ICH in the right frontal lobe (a). The combination of hyperintensities rostral of the ICH and in the right occipital lobe (b) with a normal DWI (c) in these areas is consistent with a vasogenic edema. The alterations in the cerebellum were largely unchanged (d).

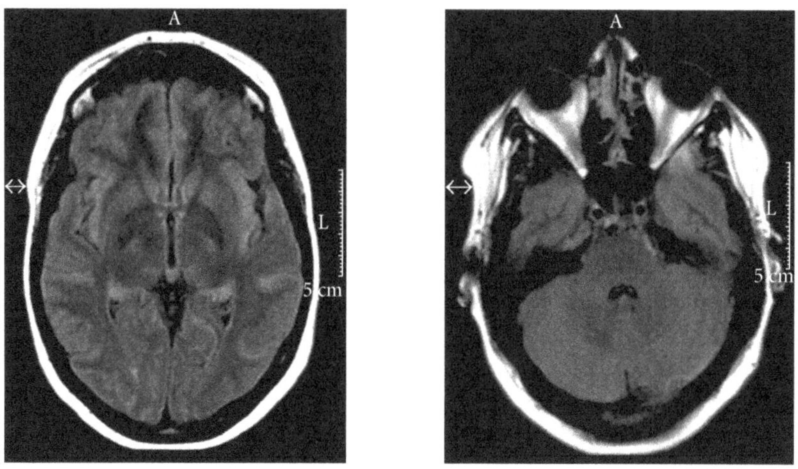

Figure 3: A followup MRI examination three months after admission shows a complete resolution of the vasogenic edema.

other causes than eclampsia. Our patient was hypertensive with systolic blood pressures up to 200 mm Hg. According to the initial diagnosis of a posterior circulation infarction, the blood pressure was not lowered, as recommended by the national and international guidelines [17, 18] for the acute phase of an ischemic stroke. In eclampsia, the blood pressure value at which antihypertensive therapy should be initiated is not clearly determined due to the lack of clinical trials that address this issue. However, lowering blood pressure in eclamptic patients is recommended when systolic blood pressure reaches or exceeds 155–160 mm Hg, since higher values are associated with the occurrence of ICH [19].

This case emphasizes the importance of considering on late onset postpartum eclampsia even some weeks after delivery, as early diagnosis and subsequent initiation of the appropriate antihypertensive and anticonvulsant therapy prevent severe complications.

References

[1] K. Seck and T. Fischer, "Diagnosis and treatment of preeclampsia: overview of international recommendations," *Zeitschrift für Geburtshilfe und Neonatologie*, vol. 213, no. 3, pp. 106–112, 2009.

[2] K. A. Douglas and C. W. G. Redman, "Eclampsia in the United Kingdom," *British Medical Journal*, vol. 309, no. 6966, pp. 1395–1400, 1994.

[3] B. Sabiri, A. Moussalit, S. Salmi, S. El Youssoufi, and M. Miguil, "Post-partum eclampsia: epidemiology and prognosis," *Journal de Gynecologie Obstetrique et Biologie de la Reproduction*, vol. 36, no. 3, pp. 276–280, 2007.

[4] L. C. Chesley, "Blood pressure, edema and proteinuria in pregnancy. 9. Proposal for classification," *Progress in Clinical and Biological Research*, vol. 7, pp. 249–268, 1976.

[5] S. L. Lubarsky, J. R. Barton, S. A. Friedman, S. Nasreddine, K. Ramadan, and B. M. Sibai, "Late postpartum eclampsia revisited," *Obstetrics and Gynecology*, vol. 83, no. 4, pp. 502–505, 1994.

[6] R. Dziewas, F. Stogbauer, M. Freund, et al., "Late onset postpartum eclampsia: a rare and difficult diagnosis," *Journal of Neurology*, vol. 249, no. 9, pp. 1287–1291, 2002.

[7] S. T. Engelter, J. M. Provenzale, and J. R. Petrella, "Assessment of vasogenic edema in eclampsia using diffusion imaging," *Neuroradiology*, vol. 42, no. 11, pp. 818–820, 2000.

[8] W. S. Bartynski, "Posterior reversible encephalopathy syndrome—part 1: fundamental imaging and clinical features," *American Journal of Neuroradiology*, vol. 29, no. 6, pp. 1036–1042, 2008.

[9] V. Finocchi, A. Bozzao, M. Bonamini, et al., "Magnetic resonance imaging in posterior reversible encephalopathy syndrome: report of three cases and review of literature," *Archives of Gynecology and Obstetrics*, vol. 271, no. 1, pp. 79–85, 2005.

[10] A. Gass, M. Filippi, and R. I. Grossman, "The contribution of MRI in the differential diagnosis of posterior fossa damage," *Journal of the Neurological Sciences*, vol. 172, supplement 1, pp. S43–S49, 2000.

[11] J. Hinchey, C. Chaves, B. Appignani, et al., "A reversible posterior leukoencephalopathy syndrome," *The New England Journal of Medicine*, vol. 334, no. 8, pp. 494–500, 1996.

[12] G. Mello, E. Parretti, L. Marozio, et al., "Thrombophilia is significantly associated with severe preeclampsia: results of a large-scale, case-controlled study," *Hypertension*, vol. 46, no. 6, pp. 1270–1274, 2005.

[13] E. V. Kuklina, C. Ayala, and W. M. Callaghan, "Hypertensive disorders and severe obstetric morbidity in the united states," *Obstetrics and Gynecology*, vol. 113, no. 6, pp. 1299–1306, 2009.

[14] K. A Okanloma and J. Moodley, "Neurological complications associated with the pre-eclampsia/eclampsia syndrome," *International Journal of Gynecology and Obstetrics*, vol. 71, no. 3, pp. 223–225, 2000.

[15] L. Duley and D. Henderson-Smart, "Magnesium sulphate versus phenytoin for eclampsia," *Cochrane Database of Systematic Reviews*, no. 4, Article ID CD000128, 2003.

[16] L. Duley and D. Henderson-Smart, "Magnesium sulphate versus diazepam for eclampsia," *Cochrane Database of Systematic Reviews*, no. 4, Article ID CD000127, 2003.

[17] H. P. Adams Jr., G. del Zoppo, M. J. Alberts, et al., "Guidelines for the early management of adults with ischemic stroke: a guideline from the American Heart Association/American Stroke Association Stroke Council, Clinical Cardiology Council, Cardiovascular Radiology and Intervention Council, and the Atherosclerotic Peripheral Vascular Disease and Quality of Care Outcomes in Research Interdisciplinary Working Groups: the American Academy of Neurology affirms the value of this guideline as an educational tool for neurologists," *Circulation*, vol. 115, no. 20, pp. e478–e534, 2007.

[18] S. Kulkens, P. A. Ringleb, and W. Hacke, "Recommendations of the European Stroke Initiative (EUSI) for treatment of ischemic stroke—update 2003. I. Organization and acute therapy," *Nervenarzt*, vol. 75, no. 4, pp. 368–379, 2004.

[19] J. N. Martin Jr., B. D. Thigpen, R. C. Moore, C. H. Rose, J. Cushman, and W. May, "Stroke and severe preeclampsia and eclampsia: a paradigm shift focusing on systolic blood pressure," *Obstetrics and Gynecology*, vol. 105, no. 2, pp. 246–254, 2005.

13

Neurodegeneration and Glial Response after Acute Striatal Stroke: Histological Basisfor Neuroprotective Studies

Rafael R. Lima,[1] Luana N. S. Santana,[1] Rafael M. Fernandes,[1] Elder M. Nascimento,[2] Ana Carolina A. Oliveira,[1] Luanna M. P. Fernandes,[1] Enio Mauricio N. dos Santos,[1] Patrycy Assis N. Tavares,[2] Ijair Rogério dos Santos,[2] Adriano Gimarães-Santos,[2] and Walace Gomes-Leal[2]

[1]*Institute of Biological Sciences, Laboratory of Functional and Structural Biology, Federal University of Pará, 66075-900 Belém, PA, Brazil*

[2]*Institute of Biological Sciences, Laboratory of Experimental Neuroprotection and Neuroregeneration, Federal University of Pará, 66075-900 Belém, PA, Brazil*

Correspondence should be addressed to Rafael R. Lima; rafalima@ufpa.br

Academic Editor: Michael D. Coleman

Stroke is a leading cause of death and neurological disability worldwide and striatal ischemic stroke is frequent in humans due to obstruction of middle cerebral artery. Several pathological events underlie damage progression and a comprehensive description of the pathological features following experimental stroke in both acute and chronic survival times is a necessary step for further functional studies. Here, we explored the patterns of microglial activation, astrocytosis, oligodendrocyte damage, myelin impairment, and Nogo-A immunoreactivity between 3 and 30 postlesion days (PLDs) after experimental striatal stroke in adult rats induced by microinjections of endothelin-1 (ET-1). The focal ischemia induced tissue loss concomitant with intense microglia activation between 3 and 14 PLDs (maximum at 7 PLDs), decreasing afterward. Astrocytosis was maximum around 7 PLDs. Oligodendrocyte damage and Nogo-A upregulation were higher at 3 PLDs. Myelin impairment was maximum between 7 and 14 PLDs. Nogo-A expression was higher in the first week in comparison to control. The results add important histopathological features of ET-1 induced stroke in subacute and chronic survival times. In addition, the establishment of the temporal evolution of these neuropathological events is an important step for future studies seeking suitable neuroprotective drugs targeting neuroinflammation and white matter damage.

1. Introduction

Stroke is a devastating condition and a leading cause of death and functional disability worldwide [1, 2]. This central nervous system (CNS) disorder is characterized by obstruction of blood vessels (ischemic stroke) or their rupture (hemorrhagic stroke) leading to metabolic collapse and a multitude of secondary mechanisms, including excitotoxicity, inflammation, metabolic acidosis, apoptosis, periinfarct depolarization, and oxidative stress [1, 2].

Following stroke an intense inflammatory response takes place, characterized by recruitment of neutrophils [3, 4], microglial activation [3, 5–7], and astrocytosis [8, 9]. Microglia activation plays both beneficial and detrimental actions following experimental stroke [5, 10, 11]. Inhibition of microglial activation with minocycline induces conspicuous neuroprotection following focal ischemia [12–14], but other experimental reports suggest that microglia may be also beneficial following stroke [10, 15–17].

Astrocytes are activated following both acute [18, 19] and chronic [20] neural disorders. These glial cells play both detrimental and beneficial actions following stroke and spinal cord injury (SCI) [21]. Astrocyte activation may contribute to ischemic damage in the hippocampus by activation of N-methyl-D-aspartate (NMDA) extrasynaptic receptors, a phenomenon involving calcium signaling [19]. On the other hand, astrocytes seem to mediate endogenous neuroprotection following stroke, a phenomenon involving activation of a glial-specific purinergic receptor, P2Y(1)R, and inositol 1,4,5 trisphosphate IP(3)/Ca^{2++} signaling [22].

Following stroke and SCI, neuroplasticity is inhibited by white matter- (WM-) associated proteins, including Nogo-A and proteoglycans [23]. Chondroitin sulfate proteoglycans (CSPS) are associated with astrocytosis and contribute to inhibition of axonal regeneration following stroke and SCI [24]. Nogo-A is an oligodendrocyte-associated protein and a major inhibitor of axonal sprouting [25, 26]. CSPS degradation with chondroitinase ABC enhances axonal sprouting following SCI [27, 28] and stroke [29, 30]. Similar findings have been found using a neutralizing antibody against Nogo-A [31–34].

In our previous investigations, we have described the patterns of microglial activation [3, 4, 12, 35], astrocytosis [18], and WM damage [3, 4, 35, 36] using experimental models of stroke, excitotoxicity, and SCI. Nevertheless, the pathological events were described up to 7 days from the disease onset. It has been suggested that WM damage with concomitant neuroinflammation is a long-lasting phenomenon even following human stroke [37]. In addition, it has been reported that the expression of Nogo-A is associated with inhibition of neuroplasticity following experimental stroke [31, 32].

Middle cerebral artery occlusion (MCAO) is a common pathological event in human stroke in which striatum and parietal cortex are damaged [37]. A comprehensive descriptive study on the basic neuropathology in both acute and chronic survival times following experimental striatal stroke is a fundamental step for future investigations seeking for neuroprotective and neuroregenerative therapies. In this study, we describe the patterns of microglia activation, astrocytosis, oligodendrocyte damage, Nogo-A immunoreactivity, and myelin impairment from 3 days to 30 days following focal ischemia induced by microinjections of endothelin-1 (ET-1) into the rat striatum.

2. Material and Methods

2.1. Experimental Animals. Male adult Wistar rats (290–300 g) were obtained from the Central Animal Facility in the Federal University of Pará. All animals were housed under standard conditions with food and water available *ad libitum*.

2.2. Ethics Statement. All procedures were approved by the Ethics Committee on Experimental Animals of the Federal University of Pará (CEPAE-UFPA), under license BIO 038-12. All experimental procedures followed the Principles of laboratory animal care (NIH Publication number 86-23, revised 1985). All efforts were made to avoid animal suffering and distress.

2.3. Stroke Model. Animals were deeply anesthetized with an intraperitoneal injection of a mixture of ketamine hydrochloride (90 mg/kg, i.p.) and xylazine hydrochloride (10 mg/kg, i.p.) and positioned in a stereotaxic apparatus after abolishment of their corneal reflex. After craniotomy, 80 pMol of ET-1 (Sigma-Aldrich, USA) in 1 μL of sterile saline was injected into the rat striatum ($N = 5$ per survival time) over a period of 2 min using a glass capillary micropipette. The pipette was left in place for 3 min before being slowly withdrawn. Control animals were injected with the same volume of sterile saline ($N = 12$). We used the following stereotaxic coordinates for the injection (in millimeters relative to bregma): 2.5 mm lateral; 1.2 mm posterior; and 4.5 mm below from the pial surface. After surgery, animals were allowed to rest in their cages (maximum 4 animals per cage) with water and food *ad libitum* until postlesion days (PLDs) 3, 7, 14, and 30. This stroke model was established in our previous reports [3, 13]. The mortality rate is less than 5% in this stroke model.

2.4. Perfusion and Histological Procedures. Following the described survival times, animals were deeply anesthetized with ketamine hydrochloride (90 mg/kg, i.p.) and xylazine hydrochloride (10 mg/kg, i.p.) and transcardially perfused with heparinized 0.9% phosphate-buffered saline (PBS) followed by 4% paraformaldehyde in 0.2 M phosphate buffer. Surgical manipulation was performed only after both corneal and the paw withdraw reflexes were abolished. Brains were removed from the skull, post-fixed for 24 h in the same fixative, and cryoprotected in increasing concentrations of sucrose–glycerol solutions over 7 days. The brains were then frozen in TissueTek and sectioned in order to obtain 20 and 50 μm coronal sections using a cryostat (Carl Zeiss/Micron, Germany). Sections were mounted onto gelatinized slides and air-dried for 24 h. Slides were stored in a freezer at −20°C for posterior histopathological analysis.

2.5. Gross Histopathology and Immunohistochemistry. The ischemic lesion area was visualized in coronal sections (50 μm thick) stained with cresyl violet. The site of ET-1 injection was recognized by tissue pallor associated with loss of cell bodies as described in our previous studies [3, 13, 38].

To analyze microglial activation, we resorted to standard immunohistochemical procedures. Activated microglia/macrophages were labeled using the antibody anti-rat CD68 (clone ED1, 1 : 500, Serotec, UK), which binds to an epitope on the lysosomal membrane of activated macrophages/microglia [38–40], rabbit anti-Iba1 (1 : 1000, WAKO), an antibody that recognizes a calcium binding protein present in the cytoplasm of microglia [41–43], and mouse anti-MHC-II (1 : 100, Serotec), an antibody that recognizes the major histocompatibility complex class II molecule [7].

Based on previous reports showing that pathological oligodendrocytes become Tau-1 positive after brain trauma and ischemia [44], we used the mouse anti-Tau-1 antibody (1 : 500, Chemicon, USA) to label dephosphorylated epitopes on damaged oligodendrocytes. Normal oligodendrocytes were labeled by mouse anti-Nogo-A (1 : 100, BD Transduction Lab, USA), an antibody that recognizes Nogo-A in the rat brain [45]. Myelin impairment was evaluated using an antibody against mouse anti-myelin basic protein (MBP), an important component of the compact myelin (1 : 100, Serotec, UK) [35].

Astrocytes were immunolabeled with an antibody rabbit antiglial fibrillary acid protein (GFAP, 1 : 1000, DAKO, UK), a classical astrocyte marker [18, 46, 47].

2.6. Immunolabeling Protocol. The slide-mounted sections were removed from the freezer, kept in an oven at 37°C for 30 minutes, and rinsed in 0.1 M phosphate buffer saline (PBS) for 5 min. To improve labeling intensity, sections were treated with 0.2 M boric acid (pH 9.0) previously heated to 65°C for 25 min. This temperature was maintained constant over the treatment period. Sections were allowed to cool down for about 20 min and incubated under constant agitation in 1% hydrogen peroxide solution in methanol for 20 min. Sections were then rinsed in 0.05% PBS/Tween (Sigma-Aldrich, USA) solution for 5 min for three times and incubated with 10% normal goat (GFAP, Iba-1) or horse (CD68, MBP, MHC-II, and Tau-1, Nogo-A) serum in PBS for 1 h.

Without further rinsing, sections were then incubated overnight with primary antibody in PBS, rinsed in PBS/Tween solution for 5 min (3 times), and incubated with biotinylated goat anti-rabbit (GFAP and Iba-1) or horse anti-mouse (ED1, MBP, MHC-II, Tau-1, Nogo-A) secondary antibodies (Vector Laboratories, USA) diluted at 1:200 or 1:100 in PBS, respectively, for 2 h. As a negative control, normal sera, rather the primary antibody, were used in some sections. Sections were rinsed again for 5 min (three times) and incubated in the avidin-biotin-peroxidase complex (ABC Kit, Vector Laboratories, USA) for 2 h. Sections were rinsed four times (5 min each) and revealed with DAB. After DAB reaction, sections were rinsed two times (5 min each) in 0.1 PB, dehydrated, and coverslipped with Entellan (Merck, Germany).

2.7. Qualitative Analysis. All sections stained with the different histological methods were surveyed by light microscopy (Nikon Eclipse E200). Illustrative images from all experimental groups were obtained using a digital camera attached to the microscope (Nikon Eclipse, 50i) using the software Moticam 2500®.

2.8. Quantitative Analysis. We used coronal sections containing the damaged striatum located at 1.2 mm posterior to bregma to count the number of activated macrophages/microglia (CD68+ cells), MHC-II+ cells, pathological oligodendrocytes (Tau-1+ cells), Nogo-A+ cells, and astrocytes (GFAP+ cells) per field. Adjacent 20 μm sections anterior and posterior to the lesion site were used for immunohistochemistry and cell bodies were counted over 1.5 mm from the lesion site. The counting field was defined as a square 0.25 mm wide grid (objective, ×40) in the eyepiece of a microscope. In the ×40 objective, this grid corresponds to an area of 0.0625 mm^2. We counted 9 fields located at the dorsal striatum per section and 3 sections/animal ($N = 5$ animals per group) for all experimental groups (Figure 1).

For quantitative analysis of MBP immunolabeling, photomicrographs were segmented by Color Deconvolution plugin (Gabriel Landini, http://www.dentistry.bham.ac.uk/landinig/software/software.html) from ImageJ software version 1.33-1.34 (NIMH, NIH, Bethesda, MD, USA, https://imagej.nih.gov/ij/). After image segmentation, area values (μm) and percentual fraction of DAB staining on sections were measured [48, 49]. We evaluated 5 sections/animal ($N = 5$ animals per group). Average values were expressed as mean ± S.E.M.

2.9. Statistical Analysis. Means and standard errors were calculated for all groups of data. Comparisons between different groups were assessed by analysis of variance (ANOVA) with Tukey *post hoc* test (one-way ANOVA-Tukey). Statistical significance was accepted at $p < 0.05$. All statistical analyses were performed using the Graphpad Prism 5.0 software.

3. Results

3.1. Focal Ischemia Induced by ET-1 Microinjections into the Rat Striatum. ET-1 microinjections caused a focal ischemic damage characterized by tissue pallor, edema, intense inflammatory response, and loss of cell bodies (Figures 2(c)–2(j)). The tissue damage evolved from 1 day PLD with maximum infiltration of inflammatory cells between 3 and 7 PLDs (Figures 2(c)–2(f)). Mononuclear cells were present at 14 PLDs (Figures 2(g) and 2(h)), but there was a conspicuous decrease in their presence at 30 PLDs (Figures 2(i) and 2(j)). Control animals injected with sterile saline did not present these histopathological findings (Figures 2(a) and 2(b)).

3.2. ET-1 Microinjections Induce Progressive Astrocyte Activation in the Ischemic Striatum. In vehicle animals, astrocytes presented their normal morphology with nonhypertrophic cell bodies and a ramified pattern of their branches (Figures 3(a) and 3(b)). In ischemic animals, there was a progressive astrocyte activation starting from 3 PLDs (Figures 3(c) and 3(d)), with peak between 7 (Figures 3(e) and 3(f)) and 14 PLDs (Figures 3(g) and 3(h)) and clear reduction at 30 PLDs (Figures 3(i) and 3(j)). This activation was characterized by increased cell body volume and ramifications, mainly at 7 (Figures 3(e) and 3(f)) and 14 PLDs (Figures 3(g) and 3(h)).

One-way ANOVA revealed significant changes in the variance of the number of GFAP+ cells ($F_4 = 28.55$; $p < 0.0001$). There was a decrease in the number of GFAP+ cells at 3 PLDs (129.2 ± 5.65) compared to vehicle animals (163.2 ± 6.13; $p < 0.05$). A further decrease occurred from 3 PLDs to 7 (85.00 ± 6.06; $p < 0.001$) and 14 PLDs (78.20 ± 6.93; $p < 0.001$) PLDs. There was a rise in the number of GFAP+ cells at 30 PLDs (113.2 ± 7.38) compared to 7 and 14 PLDs.

3.3. Microinjections of ET-1 Induce Microglia Activation up to 30 Days after Focal Ischemia. Microglial activation was investigated using immunohistochemistry for 3 antibodies: Ibal, CD68, and MHC-II. In control animals, microglia displayed a ramified morphology with small Ibal+ cell bodies, which are characteristic features of resting microglia (Figures 4(a) and 4(b)). After focal ischemia, there was a progressive activation of microglia from 3 PLDs up to 14 PLDs (Figures 4(c)–4(h)). At 30 PLDs, microglia displayed morphological features of resting microglia (Figures 4(i) and 4(j)). The peak of microglia activation was around 7 PLDs (Figures 4(e) and 4(f)).

The Ibal immunohistochemistry revealed the evolution of the morphological activation of microglia in ischemic animals. At 3 PLDs, there was a decrease in ramified Ibal+ cells in the ischemic site, with increase in amoeboid and

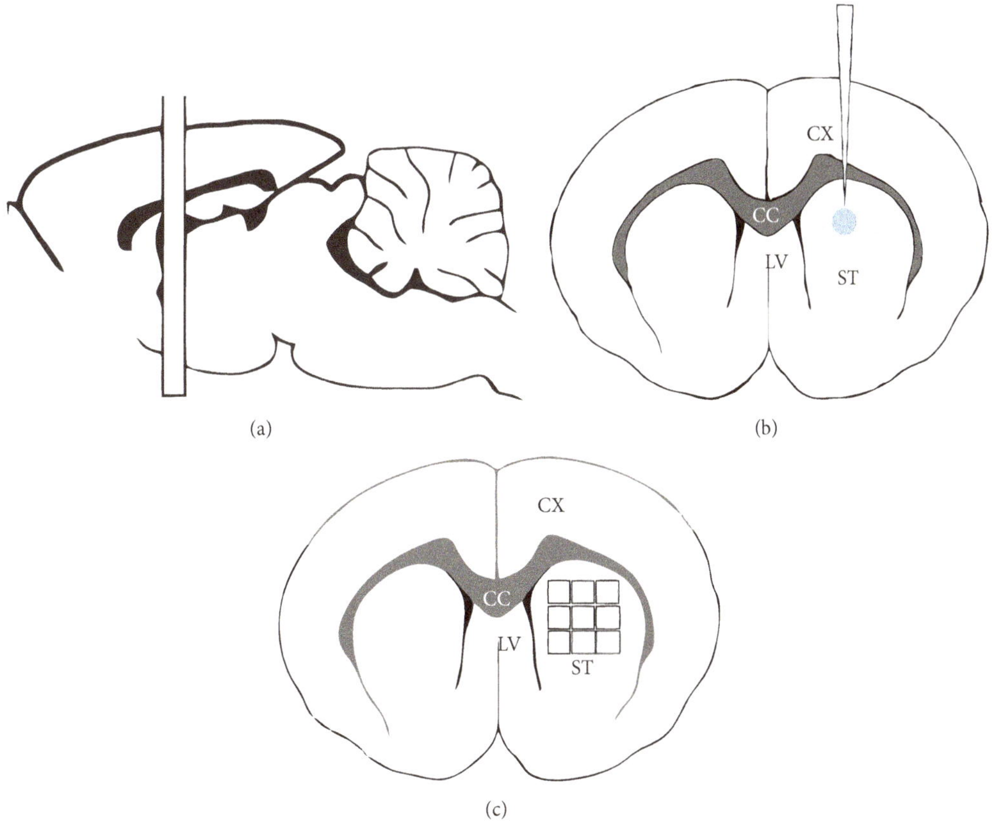

FIGURE 1: Schematic diagram illustrating the striatal injection site of ET-1 and the counting method. Drawing of a parasagittal section depicting the sectioning location (a), illustration of the ET-1 injection site in a coronal section drawing (b), and the location of the counting fields in the rat striatum (c). The squares in (c) are in scale to the counting fields they represent. CX = cortex; CC = corpus callosum; ST = striatum; LV = lateral ventricle.

round Iba1+ cells (Figures 4(c) and 4(d)). The amount of round Iba1+ cells (phagocytes) dramatically increased at the ischemic core at 7 days PLDs (Figures 4(e) and 4(f)). There was a progressive decrease in microglia activation at 14 (Figures 4(g) and 4(h)) and 30 PLDs (Figures 4(i) and 4(j)). At this later PLD, ramified Iba1+ cells were again observed in the ischemic site, despite the presence of some round and amoeboid microglia (Figures 4(i) and 4(j)).

To quantitatively describe the temporal evolution of microglia activation following striatal ischemia, we counted the number of CD68+ cells between 3 and 30 PLDs (Figure 5(k)). The temporal immunoreactivity of CD68+ cells followed that described using the anti-Iba1 antibody (Figures 5(i) and 5(j)). One-way ANOVA revealed significant changes in the variance of the number of CD68+ cells ($F_4 = 96.35$; $p < 0.0001$). The average number of CD68+ cells was 6.44 ± 0.29 cells/field in vehicle animals (Figures 5(a), 5(b), and 5(k)). Subsequent Tukey's *post hoc* comparisons indicated that this number increased to 209.70 ± 13.90, 266.40 ± 9.8, and 218.40 ± 1.69 cells/field at 3, 7, and 14 PLDs, respectively, ($p < 0.001$, Figure 5(k)). There was a considerable decrease in the number of CD68+ cells at 30 PLDs (140.70 ± 7.14; $p < 0.001$), but it remained elevated in comparison to control animals (6.44 ± 0.29; $p < 0.001$, Figures 5(i)–5(k)).

After ET-1 microinjections, there was a progressive expression of MHC-II in the ischemic striatum. The temporal profile of MHC-II expression was similar to those described with Iba1 and CD68, with maximum number of cells at 7 PLDs (Figures 5(l)–5(u) and 5(v)). MHC-II+ cells displayed morphology of activated round microglia (Figures 5(n)–5(u)). The average number of MHC-II+ cells was 5.77 ± 1.06 cells/field in control animals (Figure 5(v)).

One-way ANOVA revealed significant changes in the variance of the number of MHC-II+ cells ($F_4 = 153.1$; $p < 0.0001$). *Post hoc* comparisons indicated that there was a progressive increase in the number of MHC-II+ cells per field at 3 and 7 PLDs, (201.26 ± 1.54; 236.57 ± 14.58; $p < 0.001$, Figure 5(v)). These numbers decreased at 14 and 30 PLDs, respectively (86.20 ± 2.69; 73.20 ± 1.98, $p < 0.001$, Figure 5(v)). All ischemic groups statistically differed from control animals. There was no statistical difference between 14 and 30 PLDs ($p > 0.05$, ANOVA-Tukey).

3.4. Microinjections of ET-1 Induced Progressive Impairment of MBP Immunoreactivity in the Ischemic Striatum. The immunolabeling of the myelin sheath was performed using an anti-MBP antibody [35]. One-way ANOVA revealed significant changes in the variance of the values for MBP

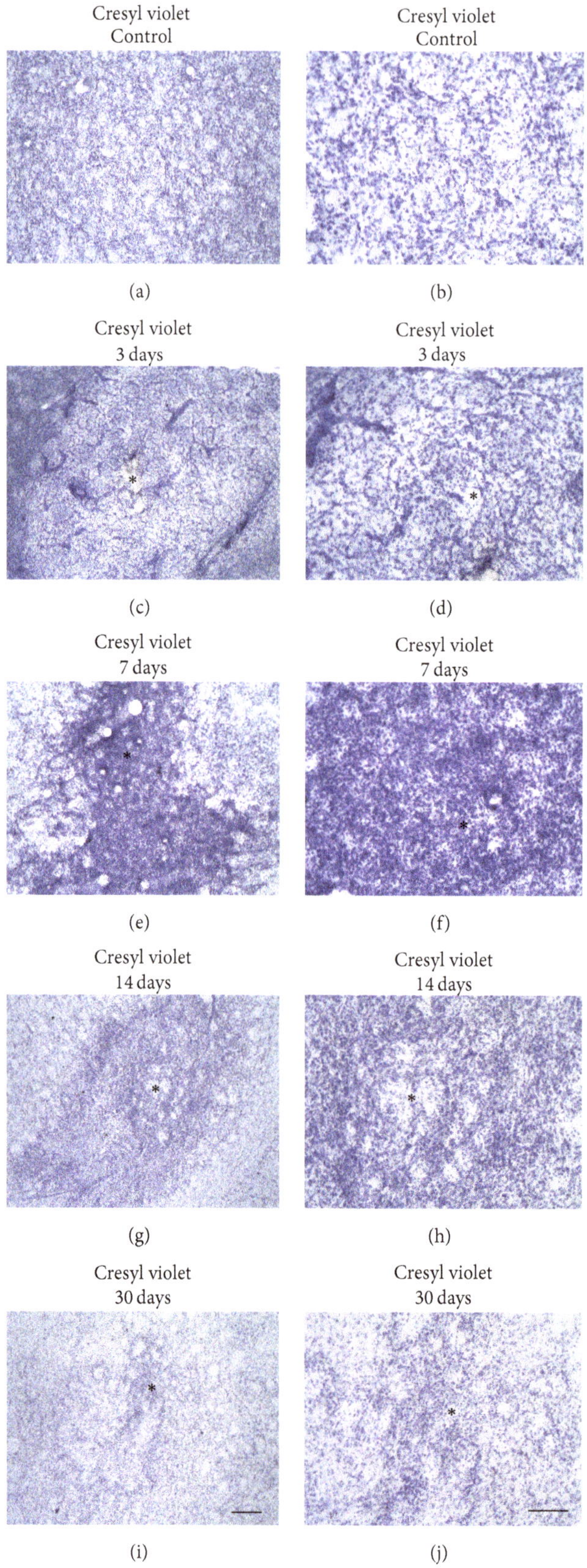

FIGURE 2: Gross histopathology after ET-1 microinjections revealed by cresyl violet staining. Control animal injected with sterile saline (a-b) or ischemic animals injected with ET-1 at 3 (c-d), 7 (e-f), 14 (g-h), and 30 (i-j) PLDs. Asterisks are in the lesion epicenter. Scale bars: (a), (c), (e), (g), and (i) (200 μm) and (b), (d), (f), (h), and (j) (100 μm).

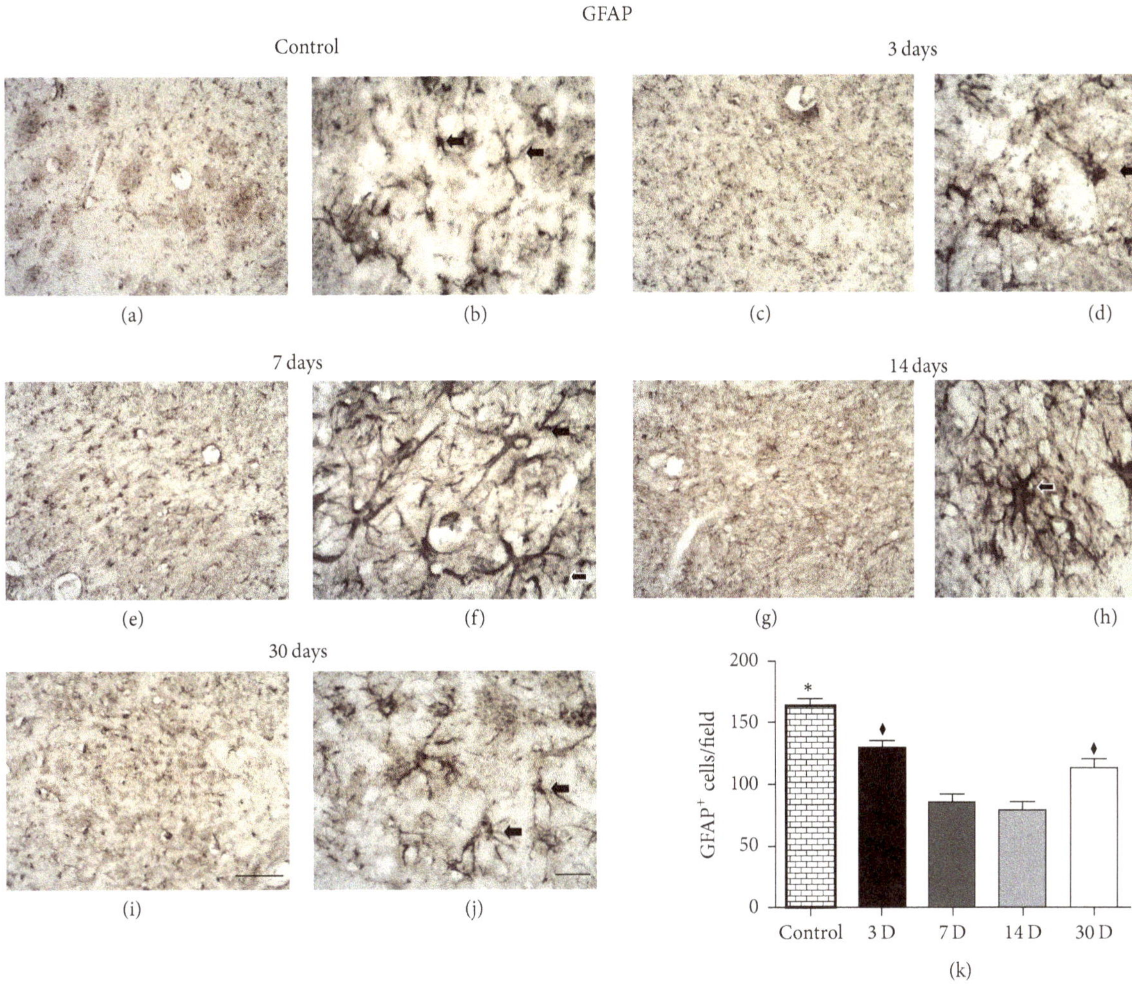

FIGURE 3: Progressive astrocyte activation after striatal focal ischemia. Control animal injected with sterile saline (a-b) or ischemic animals injected with ET-1 at 3 (c-d), 7 (e-f), 14 (g-h), and 30 (i-j) PLDs. Maximum astrocyte activation occurred around 7 and 14 PLDs. The cell density was smaller at 7 and 14 PLDs. $^{*}p < 0.05$ compared to others groups; $^{\blacklozenge}p < 0.05$ compared to 7 and 14 PLDs. Arrows point to astrocytes in the higher power images. Scale bars: (a), (c), (e), (g), and (i) (100 μm) and (b), (d), (f), (h), and (j) (20 μm).

immunoreactivity in the striatum of ischemic animals ($F_4 = 28.97$; $p < 0.0001$). Subsequent Tukey's *post hoc* comparisons indicated that there was a progressive impairment of MBP immunoreactivity after focal ischemia in the rat striatum from 3 days (12.67 ± 0.59; $p < 0.05$, Figure 6(b)) up to 30 days (9.71 ± 0.54; $p < 0.001$, Figure 6(e)) PLDs. The loss of MBP immunoreactivity was maximum at 7 (8.01 ± 0.57; $p < 0.001$, Figure 6(c)) and 14 PLDs (8.17 ± 0.46; $p < 0.001$, Figure 6(d)), but myelin impairment could be also observed at 30 PLDs (Figure 6(e)).

3.5. Microinjections of ET-1 Induce Oligodendrocytes Damage after Striatal Ischemia. It has been shown that Tau-1 is a marker of pathological oligodendrocytes after acute damage to CNS [44, 50, 51]. Control animals expressed a small amount (3.773 ± 1.095/field) of Tau-1+ cells in the striatum (Figures 7(a), 7(b), and 7(k)). Ischemic damage induced a considerable increase in Tau-1 immunoreactivity in the acute phase after focal ischemia (Figure 7). One-way ANOVA revealed significant changes in the variance of the number of Tau-1+ cells in the striatum of ischemic animals ($F_4 = 153.1$; $p < 0.0001$). Subsequent Tukey's *post hoc* comparisons indicated that the number of Tau-1+ cells/field was 33.56 ± 1.51 at 3 PLDs ($p < 0.001$, Figures 7(c), 7(d), and 7(k)). This number decreased to 14.80 ± 1.49, 2.59 ± 0.55, and 1.46 ± 0.22 at 7, 14, and 30 PLDs compared to 3 PLDs ($p < 0.001$, Figure 7(k)).

3.6. The ET-1-Induced Striatal Ischemic Damage Results in Progressive Increase in Nogo-A Immunoreactivity. Nogo-A is an oligodendrocyte-associated protein involved in the inhibition of axonal growth after acute CNS damage [31, 34]. One-way ANOVA revealed significant chances in the variance of the number of Nogo-A+ cells in the striatum of ischemic animals ($F_4 = 206.2$; $p < 0.0001$). Subsequent Tukey's *post hoc* comparisons indicated that microinjections of ET-1 induced progressive increase in the number of Nogo-A+ cells with peak around 3 PLDs (267.59 ± 5.69; $p < 0.001$), with subsequent decrease at 7 (193.8 ± 3.980; $p < 0.001$), 14 (137.9 ± 137.9; $p < 0.001$), and 30 (112.8 ± 3.39; $p < 0.001$)

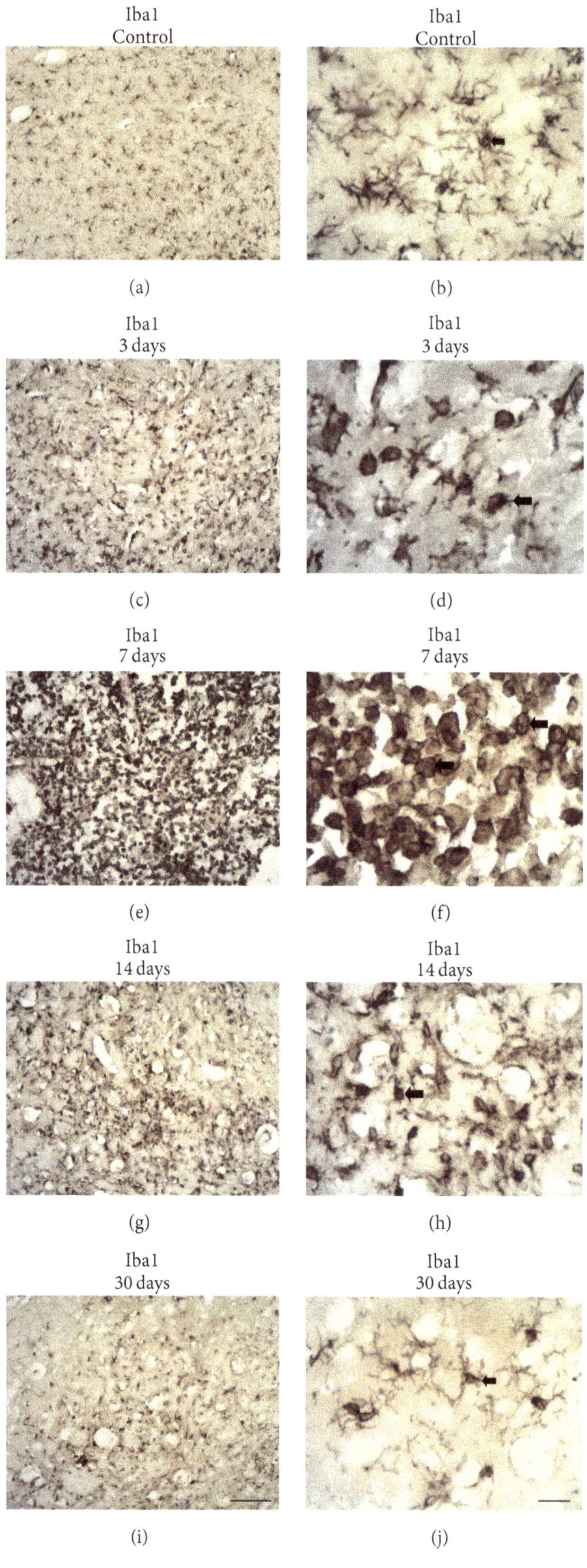

FIGURE 4: Progressive microglia activation after striatal focal ischemia revealed by Iba1 immunohistochemistry. Ramified microglia in a control animal injected with sterile saline (a-b). Morphological activation of microglia at 3 (c-d), 7 (e-f), 14 (g-h), and 30 (i-j) PLDs. Maximum activation occurred around 7 PLDs (e-f). Microglia activation decreased by 30 PLDs (i-j). Arrows point to Iba1+ ramified microglia (b, j) or round macrophages (d, f, h). Scale bars: (a), (c), (e), (g), and (i) (100 μm) and (b), (d), (f), (h), and (j) (20 μm).

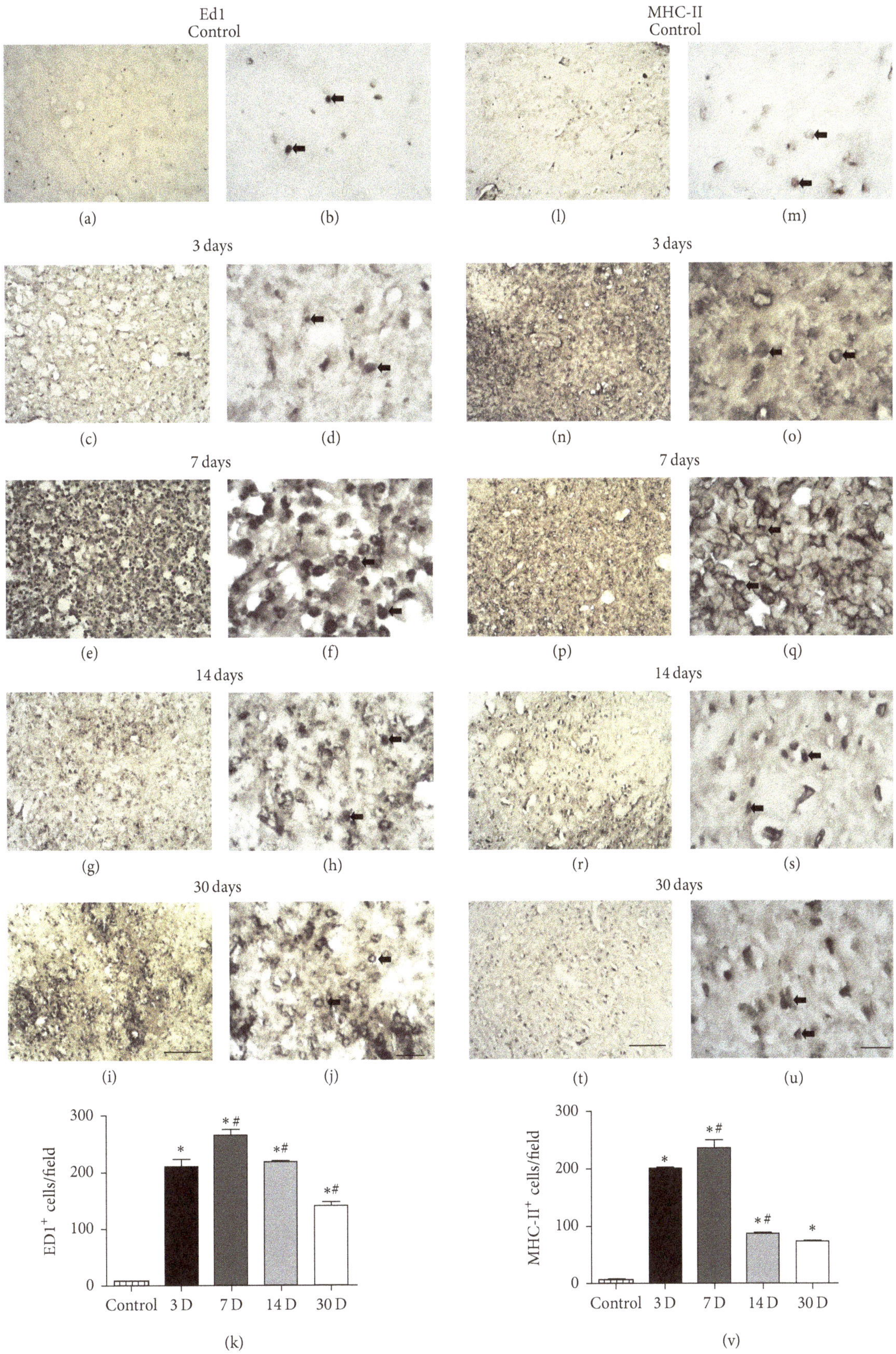

FIGURE 5: Microglia activation revealed by anti-CD68 and MHC-II immunohistochemistry. Control animals injected with sterile saline (a-b, l-m). Morphological activation of CD68+ or MHC-II+ microglia at 3 (c-d, n-o), 7 (e-f, p-q), 14 (g-h, r-s), and 30 (i-j, t-u) PLDs. Both techniques are labeled activated round macrophages (arrows). Quantitative analysis showed maximum number of cells at 7 PLDs with decrease at later survival times (k, v). $^*p < 0.05$ compared to control; $^\#p < 0.05$ compared to previous survival time. Scale bars: (a), (c), (e), (g), (i), (l), (n), (p), (r), and (t) (100 μm) and (b), (d), (f), (h), (j), (m), (o), (q), (s), and (u) (20 μm).

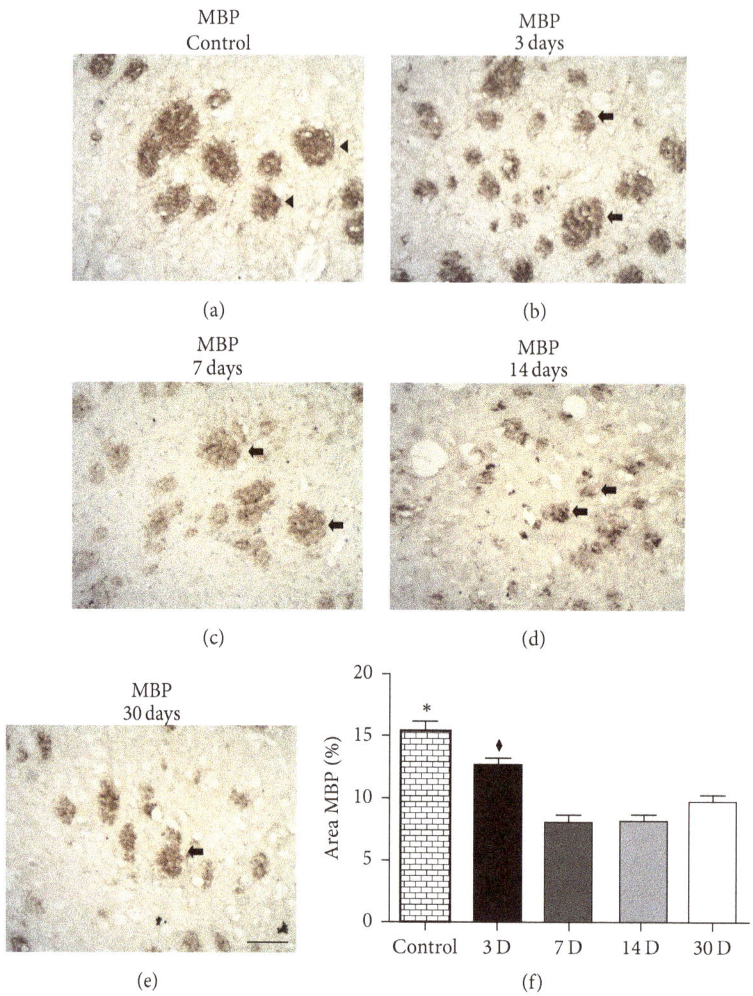

FIGURE 6: Myelin impairment revealed by anti-MBP immunohistochemistry. Control animal injected with sterile saline (a) or ischemic animals injected with ET-1 at 3 (b), 7 (c), 14 (d), and 30 (e) PLDs. There was a progressive impairment of MBP labeled WM tracts (arrows) compared to control (arrow in (a)). Quantitative analysis in (f). $^{*}p < 0.05$ compared to others groups; $^{\blacklozenge}p < 0.05$ compared to others survival time. Arrows point to WM tracts. Scale bars: 100 μm.

PLDs (Figures 7(l)–7(u)). The average number of Nogo-A+ cells in control animals was (97.11 ± 10.47). All ischemic groups statistically differed from the control animals, even at 30 PLDs (Figure 7(v)).

4. Discussion

We have investigated the patterns of glial activation and Tau-1 and Nogo-A immunoreactivity from 3 up to 30 days after microinjections of ET-1 into the striatum of adult rats. The ET-1 model of focal ischemia uses the vasoconstrictor actions of the peptide ET-1 [52, 53]. This peptide causes focal ischemic damage after microinjections into the CNS [54], which is suitable for reproducing the focal strokes frequently occurring in the human brain [55]. In addition, the ET-1 model is easily performed without the complicated surgical procedures of other stroke models like the MCAO intraluminal filament technique, which may induce hyperthermia and other surgical complications [56]. This stroke model has been used in several publications by our group [3, 4, 12, 13].

We thought it would be important to establish the temporal evolution of microglia activation, astrocytosis, oligodendrocyte damage, and Nogo-A immunoreactivity during the first month after ET-1-induced stroke, as a morphological basis for further functional studies seeking new neuroprotective drugs.

Striatal ET-1 microinjections induced progressive astrocyte activation, as revealed by GFAP immunohistochemistry. Maximum activation was present in the first two weeks with a decline at 30 PLDs. This is in agreement with a previous study using the MCAO stroke model [57]. Nevertheless, in this study, the description of GFAP immunoreactivity was incomplete. No illustrations were provided for all survival times. Here, we filled this gap providing a comprehensive description of astrocyte activation from 3 to 30 days after experimental stroke onset.

The mechanisms by which astrocytes are activated after stroke and other neural disorders are not established. The meaning of this glial cell activation has been a matter of

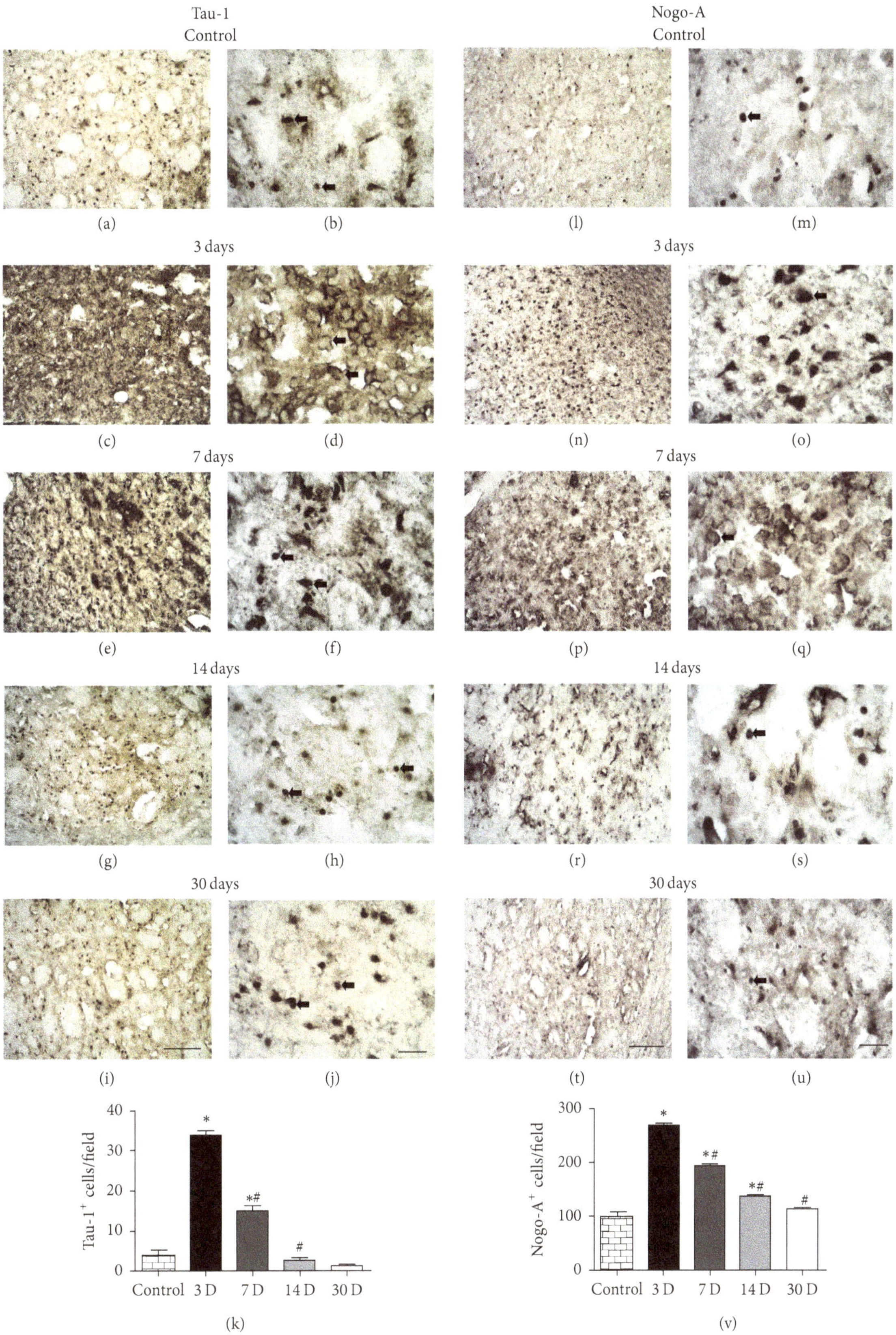

FIGURE 7: Oligodendrocyte damage (Tau-1+ cells) and increased Nogo-A immunoreactivity after focal striatal ischemia. Control animals injected with sterile saline (a-b, l-m). Tau-1 and Nogo-A+ cells at 3 (c-d, n-o), 7 (e-f, p-q), 14 (g-h, r-s), and 30 (i-j, t-u) PLDs. Quantitative analysis showed maximum numbers of Tau-1 and Nogo-A+ cells at 3 PLDs (k, v). There is a long-lasting increase in the number of Nogo-A+ cells up to 30 PLDs compared to control ($p < 0.05$, ANOVA-Tukey). $^{*}p < 0.05$ compared to control; $^{\#}p < 0.05$ compared to previous survival time. Scale bars: (a), (c), (e), (g), (i), (l), (n), (p), (r), and (t) (100 μm) and (b), (d), (f), (h), (j), (m), (o), (q), (s), and (u) (20 μm).

continuous debate for many years [58]. These cells are an important component of the glial scar in chronic survival times after CNS stroke and trauma [59]. The expression of proteoglycans is a biochemical barrier for axonal regeneration concomitant with a mechanical impediment imposed by intense astrocyte reaction and some degree of proliferation [8, 59]. The proliferation of these glial cells is influenced by factors including survivin [60]. Astrocytes may release deleterious molecules including the proinflammatory cytokine tumor necrosis factor-α, metalloproteinases, and reactive oxygen derived species [58, 61].

Nevertheless, astrocyte activation has also beneficial functions after stroke and other neural disorders [58, 62]. Astrocytes seem to contribute to neuroblast migration to striatum after stroke by releasing stroma-derived factor-1α (SDF-1) [63, 64] and monocyte chemoattractant protein 1 (MCP-1) [63]. This is important considering that partial replacement of neuronal loss is afforded by adult neurogenesis after striatal damage [65]. In addition, these glial cells can uptake glutamate in both physiological and ischemic conditions, buffering neurotoxicity [66]. Astrocyte may also release growth factors, including brain-derived neurotrophic factors (BDNF), contributing to neuron survival after stroke in rats [67].

There was intense microglia activation following microinjections of ET-1 into the rat striatum between 3 and 30 days after ischemic onset. Maximum activation occurred around 7 PLDs, but microglia remained activated up to 30 PLDs. These results are in agreement with previous studies using ET-1 stroke model [3, 4, 54] or MCAO [7, 68].

Microglia activation is a general response to any kind of CNS damage [11]. In nonpathological conditions, these brain resident macrophages patrol the CNS using stochastic movements of their fine branches [69, 70]. In pathological conditions like ischemia and trauma, microglia change their morphology becoming amoeboid and highly phagocytic round cells (macrophages) [11, 71]. Concomitant with morphological alterations, microglia change their genetic machinery expressing several types of receptors on their membranes, increased levels of transcription factors, and cytoplasmic enzymes [11].

We have labeled microglia using three antibodies: Iba1, ED1, and MHC-II. Iba1 immunohistochemistry allowed labeling the general population of microglial cells [41]. ED1 and MHC-II labeled a population of activated microglia [7, 39]. ED1 and MHC-II+ cells comprise both macrophages derived from the resident microglia and blood-borne macrophages [72]. These markers do not differentiate the origin of activate macrophages present in the ischemic striatum. It has been shown, using chimeric animals, that resident microglia first respond to the damage followed by hematogenous macrophages [72, 73].

The reasons by which microglia are both detrimental and beneficial after stroke are unknown. Recently, we have hypothesized these glial cells might be beneficial and/or detrimental in different pathological niches following striatal ischemia, a phenomenon likely determined by different concentrations of specific ligands along the pathological environment, which might act on different receptors in the microglia membrane [11]. This is in agreement with a recent study showing that M1 and M2 microglia phenotypes are present in the ischemic striatum following MCAO [74].

Microinjections of ET-1 into the rat striatum induced damage of oligodendrocytes (maximum at 3 PLD) and progressive myelin impairment (maximum between 7 and 14 PLDs). It seems that myelin impairment follows damage to oligodendrocyte cell bodies. It has been shown that oligodendrocytes present structural changes in their cytoskeleton (dephosphorylation) following ischemia, excitotoxicity, and trauma, which is visualized as an increased immunoreactivity for Tau-1 [44, 50, 75]. Tau-1 immunoreactivity has been frequently used as a specific marker of damaged oligodendrocytes [51, 54, 76]. We [51] and other authors have shown that this pathological phenomenon occurs in the acute phase after stroke [54, 76], which is in agreement with the present results. In addition, damage to axonal cylinder may precede both oligodendrocyte damage and myelin impairment. It has been shown that damage to axonal cylinder occurs in an early time point (6 hours) after focal striatal damage induced by ET-1 [72].

The increased immunoreactivity for Tau-1 in oligodendrocytes may be an early event underlying oligodendrocyte pathology [77]. It has been shown that oligodendrocytes but not astrocytes are labeled by Tau-1 after ischemia [77]. The increased immunoreactivity for Tau-1 in oligodendrocytes may represent an attempt to preserve oligodendrocyte cytoskeleton likely from free radicals-mediated damage [51]. This is in agreement with a previous report showing that Tau protein is fundamental for microtubule assembly [78] and that this structure is especially vulnerable to ischemia induced oxidative stress [75, 79]. The decrease in the number of Tau-1+ cells in later survival times in this study may be due to the loss of oligodendrocytes by apoptosis. This hypothesis is supported by a previous report of our group showing that striatal oligodendrocytes become apoptotic in later survival times following excitotoxic damage and that minocycline treatment decreases the number of Tau-1+ cells and partially reverses the apoptotic damage [51]. Several other authors have shown that oligodendrocytes undergo apoptosis following acute neural disorders [80–82]. Further studies should be performed to investigate the mechanisms by which oligodendrocytes are damaged after stroke and to address the therapeutic potential of neuroprotective drugs in reducing the WM demise.

The results show an increased number of Nogo-A+ cells in the acute phase after ET-1 induced stroke. This number remained elevated up to 30 days compared to nonischemic animals. This is in agreement with previous report using the MCAO filament model [45, 83]. The expression of Nogo-A in both neurons and oligodendrocytes is correlated with reduced neuroplasticity after SCI [25, 34, 84] and stroke [31, 83, 85]. Both early and delayed treatments of animals with monoclonal antibodies against Nogo-A increase neuroplasticity in these acute neural disorders [25, 31, 32, 34, 83–85]. Nevertheless, Nogo-A may also be involved in the survival of neurons after ischemia [33]. It follows that the increased expression of Nogo-A in the ischemic striatum can be related to both detrimental and beneficial actions. Further studies should consider this dual role of Nogo-A before the use of experimental approaches to neutralize the action of this protein.

5. Conclusion

Microinjections of ET-1 into the rat striatum induced conspicuous tissue loss, concomitant with progressive microglia and astrocyte activation, myelin impairment, oligodendrocyte damage, and Nogo-A up regulation. These pathological events were described from 3 to 30 days after ET-1-induced focal striatal ischemia. The establishment of the temporal evolution of these neuropathological events is an important step for future studies in which the manipulation of neuroinflammation and Nogo-A expression may be performed to enhance neuroprotection (in gray and white matter), adult neurogenesis, and functional recovery following striatal ischemic damage. We are addressing these issues in undergoing investigations.

Competing Interests

The authors declare that they have no competing interests.

Authors' Contributions

Rafael R. Lima and Luana N. S. Santana contributed equally to this work. Walace Gomes-Leal, Rafael R. Lima, and Luana N. S. Santana conceived the study, participated in the experimental design, and wrote the manuscript. Enio Mauricio N. dos Santos, Ijair Rogério dos Santos, and Adriano Gimarães-Santos performed stroke analyses. Ana Carolina A. Oliveira, Luanna M. P. Fernandes, and Patrycy Assis N. Tavares performed immunohistochemistry. Elder M. Nascimento contributed to quantitative analysis. All authors read and approved the final manuscript.

Acknowledgments

This work was supported by the Brazilian National Council for Scientific and Technological Development (CNPq) and Fundação de Amparo A Pesquisa do Estado do Pará (FAPESPA). W. Gomes-Leal is a principal investigator in the Ministry of Science and Technology (MCT; Grant no. 573872/2008-2), Ministry of Health (MS) and CNPq (Edital CT-Biotecnologia/MCT/CNPq/MS/SCTIE/DECIT no. 17/2008), and FAPESPA (PRONEX-FAPESPA-CNPQ-Edital 012-2009). Rafael R. Lima is investigator from CNPq (Edital MCTI/CNPQ/Universal 14/2014).

References

[1] M. A. Moskowitz, E. H. Lo, and C. Iadecola, "The science of stroke: mechanisms in search of treatments," *Neuron*, vol. 67, no. 2, pp. 181–198, 2010.

[2] E. H. Lo and M. Ning, "Mechanisms and challenges in translational stroke research," *Journal of Investigative Medicine*, vol. 64, no. 4, pp. 827–829, 2016.

[3] R. D. Souza-Rodrigues, A. M. R. Costa, R. R. Lima, C. D. Dos Santos, C. W. Picanço-Diniz, and W. Gomes-Leal, "Inflammatory response and white matter damage after microinjections of endothelin-1 into the rat striatum," *Brain Research*, vol. 1200, pp. 78–88, 2008.

[4] C. D. Dos Santos, C. W. Picanço-Diniz, and W. Gomes-Leal, "Differential patterns of inflammatory response, axonal damage and myelin impairment following excitotoxic or ischemic damage to the trigeminal spinal nucleus of adult rats," *Brain Research*, vol. 1172, no. 1, pp. 130–144, 2007.

[5] M. Tóth, P. Little, F. Arnberg et al., "Acute neuroinflammation in a clinically relevant focal cortical ischemic stroke model in rat: longitudinal positron emission tomography and immunofluorescent tracking," *Brain Structure and Function*, vol. 221, no. 3, pp. 1279–1290, 2016.

[6] Z. Zhang, Z. Zhang, H. Lu, Q. Yang, H. Wu, and J. Wang, "Microglial polarization and inflammatory mediators after intracerebral hemorrhage," *Molecular Neurobiology*, 2016.

[7] P. Thored, U. Heldmann, W. Gomes-Leal et al., "Long-term accumulation of microglia with proneurogenic phenotype concomitant with persistent neurogenesis in adult subventricular zone after stroke," *Glia*, vol. 57, no. 8, pp. 835–849, 2009.

[8] G. E. Barreto, X. Sun, L. Xu, and R. G. Giffard, "Astrocyte proliferation following stroke in the mouse depends on distance from the infarct," *PLoS ONE*, vol. 6, no. 11, Article ID e27881, 2011.

[9] P. Cordeau Jr., M. Lalancette-Hébert, Y. C. Weng, and J. Kriz, "Live imaging of neuroinflammation reveals sex and estrogen effects on astrocyte response to ischemic injury," *Stroke*, vol. 39, no. 3, pp. 935–942, 2008.

[10] Z. Chen and B. D. Trapp, "Microglia and neuroprotection," *Journal of Neurochemistry*, vol. 136, supplement 1, pp. 10–17, 2016.

[11] W. Gomes-Leal, "Microglial physiopathology: How to explain the dual role of microglia after acute neural disorders?" *Brain and Behavior*, vol. 2, no. 3, pp. 345–356, 2012.

[12] E. C. S. Franco, M. M. Cardoso, A. Gouvêia, A. Pereira, and W. Gomes-Leal, "Modulation of microglial activation enhances neuroprotection and functional recovery derived from bone marrow mononuclear cell transplantation after cortical ischemia," *Neuroscience Research*, vol. 73, no. 2, pp. 122–132, 2012.

[13] M. M. Cardoso, E. C. S. Franco, C. C. De Souza, M. C. Da Silva, A. Gouveia, and W. Gomes-Leal, "Minocycline treatment and bone marrow mononuclear cell transplantation after endothelin-1 induced striatal ischemia," *Inflammation*, vol. 36, no. 1, pp. 197–205, 2013.

[14] J. Yrjänheikki, T. Tikka, R. Keinänen, G. Goldsteins, P. H. Chan, and J. Koistinaho, "A tetracycline derivative, minocycline, reduces inflammation and protects against focal cerebral ischemia with a wide therapeutic window," *Proceedings of the National Academy of Sciences of the United States of America*, vol. 96, no. 23, pp. 13496–13500, 1999.

[15] M. Lalancette-Hébert, G. Gowing, A. Simard, C. W. Yuan, and J. Kriz, "Selective ablation of proliferating microglial cells exacerbates ischemic injury in the brain," *Journal of Neuroscience*, vol. 27, no. 10, pp. 2596–2605, 2007.

[16] J. Neumann, M. Gunzer, H. O. Gutzeit, O. Ullrich, K. G. Reymann, and K. Dinkel, "Microglia provide neuroprotection after ischemia," *The FASEB Journal*, vol. 20, no. 6, pp. 714–716, 2006.

[17] J. Neumann, S. Sauerzweig, R. Rönicke et al., "Microglia cells protect neurons by direct engulfment of invading neutrophil granulocytes: a new mechanism of CNS immune privilege," *The Journal of Neuroscience*, vol. 28, no. 23, pp. 5965–5975, 2008.

[18] W. Gomes-Leal, D. J. Corkill, M. A. Freire, C. W. Picanço-Diniz, and V. H. Perry, "Astrocytosis, microglia activation, oligodendrocyte degeneration, and pyknosis following acute spinal cord injury," *Experimental Neurology*, vol. 190, no. 2, pp. 456–467, 2004.

[19] Q.-P. Dong, J.-Q. He, and Z. Chai, "Astrocytic Ca^{2+} waves mediate activation of extrasynaptic NMDA receptors in hippocampal neurons to aggravate brain damage during ischemia," *Neurobiology of Disease*, vol. 58, pp. 68–75, 2013.

[20] A. Minagar, P. Shapshak, R. Fujimura, R. Ownby, M. Heyes, and C. Eisdorfer, "The role of macrophage/microglia and astrocytes in the pathogenesis of three neurologic disorders: HIV-associated dementia, Alzheimer disease, and multiple sclerosis," *Journal of the Neurological Sciences*, vol. 202, no. 1-2, pp. 13–23, 2002.

[21] G. R. Choudhury and S. Ding, "Reactive astrocytes and therapeutic potential in focal ischemic stroke," *Neurobiology of Disease*, vol. 85, pp. 234–244, 2016.

[22] W. Zheng, L. Talley Watts, D. M. Holstein, J. Wewer, and J. D. Lechleiter, "P2Y1R-initiated, IP3R-dependent stimulation of astrocyte mitochondrial metabolism reduces and partially reverses ischemic neuronal damage in mouse," *Journal of Cerebral Blood Flow and Metabolism*, vol. 33, no. 4, pp. 600–611, 2013.

[23] G. Yiu and Z. He, "Glial inhibition of CNS axon regeneration," *Nature Reviews Neuroscience*, vol. 7, no. 8, pp. 617–627, 2006.

[24] C. M. Galtrey and J. W. Fawcett, "The role of chondroitin sulfate proteoglycans in regeneration and plasticity in the central nervous system," *Brain Research Reviews*, vol. 54, no. 1, pp. 1–18, 2007.

[25] M. S. Chen, A. B. Huber, M. E. Van Der Haar et al., "Nogo-A is a myelin-associated neurite outgrowth inhibitor and an antigen for monoclonal antibody IN-1," *Nature*, vol. 403, no. 6768, pp. 434–439, 2000.

[26] T. Wang, J.-Q. Xiong, X.-B. Ren, and W. Sun, "The role of Nogo-A in neuroregeneration: a review," *Brain Research Bulletin*, vol. 87, no. 6, pp. 499–503, 2012.

[27] E. J. Bradbury, L. D. F. Moon, R. J. Popat et al., "Chondroitinase ABC promotes functional recovery after spinal cord injury," *Nature*, vol. 416, no. 6881, pp. 636–640, 2002.

[28] E. J. Bradbury and L. M. Carter, "Manipulating the glial scar: chondroitinase ABC as a therapy for spinal cord injury," *Brain Research Bulletin*, vol. 84, no. 4-5, pp. 306–316, 2011.

[29] J. J. Hill, K. Jin, X. O. Mao, L. Xie, and D. A. Greenberg, "Intracerebral chondroitinase ABC and heparan sulfate proteoglycan glypican improve outcome from chronic stroke in rats," *Proceedings of the National Academy of Sciences of the United States of America*, vol. 109, no. 23, pp. 9155–9160, 2012.

[30] S. Soleman, P. K. Yip, D. A. Duricki, and L. D. F. Moon, "Delayed treatment with chondroitinase ABC promotes sensorimotor recovery and plasticity after stroke in aged rats," *Brain*, vol. 135, no. 4, pp. 1210–1223, 2012.

[31] A. B. Seymour, E. M. Andrews, S.-Y. Tsai et al., "Delayed treatment with monoclonal antibody IN-1 1 week after stroke results in recovery of function and corticorubral plasticity in adult rats," *Journal of Cerebral Blood Flow and Metabolism*, vol. 25, no. 10, pp. 1366–1375, 2005.

[32] C. M. Papadopoulos, S.-Y. Tsai, J. L. Cheatwood et al., "Dendritic plasticity in the adult rat following middle cerebral artery occlusion and Nogo-a neutralization," *Cerebral Cortex*, vol. 16, no. 4, pp. 529–536, 2006.

[33] E. Kilic, A. Elali, U. Kilic et al., "Role of Nogo-A in neuronal survival in the reperfused ischemic brain," *Journal of Cerebral Blood Flow and Metabolism*, vol. 30, no. 5, pp. 969–984, 2010.

[34] L. Schnell and M. E. Schwab, "Axonal regeneration in the rat spinal cord produced by an antibody against myelin-associated neurite growth inhibitors," *Nature*, vol. 343, no. 6255, pp. 269–272, 1990.

[35] R. R. Lima, J. Guimaraes-Silva, J. L. Oliveira et al., "Diffuse axonal damage, myelin impairment, astrocytosis and inflammatory response following microinjections of NMDA into the rat striatum," *Inflammation*, vol. 31, no. 1, pp. 24–35, 2008.

[36] W. Gomes-Leal, D. J. Corkill, and C. W. Picanço-Diniz, "Systematic analysis of axonal damage and inflammatory response in different white matter tracts of acutely injured rat spinal cord," *Brain Research*, vol. 1066, no. 1-2, pp. 57–70, 2005.

[37] A. Thiel and W.-D. Heiss, "Imaging of microglia activation in stroke," *Stroke*, vol. 42, no. 2, pp. 507–512, 2011.

[38] G. B. Oliveira, E. D. A. Fontes Jr., S. De Carvalho et al., "Minocycline mitigates motor impairments and cortical neuronal loss induced by focal ischemia in rats chronically exposed to ethanol during adolescence," *Brain Research*, vol. 1561, pp. 23–34, 2014.

[39] C. D. Dijkstra, E. A. Döpp, P. Joling, and G. Kraal, "The heterogeneity of mononuclear phagocytes in lymphoid organs: distinct macrophage subpopulations in rat recognized by monoclonal antibodies ED1, ED2 and ED3," *Advances in Experimental Medicine and Biology*, vol. 186, pp. 409–419, 1985.

[40] R. S. Lopes, M. M. Cardoso, A. O. Sampaio et al., "Indomethacin treatment reduces microglia activation and increases numbers of neuroblasts in the subventricular zone and ischaemic striatum after focal ischaemia," *Journal of Biosciences*, vol. 41, no. 3, pp. 381–394, 2016.

[41] D. Ito, Y. Imai, K. Ohsawa, K. Nakajima, Y. Fukuuchi, and S. Kohsaka, "Microglia-specific localisation of a novel calcium binding protein, Iba1," *Molecular Brain Research*, vol. 57, no. 1, pp. 1–9, 1998.

[42] A. C. A. Oliveira, M. C. S. Pereira, L. N. D. S. Santana et al., "Chronic ethanol exposure during adolescence through early adulthood in female rats induces emotional and memory deficits associated with morphological and molecular alterations in hippocampus," *Journal of Psychopharmacology*, vol. 29, no. 6, pp. 712–724, 2015.

[43] F. B. Teixeira, L. N. D. S. Santana, F. R. Bezerra et al., "Chronic ethanol exposure during adolescence in rats induces motor impairments and cerebral cortex damage associated with oxidative stress," *PLoS ONE*, vol. 9, no. 6, Article ID e101074, 2014.

[44] E. A. Irving, J. Nicoll, D. I. Graham, and D. Dewar, "Increased tau immunoreactivity in oligodendrocytes following human stroke and head injury," *Neuroscience Letters*, vol. 213, no. 3, pp. 189–192, 1996.

[45] J. L. Cheatwood, A. J. Emerick, M. E. Schwab et al., "Nogo-a expression after focal ischemic stroke in the adult rat," *Stroke*, vol. 39, no. 7, pp. 2091–2098, 2008.

[46] E. A. Fontes-Júnior, C. S. Maia, L. M. Fernandes et al., "Chronic alcohol intoxication and cortical ischemia: study of their comorbidity and the protective effects of minocycline," *Oxidative Medicine and Cellular Longevity*, vol. 2016, Article ID 1341453, 10 pages, 2016.

[47] A. F. Silva Jr., M. S. S. Aguiar, O. S. Carvalho Jr. et al., "Hippocampal neuronal loss, decreased GFAP immunoreactivity and cognitive impairment following experimental intoxication of rats with aluminum citrate," *Brain Research*, vol. 1491, pp. 23–33, 2013.

[48] N. C. Fagundes, L. M. Fernandes, R. S. Paraense et al., "Binge drinking of ethanol during adolescence induces oxidative damage and morphological changes in salivary glands of female rats," *Oxidative Medicine and Cellular Longevity*, vol. 2016, Article ID 7323627, 11 pages, 2016.

[49] L. M. P. Fernandes, F. B. Teixeira, S. M. A. Junior, J. D. J. V. Pinheiro, C. D. S. F. Maia, and R. R. Lima, "Immunohistochemical changes and atrophy after chronic ethanol intoxication in rat salivary glands," *Histology and Histopathology*, vol. 30, no. 9, pp. 1069–1078, 2015.

[50] E. A. Irving, D. L. Bentley, and A. A. Parsons, "Assessment of white matter injury following prolonged focal cerebral ischaemia in the rat," *Acta Neuropathologica*, vol. 102, no. 6, pp. 627–635, 2001.

[51] J. S. Guimarães, M. A. M. Freire, R. R. Lima, C. W. Picanço-Diniz, A. Pereira, and W. Gomes-Leal, "Minocycline treatment reduces white matter damage after excitotoxic striatal injury," *Brain Research*, vol. 1329, pp. 182–193, 2010.

[52] K. Fuxe, A. Cintra, B. Andbjer, E. Anggard, M. Goldstein, and L. F. Agnati, "Centrally administered endothelin-1 produces lesions in the brain of the male rat," *Acta Physiologica Scandinavica*, vol. 137, no. 1, pp. 155–156, 1989.

[53] L. F. Agnati, M. Zoli, M. Kurosawa et al., "A new model of focal brain ischemia based on the intracerebral injection of endothelin-1," *Italian Journal of Neurological Sciences*, vol. 12, no. 3, supplement 11, pp. 49–53, 1991.

[54] P. M. Hughes, D. C. Anthony, M. Ruddin et al., "Focal lesions in the rat central nervous system induced by endothelin-1," *Journal of Neuropathology and Experimental Neurology*, vol. 62, no. 12, pp. 1276–1286, 2003.

[55] H. Delavaran, H. Sjunnesson, A. Arvidsson et al., "Proximity of brain infarcts to regions of endogenous neurogenesis and involvement of striatum in ischaemic stroke," *European Journal of Neurology*, vol. 20, no. 3, pp. 473–479, 2013.

[56] Q. Zhao, H. Memezawa, M.-L. Smith, and B. K. Siejö, "Hyperthermia complicates middle cerebral artery occlusion induced by an intraluminal filament," *Brain Research*, vol. 649, no. 1-2, pp. 253–259, 1994.

[57] R. K. Clark, E. V. Lee, C. J. Fish et al., "Development of tissue damage, inflammation and resolution following stroke: An Immunohistochemical and Quantitative Planimetric Study," *Brain Research Bulletin*, vol. 31, no. 5, pp. 565–572, 1993.

[58] A. Buffo, C. Rolando, and S. Ceruti, "Astrocytes in the damaged brain: molecular and cellular insights into their reactive response and healing potential," *Biochemical Pharmacology*, vol. 79, no. 2, pp. 77–89, 2010.

[59] G. Stoll, S. Jander, and M. Schroeter, "Inflammation and glial responses in ischemic brain lesions," *Progress in Neurobiology*, vol. 56, no. 2, pp. 149–171, 1998.

[60] S. Sukumari-Ramesh, C. H. Alleyne, and K. M. Dhandapani, "Astrocyte-specific expression of survivin after intracerebral hemorrhage in mice: a possible role in reactive gliosis?" *Journal of Neurotrauma*, vol. 29, no. 18, pp. 2798–2804, 2012.

[61] H. Neumann, R. Schweigreiter, T. Yamashita, K. Rosenkranz, H. Wekerle, and Y.-A. Barde, "Tumor necrosis factor inhibits neurite outgrowth and branching of hippocampal neurons by a Rho-dependent mechanism," *The Journal of Neuroscience*, vol. 22, no. 3, pp. 854–862, 2002.

[62] G. Barreto, R. E. White, Y. Ouyang, L. Xu, and R. G. Giffard, "Astrocytes: targets for neuroprotection in stroke," *Central Nervous System Agents in Medicinal Chemistry*, vol. 11, no. 2, pp. 164–173, 2011.

[63] Y.-P. Yan, K. A. Sailor, B. T. Lang, S.-W. Park, R. Vemuganti, and R. J. Dempsey, "Monocyte chemoattractant protein-1 plays a critical role in neuroblast migration after focal cerebral ischemia," *Journal of Cerebral Blood Flow & Metabolism*, vol. 27, no. 6, pp. 1213–1224, 2007.

[64] P. Thored, A. Arvidsson, E. Cacci et al., "Persistent production of neurons from adult brain stem cells during recovery after stroke," *Stem Cells*, vol. 24, no. 3, pp. 739–747, 2006.

[65] A. Arvidsson, T. Collin, D. Kirik, Z. Kokaia, and O. Lindvall, "Neuronal replacement from endogenous precursors in the adult brain after stroke," *Nature Medicine*, vol. 8, no. 9, pp. 963–970, 2002.

[66] O. P. Ottersen, J. H. Laake, W. Reichelt, F.-M. Haug, and R. Torp, "Ischemic disruption of glutamate homeostasis in brain: quantitative immunocytochemical analyses," *Journal of Chemical Neuroanatomy*, vol. 12, no. 1, pp. 1–14, 1996.

[67] Y. Béjot, A. Prigent-Tessier, C. Cachia et al., "Time-dependent contribution of non neuronal cells to BDNF production after ischemic stroke in rats," *Neurochemistry International*, vol. 58, no. 1, pp. 102–111, 2011.

[68] T. Morioka, A. N. Kalehua, and W. J. Streit, "Characterization of microglial reaction after middle cerebral artery occlusion in rat brain," *Journal of Comparative Neurology*, vol. 327, no. 1, pp. 123–132, 1993.

[69] A. Nimmerjahn, F. Kirchhoff, and F. Helmchen, "Neuroscience: resting microglial cells are highly dynamic surveillants of brain parenchyma in vivo," *Science*, vol. 308, no. 5726, pp. 1314–1318, 2005.

[70] D. Davalos, J. Grutzendler, G. Yang et al., "ATP mediates rapid microglial response to local brain injury in vivo," *Nature Neuroscience*, vol. 8, no. 6, pp. 752–758, 2005.

[71] W. J. Streit, "Microglia and the response to brain injury," *Ernst Schering Research Foundation Workshop*, no. 39, pp. 11–24, 2002.

[72] M. Schilling, M. Besselmann, M. Müller, J. K. Strecker, E. B. Ringelstein, and R. Kiefer, "Predominant phagocytic activity of resident microglia over hematogenous macrophages following transient focal cerebral ischemia: an investigation using green fluorescent protein transgenic bone marrow chimeric mice," *Experimental Neurology*, vol. 196, no. 2, pp. 290–297, 2005.

[73] M. Schroeter, S. Jander, I. Huitinga, O. W. Witte, and G. Stoll, "Phagocytic response in photochemically induced infarction of rat cerebral cortex: the role of resident microglia," *Stroke*, vol. 28, no. 2, pp. 382–386, 1997.

[74] X. Hu, P. Li, Y. Guo et al., "Microglia/macrophage polarization dynamics reveal novel mechanism of injury expansion after focal cerebral ischemia," *Stroke*, vol. 43, no. 11, pp. 3063–3070, 2012.

[75] E. A. Irving, K. Yatsushiro, J. McCulloch, and D. Dewar, "Rapid alteration of tau in oligodendrocytes after focal ischemic injury in the rat: involvement of free radicals," *Journal of Cerebral Blood Flow and Metabolism*, vol. 17, no. 6, pp. 612–622, 1997.

[76] M. M. Gresle, B. Jarrott, N. M. Jones, and J. K. Callaway, "Injury to axons and oligodendrocytes following endothelin-1-induced middle cerebral artery occlusion in conscious rats," *Brain Research*, vol. 1110, no. 1, pp. 13–22, 2006.

[77] V. Valeriani, D. Dewar, and J. McCulloch, "Quantitative assessment of ischemic pathology in axons, oligodendrocytes, and neurons: attenuation of damage after transient ischemia," *Journal of Cerebral Blood Flow & Metabolism*, vol. 20, no. 5, pp. 765–771, 2000.

[78] M. D. Weingarten, A. H. Lockwood, S. Y. Hwo, and M. W. Kirschner, "A protein factor essential for microtubule assembly," *Proceedings of the National Academy of Sciences of the United States of America*, vol. 72, no. 5, pp. 1858–1862, 1975.

[79] E. McCracken, V. Valeriani, C. Simpson, T. Jover, J. McCulloch, and D. Dewar, "The lipid peroxidation by-product 4-hydroxynonenal is toxic to axons and oligodendrocytes," *Journal of Cerebral Blood Flow and Metabolism*, vol. 20, no. 11, pp. 1529–1536, 2000.

[80] G. L. Li, M. Farooque, A. Holtz, and Y. Olsson, "Apoptosis of oligodendrocytes occurs for long distances away from the primary injury after compression trauma to rat spinal cord," *Acta Neuropathologica*, vol. 98, no. 5, pp. 473–480, 1999.

[81] J. C. Gensel, C. A. Tovar, J. C. Bresnahan, and M. S. Beattie, "Topiramate treatment is neuroprotective and reduces oligodendrocyte loss after cervical spinal cord injury," *PLoS ONE*, vol. 7, no. 3, Article ID e33519, 2012.

[82] R. P. Skoff, D. A. Bessert, J. D. E. Barks, D. Song, M. Cerghet, and F. S. Silverstein, "Hypoxic-ischemic injury results in acute disruption of myelin gene expression and death of oligodendroglial precursors in neonatal mice," *International Journal of Developmental Neuroscience*, vol. 19, no. 2, pp. 197–208, 2001.

[83] C. Wiessner, F. M. Bareyre, P. R. Allegrini et al., "Anti-Nogo-A antibody infusion 24 hours after experimental stroke improved behavioral outcome and corticospinal plasticity in normotensive and spontaneously hypertensive rats," *Journal of Cerebral Blood Flow and Metabolism*, vol. 23, no. 2, pp. 154–165, 2003.

[84] P. Freund, E. Schmidlin, T. Wannier et al., "Anti-Nogo-A antibody treatment promotes recovery of manual dexterity after unilateral cervical lesion in adult primates—re-examination and extension of behavioral data," *European Journal of Neuroscience*, vol. 29, no. 5, pp. 983–996, 2009.

[85] A. B. Seymour, E. M. Andrews, S.-Y. Tsai et al., "Delayed treatment with monoclonal antibody IN-1 1 week after stroke results in recovery of function and corticorubral plasticity in adult rats," *Journal of Cerebral Blood Flow & Metabolism*, vol. 25, no. 10, pp. 1366–1375, 2005.

14

Apixaban in Comparison to Warfarin for Stroke Prevention in Nonvalvular Atrial Fibrillation: A Systematic Review and Meta-Analysis of Observational Studies

Muhammad U. Siddiqui,[1] David Scalzitti,[2] and Zunaira Naeem[3]

[1]*Department of Medicine, Marshfield Clinic, Rice Lake, WI 54701, USA*
[2]*Department of Biostatistics, George Washington University, Washington, DC 20052, USA*
[3]*Department of Medicine, Marshfield Clinic, Chippewa Falls, WI 54721, USA*

Correspondence should be addressed to Muhammad U. Siddiqui; siddiqi.umer@gmail.com

Academic Editor: Luigina Guasti

Introduction. Atrial fibrillation leads to increased risk of systemic embolism and stroke. To decrease these adverse events, anticoagulation is routinely prescribed. Nonvitamin K anticoagulants like apixaban and rivaroxaban are becoming popular and being used more frequently nowadays. We here compare the efficacy and safety of apixaban with those of warfarin. *Methods and Analysis.* This systematic review aims to assess the efficacy and safety of apixaban compared to those of warfarin. Eligible participants were adults diagnosed with nonvalvular atrial fibrillation. The intervention was apixaban, and the comparator was warfarin. The primary efficacy endpoint is the first admission with systemic embolism or stroke, and the primary safety outcome is the occurrence of major bleeding. Relevant studies were searched in the Cochrane Central Register of Controlled Trials, MEDLINE, PubMed, and clinicaltrials.gov. After being independently reviewed by two authors, five articles were included in the systematic review. The risk of bias of included studies was assessed using the Cochrane risk of bias tool and SIGN methodology. The RevMan software was used to assess the effect size and perform meta-analysis. *Results.* Apixaban was found to be superior to warfarin in terms of safety (RR 0.58; CI 0.52–0.66) but not superior to warfarin in terms of efficacy (RR 0.93; CI 0.70–1.24). *Conclusion.* Apixaban is superior to warfarin in terms of safety, but no difference in efficacy is noted. The choice of anticoagulation should be individualized based on the risk factor profile of the patient.

1. Introduction

1.1. Background. Atrial fibrillation (AF) is an irregular heart rhythm. It is considered the most common cardiac arrhythmia and increases the risk of strokes by fivefold [1]. In order to prevent strokes, anticoagulants are routinely prescribed, particularly in population with the CHA_2DS_2-VASc score greater than or equal to 2 [2]. CHA_2DS_2-VASc and $CHADS_2$ risk models are preferred tools to estimate the risk of embolic strokes in patients with atrial fibrillation [3, 4]. The CHA_2DS_2-VASc tool assigns a score of 0, 1, or >2 to the individuals with atrial fibrillation. The benefits of anticoagulation significantly outweigh the risk in almost all patients with nonvalvular atrial fibrillation with a CHA_2DS_2-VASc score equal to or greater than 2 [2, 5]. Warfarin reduces the risk of strokes by 68% and however requires regular international normalized ratio testing and has frequent interactions with multiple drugs and food. In recent years, researchers have overcome these shortcomings by introducing a new class of anticoagulants called nonvitamin K oral anticoagulants (NOACs). Clinical trials have demonstrated that NOACs are equivalent to warfarin in effectiveness and safety and therefore are now routinely used in practice [6–9].

Among the NOACs, there are factor Xa inhibitors (apixaban, rivaroxaban, and edoxaban). A 2014 Cochrane review compared factor Xa inhibitors to warfarin and identified lower rates of strokes and bleeding with factor Xa inhibitors [10]. This review did not compare the efficacy and safety of different agents among factor Xa inhibitors with each other. To answer this question, head-to-head trials are required which are lacking. Hence, investigators have tried to answer this question by performing network analysis and indirectly comparing these agents [11, 12]. These trials found similar effectiveness in preventing strokes but found lower risk of major bleeding with apixaban. Due to lack of direct comparison, these results are not fully incorporated in clinical practice and the decision is left up to the clinician's preference.

As NOACs are becoming popular and more frequently used, new trials and evidence are constantly being reported. A systematic review of observational studies recently reported a low risk of stroke/systemic embolism and major bleeding with apixaban when compared to warfarin [13]. In order to further scrutinize and incorporate this new evidence in clinical practice, we decided to perform a combined systematic review of randomized and nonrandomized controlled trials to find if both regular-dose apixaban (5 mg) and reduced-dose apixaban (2.5 mg) are superior/noninferior to warfarin in terms of efficacy and safety.

1.2. Objectives. The objectives of this study are to determine efficacy and safety of apixaban in comparison to those of warfarin for preventing strokes in patients of 18 years old and above with nonvalvular atrial fibrillation.

2. Methods

2.1. Eligibility Criteria. This review included randomized controlled trials (RCTs) and non-RCTs (case-control and cohort) comparing efficacy and safety of apixaban vs those of warfarin in patients with nonvalvular atrial fibrillation. Studies with participants 18 years or older with nonvalvular atrial fibrillation using apixaban or warfarin to prevent stroke were included (Table S1). Inclusion criteria included a minimum 6-month continuous follow-up after initiation of apixaban or warfarin. Patients were also required to have AF diagnosis (International Classification of Disease, 9th Revision, diagnosis code 427.1) at baseline. Patients on dialysis and having valvular atrial fibrillation were excluded from the study.

The first admission with stroke or systemic embolism was considered the primary efficacy outcome. The first admission with major bleeding (gastrointestinal bleeding, intracranial bleeding, and bleeding from other sites) was the primary safety outcome.

2.2. Search Strategy. We performed a systemic search on February 7, 2018, on the following databases to search for relevant articles:

(1) MEDLINE (Ovid)
(2) Cochrane Central Register of Controlled Trials
(3) PubMed
(4) Clinicaltrials.gov

The keywords that were used to perform searches included atrial fibrillation AND stroke prevention/control AND apixaban OR factor Xa inhibitors OR pyridines AND warfarin. The keywords were inserted in the medical term (MeSH) search bar, available in the MEDLINE and Cochrane registry. They were then combined using AND/OR, as described earlier. To search for grey literatures and unpublished articles, we used the above-mentioned keywords to perform search in clinicaltrials.gov. Once search was performed, the articles were exported to legacy RefWorks. A search for duplicates was performed in RefWorks, and duplicate articles were removed.

2.3. Data Collection and Analysis. Two review authors (MUS and ZN) independently reviewed full text of the articles selected for eligibility. If there were any disagreements, a third review author (DS) was asked to arbitrate. A data collection form was created on Microsoft Word and was shared with the second author. The data regarding study characteristics, intervention, comparison, and outcomes were documented on the form (Tables S1–S3). Two authors independently extracted outcome data on a standardized data extraction tool. Any disagreements were resolved by discussion. One author transferred data into Review Manager (RevMan).

2.4. Assessment of Risk of Bias. Risk of bias for each study was assessed by two authors independently using the criteria outlined in the Cochrane Handbook for Systematic Reviews of Interventions. Any disagreements were resolved by discussion. For RCTs, the Cochrane risk of bias tool for RCTs was utilized (Table S4). For cohort studies, the SIGN methodology was utilized to assess the risk of bias (Table S5). Each potential source of bias was graded as high, low, or moderate.

2.5. Data Synthesis. The statistical analysis was undertaken using Review Manager (RevMan) version 5.3 (The Cochrane Collaboration 2014, Nordic Cochrane Centre, Copenhagen, Denmark). Outcomes from each study were pooled and compared using a random-effects model according to the heterogeneity between all included studies. The treatment effect was reported as risk ratio (RR) and 95% confidence interval (CI). The I^2 statistic was quantified to measure heterogeneity, and the Mantel–Haenszel (M-H) random-effects model was used. A p value <0.05 was considered statistically significant.

3. Results

3.1. Study Selection. One hundred two potential articles were found after search (Figure 1). One author independently screened titles and abstracts of the articles. A PRISMA flow diagram (Figure 1) is included for details. The full texts of 15 articles were retrieved for assessment of eligibility. 10 articles were excluded after the full-text review. Among excluded articles, 3 were found to be in Russian language, 4 articles

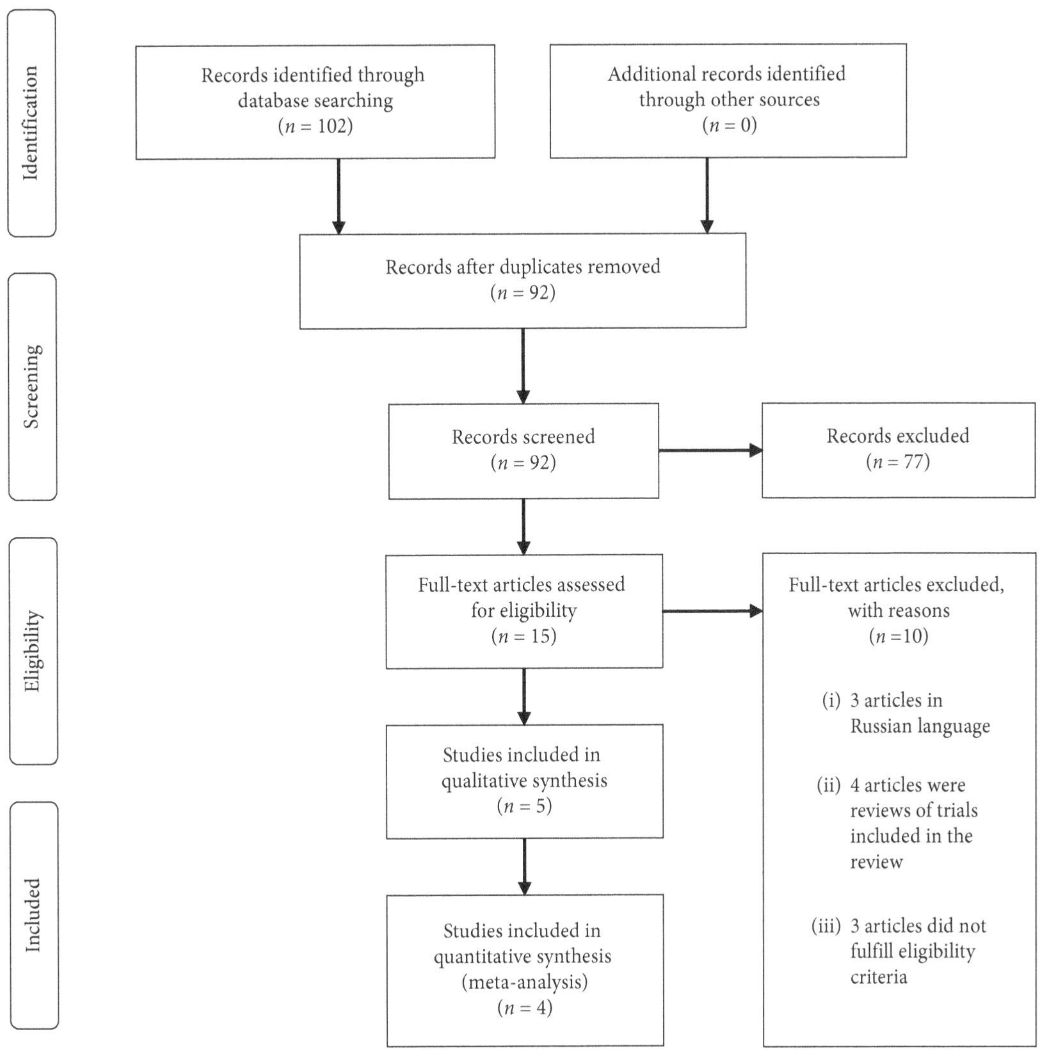

Figure 1: PRISMA flow diagram.

were reviews of studies already included in the meta-analysis, and the other excluded articles did not fulfill the inclusion criteria. 5 articles were selected to perform the systematic review [8, 14–17]. The second author (ZN) reviewed these five articles independently to assess eligibility. If there were any disagreements, the third review author (DS) was asked to arbitrate.

3.2. Study Characteristics. Overall, 65199 patients were treated with apixaban in the included five studies. Four among five studies were observational cohort studies [14–17], while one study was a randomized controlled trial [8]. The one randomized controlled trial was published in 2011 [8], and the four observational cohort studies were published between 2016 and 2018 [14–17]. Two studies were conducted in the United States [8, 15], whereas three studies were conducted in Europe [14, 16, 17]. The baseline characteristics were consistent in all the studies. Three studies reported age data using median and interquartile range (IQR) [8, 14, 17]. Since these three studies had large sample size, they were considered symmetrically distributed. Therefore, the median was estimated to be equal to mean, and the IQR was divided by 1.35 to estimate standard deviation. The mean age of patients taking apixaban ranged between 68.6 and 71.7 in three studies [8, 14, 15]. Two studies separately reported patients taking reduced-dose apixaban [15, 16]. Patients on reduced-dose apixaban are usually older with more comorbidities. Hence, in these two studies, the mean age of patients on reduced-dose apixaban ranged between 82.5 and 83.5. One study included patients taking both low- and high-dose apixaban but did not perform a subgroup analysis in terms of the dose being utilized [17]. The mean age of the apixaban group in this study was 76.

3.3. Risk of Bias Evaluation. A risk of bias evaluation was performed using the Cochrane risk of bias tool (Table S4) for randomized trials [8] and the SIGN tool (Table S5) for observational cohort studies [14–17]. All five studies overall reported a low risk of bias (Figure 2). We did not find significant publication bias in the main primary outcome, for comparison between apixaban and warfarin.

STUDY	Selection bias	Attrition bias	Performance bias	Detection bias	Reporting bias	Overall bias
Granger et al.	Low	Low	Low	Low	Low	Low
Larsen et al.	High	Low	Low	Low	Low	Moderate
Li et al.	Low	Low	Low	Low	Low	Low
Nielsen et al.	High	Low	Moderate	Low	Low	Moderate
Staerk et al.	Low	Low	Low	Low	Low	Low

FIGURE 2: Risk of bias.

Study or subgroup	Apixaban Events	Apixaban Total	Warfarin Events	Warfarin Total	Weight	Risk ratio M-H, random, 95% CI
Li et al.	400	38427	603	38427	25.4%	0.66 [0.59, 0.75]
Nielson et al.	236	4400	1686	38893	25.2%	1.24 [1.08, 1.41]
Larson et al.	225	6353	1447	35436	25.1%	0.87 [0.76, 1.00]
Stark et al.	171	6899	419	18094	24.2%	1.07 [0.90, 1.28]
Granger et al.	212	9120	265	9081	0.0%	0.80 [0.67, 0.95]
Total (95% CI)		56079		130850	100.0%	0.93 (0.70, 1.24)
Total events	1032		4155			

Heterogeneity: $tau^2 = 0.08$; $chi^2 = 48.84$; $df = 3$ ($p < 0.00001$); $I^2 = 94\%$

Test for overall effect: $Z = 0.48$ ($p = 0.63$)

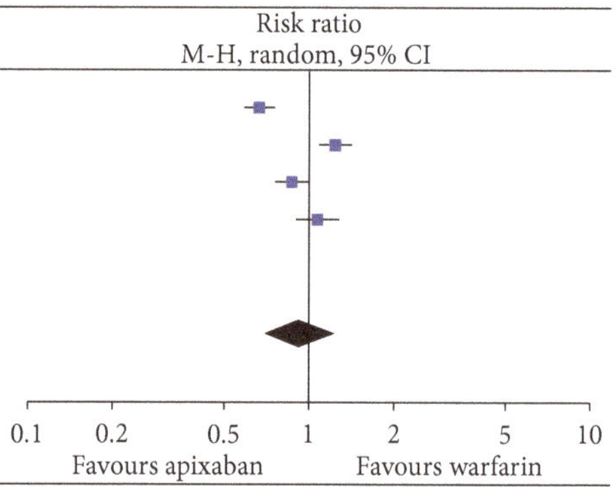

FIGURE 3: Efficacy with only nonrandomized trials.

3.4. Study Results. Risk ratio was used as a summary measure. In two studies [8, 15] comparing apixaban with warfarin, apixaban was associated with a lower risk of stroke and systemic embolism. Three studies [14, 16, 17] showed no difference in the risk of stroke and systemic embolism.

Apixaban was associated with a lower risk of major bleeding compared to warfarin in three studies [8, 14, 15]. One study [16] did not show any difference in the risk of major bleeding.

3.5. Meta-Analysis of Selected Studies. We only analyzed the four observational studies for the meta-analysis [14–17] and excluded the trial conducted by Granger et al. since it was a randomized trial. We compared the meta-analysis results with the findings from the only randomized trial [8] for similarities/differences.

3.5.1. Efficacy Outcome. In our analysis of nonrandomized trials, there was no difference in reducing stroke and/or systemic embolism when comparing apixaban with Coumadin (risk ratio, 0.93; 95% confidence interval (95% CI), 0.70–1.24; Figure 3). Analysis can be interpreted as clinically favoring apixaban over warfarin, and however, as mentioned earlier, the results were not statistically significant.

The result was slightly different from that of the randomized trial of Granger et al. which similarly to our meta-analysis found that apixaban is better in reducing strokes/SE in relation to warfarin. However, in contrast to our meta-analysis, the result was statistically significant.

3.5.2. Safety Outcome. Analysis of nonrandomized trials for major bleeding identified a statistically significant difference favoring apixaban when compared to warfarin (risk ratio, 0.58; 95% confidence interval (95% CI), 0.52–0.66; Figure 4).

The result was similar to that of the randomized trial by Granger et al. When it comes to major bleeding, a significant difference was noted favoring apixaban over warfarin in the trial performed by Granger et al.

3.5.3. Heterogeneity. An increased level of statistical heterogeneity was noted in the meta-analysis for both the outcomes. Lack of randomization in the four observational studies [14–17] is one possible reason for heterogeneity. Two included trials separately reported the comparison between reduced-dose apixaban (2.5 mg) and warfarin [15, 16]. Reduced-dose apixaban is used in older population with age >80 years, and therefore, the mean age of study population in the reduced-dose apixaban trials was 82.5–83.5. It is well known that the risk of stroke, death, and major bleeding

Study or subgroup	Apixaban Events	Apixaban Total	Warfarin Events	Warfarin Total	Weight	Risk ratio M-H, random, 95% CI
Larson et al.	109	6353	1198	35436	24.1%	0.51 [0.42, 0.62]
Li et al.	751	38427	1303	38427	45.6%	0.58 [0.53, 0.63]
Nielson et al.	160	4400	2136	38893	30.3%	0.66 [0.57, 0.78]
Granger et al.	327	9088	462	9052	0.0%	0.70 [0.61, 0.81]
Total (95% CI)		49180		112756	100.0%	0.58 [0.52, 0.66]
Total events	1020		4637			

Heterogeneity: $tau^2 = 0.01$; $chi^2 = 4.53$; $df = 2$ ($p = 0.10$); $I^2 = 56\%$

Test for overall effect: $Z = 8.56$ ($p < 0.00001$)

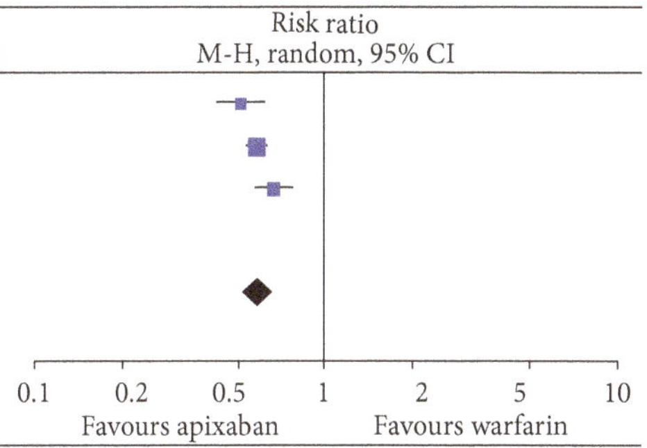

FIGURE 4: Safety with only nonrandomized trials.

increases with increased age [18]. Therefore, the increased mean age in the reduced-dose apixaban trials also contributed to the statistical heterogeneity.

4. Discussion

We reviewed five studies to determine efficacy of apixaban compared to that of warfarin and reviewed four studies to compare the safety profile of apixaban vs that of warfarin. However, the meta-analysis was performed using only observational studies [14–17]. The total number of patients who have their bleeding and thromboembolic risk assessed was >49000. The study denotes that patients who were taking warfarin had more bleeding events when compared to those who were on apixaban, and the result was statistically significant. However, there was no statistical difference between thromboembolic events in both arms. Previous meta-analysis performed by Proietti et al. favored apixaban over warfarin both in terms of efficacy and safety. However, the results for efficacy were statistically nonsignificant [13] similar to our conclusion. They further performed subgroup analysis and found that, in the reduced-dose apixaban group, the reduction in thromboembolic diseases was statistically significant. Proietti et al. did not include the phase III ARISTOTLE trial [8] comparing apixaban and warfarin in contrast to our systemic review. The ARISTOTLE landmark trial found that apixaban had statistically significant reduction in stroke/systemic embolism as well as major bleeding when compared to warfarin.

Out trial further reinforces the superiority of apixaban over warfarin. To date, there is only one randomized controlled trial on this topic [8]. Several nonrandomized cohort studies have however been reported. Though there is paucity of randomized trials, the trials so far performed have clearly shown clinical benefits of apixaban over warfarin. Other NOACs have shown similar superiority over warfarin. Therefore, NOACs are now being used more frequently in the real-world setting and being preferred over warfarin [13, 19]. Given mounting evidence, the guidelines have changed in favor of NOACs over warfarin [20].

Though the result of this meta-analysis is consistent with that of similar previous studies, an individualized approach should be exercised in managing each patient. This meta-analysis did not include patients who had valvular atrial fibrillation or patients who were on dialysis, and therefore, the results from this study cannot be applied on them. Having said that, Granger et al. performed subgroup analysis and found that apixaban was safer and caused less major bleeding episodes in patients with severe renal impairment when compared to warfarin. Apixaban was also found to have similar efficacy but a better safety profile in patients with diabetes mellitus [8]. Our meta-analysis had two trials that compared reduced-dose apixaban with warfarin [15, 16]. As described in Methods, reduced-dose apixaban is used in elderly population or patients with kidney disease [8]. Nielsen et al. compared reduced-dose apixaban with warfarin and found more thromboembolic and major bleeding events with apixaban. The ORBIT-AF II trial (Outcome Registry for Better Informed Treatment of Atrial Fibrillation Phase II trial) showed that 11.8% of patients with atrial fibrillation are undertreated with reduced-dose apixaban, and this leads to worse outcomes [21].

The four nonrandomized observational studies in our meta-analysis did not provide data on international normalized ratio (INR) values for the patients taking warfarin as this information was not available in the dataset. Granger et al. reported that the INR was in the therapeutic range (2.0 to 3.0) in the warfarin group for a mean of 62.2% of the time. Since the therapeutic window of warfarin is narrow, clinicians and researchers may argue that the favorable profile of apixaban when compared to warfarin may be due to poor quality of INR control. However, Wallentin et al. found apixaban to be more efficacious with a better safety profile than warfarin regardless of the centre's or patient's quality of INR control [22].

Overall, there was a low risk of bias associated with all the included studies (Figure 2). Given four out of the five included trials were nonrandomized studies, there is always a risk of selection bias. Two trials were noted to have a high selection bias [14, 16]. One trial was noted to have a moderate risk of performance bias [16]. Future randomized trials may be able to amend these drawbacks. All the trials reported a low risk of attrition, detection, and reporting biases. The one randomized trial included in our meta-analysis did not describe the method utilized for random sequence generation mildly affecting the quality of evidence [8].

Compared to previous meta-analysis, we have included the one randomized trial published to date in our systematic review. The outcomes however have remained the same.

Similar to previous meta-analysis, regular-dose apixaban is found to have similar efficacy but better safety compared to warfarin. The effectiveness of reduced-dose apixaban is still debatable and needs further research. Our review agrees with previous similar reviews and further reinforces the favorable profile of apixaban when compared to warfarin.

5. Limitations

There are a few limitations in our review: First, we were unable to verify participant compliance with assigned medication. Second, there are lack of randomized trials and better quality of evidence. The included studies had increased heterogeneity, confirmed by large I^2 values. Finally, due to lack of resources, we were unable to perform the search in EMBASE. Hence, it is possible that there are other studies matching our inclusion criteria that are not included in our meta-analysis.

6. Conclusion

In this systematic review and meta-analysis, apixaban was associated with a better safety profile when compared to warfarin with less major bleeding events. The analysis also favored apixaban in terms of reducing strokes/systemic embolism, and however, this result was not statistically significant. Our analysis included the only randomized trial performed on this topic, and the results are consistent with those of previous systematic reviews. This review further reinforces the superiority of apixaban in comparison to warfarin in patients with nonvalvular atrial fibrillation.

Conflicts of Interest

The authors have no conflicts of interest to report.

Supplementary Materials

Supplementary Table 1: PICO characteristics of the studies included in the systematic review and meta-analysis. Supplementary Table 2: baseline characteristics of the studies included in the systematic review and meta-analysis. Supplementary Table 3: outcomes of the studies included in the systematic review and meta-analysis. Supplementary Table 4: Cochrane risk of bias tool for randomized controlled trials. Supplementary Table 5: SIGN risk of bias tool for nonrandomized controlled trials. (*Supplementary Materials*)

References

[1] P. A. Wolf, R. D. Abbott, and W. B. Kannel, "Atrial fibrillation as an independent risk factor for stroke: the Framingham study," *Stroke*, vol. 22, no. 8, pp. 983–988, 1991.

[2] L. Friberg, M. Rosenqvist, and G. Y. H. Lip, "Net clinical benefit of warfarin in patients with atrial fibrillation," *Circulation*, vol. 125, no. 19, pp. 2298–2307, 2012.

[3] H. A. van den Ham, O. H. Klungel, D. E. Singer, H. G. M. Leufkens, and T. P. van Staa, "Comparative performance of ATRIA, CHADS2, and CHA2DS2-VASc risk scores predicting stroke in patients with atrial fibrillation," *Journal of the American College of Cardiology*, vol. 66, no. 17, pp. 1851–1859, 2015.

[4] T. P. van Staa, E. Setakis, G. L. Di Tanna, D. A. Lane, and G. Y. H. Lip, "A comparison of risk stratification schemes for stroke in 79 884 atrial fibrillation patients in general practice," *Journal of Thrombosis and Haemostasis*, vol. 9, no. 1, pp. 39–48, 2011.

[5] D. E. Singer, Y. Chang, M. C. Fang et al., "Should patient characteristics influence target anticoagulation intensity for stroke prevention in nonvalvular atrial fibrillation?," *Circulation: Cardiovascular Quality and Outcomes*, vol. 2, no. 4, pp. 297–304, 2009.

[6] S. J. Connolly, M. D. Ezekowitz, S. Yusuf et al., "Dabigatran versus warfarin in patients with atrial fibrillation," *New England Journal of Medicine*, vol. 361, no. 12, pp. 1139–1151, 2009.

[7] R. P. Giugliano, C. T. Ruff, E. Braunwald et al., "Edoxaban versus warfarin in patients with atrial fibrillation," *New England Journal of Medicine*, vol. 369, no. 22, pp. 2093–2104, 2013.

[8] C. B. Granger, J. H. Alexander, J. J. V. McMurray et al., "Apixaban versus warfarin in patients with atrial fibrillation," *New England Journal of Medicine*, vol. 365, no. 11, pp. 981–992, 2011.

[9] M. R. Patel, K. W. Mahaffey, J. Garg et al., "Rivaroxaban versus warfarin in nonvalvular atrial fibrillation," *New England Journal of Medicine*, vol. 365, no. 10, pp. 883–891, 2011.

[10] K. M. B. Slot and E. Berge, "Factor Xa inhibitors versus vitamin K antagonists for preventing cerebral or systemic embolism in patients with atrial fibrillation," *Cochrane Database of Systematic Reviews*, vol. 6, no. 3, article CD008980, 2018.

[11] J. Harenberg, S. Marx, H. C. Diener et al., "Comparison of efficacy and safety of dabigatran, rivaroxaban and apixaban in patients with atrial fibrillation using network meta-analysis," *International Angiology*, vol. 31, no. 4, pp. 330–339, 2012.

[12] L. G. Tereshchenko, C. A. Henrikson, J. Cigarroa, and J. S. Steinberg, "Comparative effectiveness of interventions for stroke prevention in atrial fibrillation: a network meta-analysis," *Journal of the American Heart Association*, vol. 5, no. 5, 2016.

[13] M. Proietti, I. Romanazzi, G. F. Romiti, A. Farcomeni, and G. Y. H. Lip, "Real-world use of apixaban for stroke prevention in atrial fibrillation," *Stroke*, vol. 49, no. 1, pp. 98–106, 2018.

[14] T. B. Larsen, F. Skjoth, P. B. Nielsen, J. N. Kjaeldgaard, and G. Y. H. Lip, "Comparative effectiveness and safety of non-vitamin K antagonist oral anticoagulants and warfarin in patients with atrial fibrillation: propensity weighted nationwide cohort study," *BMJ*, vol. 353, p. i3189, 2016.

[15] X. Li, A. Keshishian, M. Hamilton et al., "Apixaban 5 and 2.5 mg twice-daily versus warfarin for stroke prevention in nonvalvular atrial fibrillation patients: comparative effectiveness and safety evaluated using a propensity-score-matched approach," *PLoS One*, vol. 13, no. 1, Article ID e0191722, 2018.

[16] P. B. Nielsen, F. Skjøth, M. Søgaard, J. N. Kjældgaard, G. Y. H. Lip, and T. B. Larsen, "Effectiveness and safety of

reduced dose non-vitamin K antagonist oral anticoagulants and warfarin in patients with atrial fibrillation: propensity weighted nationwide cohort study," *BMJ*, vol. 356, p. j510, 2017.

[17] L. Staerk, E. L. Fosbøl, G. Y. H. Lip et al., "Ischaemic and haemorrhagic stroke associated with non-vitamin K antagonist oral anticoagulants and warfarin use in patients with atrial fibrillation: a nationwide cohort study," *European Heart Journal*, vol. 38, no. 12, pp. 907–915, 2017.

[18] S. Halvorsen, D. Atar, H. Yang et al., "Efficacy and safety of apixaban compared with warfarin according to age for stroke prevention in atrial fibrillation: observations from the ARISTOTLE trial," *European Heart Journal*, vol. 35, no. 28, pp. 1864–1872, 2014.

[19] K. Gadsbøll, L. Staerk, E. L. Fosbøl et al., "Increased use of oral anticoagulants in patients with atrial fibrillation: temporal trends from 2005 to 2015 in Denmark," *European Heart Journal*, vol. 8, pp. 899–906, 2017.

[20] L. Macle, J. Cairns, K. Leblanc et al., "2016 focused update of the Canadian cardiovascular society guidelines for the management of atrial fibrillation," *Canadian Journal of Cardiology*, vol. 32, no. 10, pp. 1170–1185, 2016.

[21] B. A. Steinberg, P. Shrader, L. Thomas et al., "Off-label dosing of non-vitamin K antagonist oral anticoagulants and adverse outcomes," *Journal of the American College of Cardiology*, vol. 68, no. 24, pp. 2597–2604, 2016.

[22] L. Wallentin, R. D. Lopes, M. Hanna et al., "Efficacy and safety of apixaban compared with warfarin at different levels of predicted international normalized ratio control for stroke prevention in atrial fibrillation," *Circulation*, vol. 127, no. 22, pp. 2166–2176, 2013.

15

Type 2 Diabetic Patients with IschemicStroke: Decreased Insulin Sensitivity and Decreasesin Antioxidant Enzyme Activity are Relatedto Different Stroke Subtypes

Aleksandra Jotic,[1] Nadezda Covickovic Sternic,[2] Vladimir S. Kostic,[2] Katarina Lalic,[1] Tanja Milicic,[1] Milija Mijajlovic,[2] Ljiljana Lukic,[1] Milorad Civcic,[1] Emina Colak,[3] Marija Macesic,[1] Jelena P. Seferovic,[1] Sandra Aleksic,[1] and Nebojsa M. Lalic[1]

[1] *Clinic for Endocrinology, Diabetes and Metabolic Disorders, Clinical Centre of Serbia, Faculty of Medicine, University of Belgrade, Dr Subotica 13, 11000 Belgrade, Serbia*
[2] *Clinic for Neurology, Clinical Centre of Serbia, Faculty of Medicine, University of Belgrade, Dr Subotica 6, 11000 Belgrade, Serbia*
[3] *Institute of Medical Biochemistry, Clinical Centre of Serbia, Pasterova 2, 11000 Belgrade, Serbia*

Correspondence should be addressed to Nebojsa M. Lalic; nebojsa.m.lalic@gmail.com

Academic Editor: Ilias Migdalis

We analyzed (a) insulin sensitivity (IS) and (b) glutathione peroxidase (GSH-Px), glutathione reductase (GR), and superoxide dismutase (SOD) antioxidant enzyme activity in type 2 diabetic (T2D) patients with atherothrombotic infarction (ATI) (group A), lacunar infarction (LI) (B), or without stroke (C) and in nondiabetics with ATI (D), LI (E), or without stroke (F). ATI and LI were confirmed by brain imaging IS levels were determined by minimal model (Si index), and the enzyme activity by spectrophotometry. In T2D patients, Si was lower in A and B versus C (1.14 ± 0.58, 1.00 ± 0.26 versus $3.14 \pm 0.62\ \text{min}^{-1}/\text{mU/l} \times 10^4$, $P < 0.001$) and in nondiabetics in D and E versus F (3.38 ± 0.77, 3.03 ± 0.72 versus $6.03 \pm 1.69\ \text{min}^{-1}/\text{mU/l} \times 10^4$, $P < 0.001$). Also, GSH-Px and GR activities were lower in A and B versus C (GSH-Px: 21.96 ± 3.56, 22.51 ± 1.23 versus 25.12 ± 1.67; GR: 44.37 ± 3.58, 43.50 ± 2.39 versus 48.58 ± 3.67 U/gHb; $P < 0.001$) and in D and E versus F (GSH-Px: 24.75 ± 3.02, 25.57 ± 1.92 versus 28.56 ± 3.91; GR: 48.27 ± 6.81, 49.17 ± 6.24 versus 53.67 ± 3.96 U/gHb; $P < 0.001$). Decreases in Si and GR were significantly related to both ATI and LI in T2D. Our results showed that decreased IS and impaired antioxidant enzymes activity influence ischemic stroke subtypes in T2D. The influence of insulin resistance might be exerted on the level of glutathione-dependent antioxidant enzymes.

1. Introduction

It was previously suggested that atherothrombotic infarction (ATI) and lacunar infarction (LI), as two different subtypes of ischemic stroke, might also differ in the set of the relevant risk factors, with ATI being more associated to the atherogenic risk factors in contrast to LI [1]. In addition, the risk factors for both ischemic stroke subtypes remain still largely unclarified.

However, decreased insulin sensitivity (IS), that is, insulin resistance, was observed both in ATI and LI, which was frequently accompanied with compensatory hyperinsulinemia in T2D patients as well as in nondiabetics [2, 3].

Simultaneously, it has been shown that impaired balance between products of oxidative stress and the level of antioxidant enzyme activities might be the important mechanism underlying the occurrence of ischemic stroke [4]. Moreover, it was elucidated that the brain has only moderate content of glutathione-dependent enzymes, for example, glutathione peroxidase (GSH-Px), glutathione reductase (GR), and superoxide dismutase (SOD), together with the fact that the intact antioxidant defense could provide first line of protection from initiation and exacerbation of ischemic cerebral injury [5].

In addition, changes in enzymatic antioxidative defense mechanisms in patients with stroke are still controversial. Previous results implied that the majority of antioxidant enzyme activity was significantly reduced in acute ischemic stroke, possibly as a consequence of increased oxidative stress [5] while the recent finding suggested increased levels of glutathione dependent enzymes as an adaptive mechanisms during acute cerebral ischemia [6]. Finally, due to novel facts, oxidative stress can be an important component for astrocytic cell death following metabolic stress [7].

Until now, experimental studies provided evidence of an association between ischemic stroke and increased oxidative stress [8, 9], but data in humans are still heterogeneous and limited. Therefore, our study was aimed to determine IS levels and three different types of antioxidant enzyme activities GSH-Px, GR, and SOD, in T2D with ATI and LI.

2. Materials and Methods

2.1. Patients. In this study we included a total of 93 patients with T2D, ascribed to the following groups: T2D patients with ATI (group A, $N = 30$), and T2D with LI (group B, $N = 30$), and T2D without ischemic stroke (group C, $N = 33$). Simultaneously, we involved a total of 93 nondiabetics, matched with the T2D patients regarding gender and age, and also comprising the following groups: nondiabetics with ATI (group D, $N = 30$), nondiabetics with LI (group E, $N = 30$), and nondiabetics without stroke (group F, $N = 33$).

T2D was diagnosed in accordance with the criteria of the World Health Organization [10]. Diagnosis of ATI and LI was done by a neurologist due to clinical features and brain imaging methods such as cranial computerized scan and/or magnetic resonance imaging in two consecutive examinations, during the first 7 days from the appearance of ischemic stroke [11]. The patients with ATI or LI were included in the study provided that they had not shown signs of cardioembolic cerebral infarction, or coronary heart disease based on a history of myocardial infarction with definite elevation of serum cardiac enzymes or coronary angiography. T2D patients were treated with insulin therapy, and/or ingestion of antioxidant supplements and drugs, which might affect free radical and antioxidant activity potential; likewise patients who had other endocrine disease or autoimmune diseases, renal or hepatic failure, current infections, neoplasms, polycythemia, or rheumatic diseases were also excluded as well as the patients with history of trauma or operation within the last 3 months. No patient had uncontrolled hypertension, severe alcohol consumption, acute infection, or an inflammatory disease during the last 4 weeks. All the patients, with or without ATI and LI, showed the similar level of their physical activity. In addition, they were required not to smoke at least 12 hr before the tests were performed.

The patients were fully informed about the study and gave the inform consent to participate.

The study was conducted at the Clinic for Endocrinology, Diabetes and Metabolic Diseases and at the Clinic for Neurology, Clinical Centre of Serbia, Faculty of Medicine, University of Belgrade, and was approved by the Institutional Ethics Committee.

2.2. Study Design. The interview, physical examination, metabolic test, and evaluation of antioxidant enzyme activities were performed in all the patients included in the study, for each patient within the same day. The interview comprised the questions about medical conditions, current medication, and habits. Hypertension was diagnosed according to World Health Organisation criteria (systolic/diastolic blood pressure $\geq 140/\geq 90$ mm Hg) or by the use of antihypertensive agents [12].

2.3. Metabolic Evaluations. The metabolic tests were implemented at least after 6 months from the occurrence of the ischemic stroke.

The evaluation of insulin sensitivity was done by Frequently Sampled Intravenous Glucose Tolerance Test (FSIGT) with minimal model analysis [13]. Briefly, before testing, each patient was required to be at a 12 hr fasting state. During the FSIGT, 0.3 g/kg body weight of glucose was injected and the blood samples for plasma glucose (PG) and plasma insulin (PI) determination were taken immediately before and 1, 2, 3, 4, 5, 6, 7, 8, 9, 10, 12, 14, 16, 20, 23, 24, 25, 27, 30, 40, 50, 60, 70, 80, 90, 100, 120, 160, and 180 minutes after intravenous glucose stimulation. Insulin was injected as a continuous infusion 4 mU/kg/min between minutes 20 and 25 in order to avoid the effect of the potentially blunted insulin response. The insulin sensitivity index (Si) was calculated from the results of PG and PI levels by computerized minimal model analysis, using the MINMOD program (kindly provided by Dr. Richard Bergman from the University of Southern California, Los Angeles) [13].

2.4. Laboratory Analyses. Determination of the antioxidant enzymes SOD, GSH-Px, GR was conducted using the commercial assays (produced by Randox Laboratories Ltd., UK), based on spectrophotometer determination methods as described previously [14].

PG was determined by glucose oxidase method using a Beckman Glucose Analyser (Beckman Instruments, Fullerton, CA). PI was tested by radioimmunoassay (INEP, Zemun, RS, double antibody kits). Total cholesterol, HDL cholesterol, and triglyceride concentrations were determined with the chromatography method using commercial kits (produced by Boehringer Mannheim). LDL cholesterol concentrations were calculated using the Friedewald formula.

2.5. Statistical Analyses. Data are presented as mean ± SE. The categorical variables were analyzed with Kruskal-Wallis Test. The continuous variables within each subtype of ischemic stroke were analyzed with analysis of variance (ANOVA) with a post hoc Bonferroni test. Multiple logistical regression analysis was performed. Differences were considered statistically significant at $P < 0.05$. All analyses were performed with the SPSS statistical package (version 16.0 for Windows).

TABLE 1: Clinical characteristics and laboratory analyses in type 2 diabetic patients and nondiabetics with different subtypes of ishemic stroke: atherotrombotic infarction (ATI) and lacunar infarction (LI).

	Groups						
	A T2D+ ATI+	B T2D+ LI+	C T2D+ Stroke−	D T2D− ATI+	E T2D− LI+	F Healthy Controls	*P* value
n (M/F)	30 (16/14)	30 (16/14)	33 (15/18)	30 (15/15)	30 (15/15)	33 (15/18)	NS
Age (years)	56.9 ± 1.67	56.03 ± 2.51	56.42 ± 3.05	57.07 ± 2.88	56.00 ± 2.03	56.97 ± 2.42	NS
Duration of diabetes (years)	4.73 ± 1.53	5.34 ± 1.00	4.65 ± 2.01	—	—	—	NS
Duration from onset of ischaemic stroke (years)	1.23 ± 0.43	1.30 ± 0.24	—	1.03 ± 0.21	1.09 ± 0.21	—	NS
HbA1c (%)	7.39 ± 0.20	7.30 ± 0.14	7.31 ± 0.43	5.52 ± 0.31	5.37 ± 0.31	4.89 ± 0.26	NS
Total cholesterol (mmol/L)	6.98 ± 0.91	6.81 ± 0.68	7.03 ± 0.62	6.25 ± 0.71	6.15 ± 0.63	6.14 ± 0.74	NS
Triglyceride (mmol/L)	2.20 ± 0.37	2.26 ± 0.38	2.18 ± 0.26	1.90 ± 0.22	2.00 ± 0.29	1.87 ± 0.35	NS
LDL-c (mmol/L)	5.21 ± 0.42*	4.81 ± 0.14	4.47 ± 0.29	4.34 ± 0.43*	4.05 ± 0.55	3.71 ± 0.49	$P < 0.05$
HDL-c (mmol/L)	0.94 ± 0.17	1.01 ± 0.40	1.01 ± 0.15	0.99 ± 0.27	1.05 ± 0.16	1.11 ± 0.21	NS
Hypertension (*n*, %)	22 (73.3%)**	21 (70.0%)**	23 (69.7%)**	22 (73.3%)**	22 (66.7%)**	0 (0%)	$P < 0.001$
Smoking (*n*, %)	10 (33.3%)	11 (36.7%)	12 (36.4%)	10 (33.3%)	11 (36.7%)	12 (36.4%)	NS

Data are *n*, means ± SEM.
*$P < 0.05$ A versus B, C and D versus E, F.
**$P < 0.001$ A, B, C, D, E versus F.

3. Results

3.1. Clinical Characteristics. The clinical characteristics and biochemistry parameters of T2D patients and nondiabetics with ATI or LI as different subtypes of ischemic stroke are shown in Table 1. The age, gender, duration of diabetes, and duration from the onset of ischemic stroke were similar in T2D patients and nondiabetics with different subtypes of ischemic stroke, together with HbA_1c levels, implying satisfactory metabolic control before metabolic investigation was done. However, LDL-c level was significantly higher in T2D patients with ATI compared to the T2D patients with LI and T2D patients without stroke and also in nondiabetics with ATI compared to nondiabetics with LI and healthy controls. There is no difference in prevalence of hypertension in patients with T2D and ATI or LI and T2D without ischemic stroke, while it was significantly higher in nondiabetics with ATI or LI than in healthy controls. The percentage of patients who were smokers was similar in all investigated groups.

3.2. Insulin Sensitivity. We found that Si levels were significantly lower in T2D patients with ATI (group A) and LI (group B) compared to T2D patients without ischemic stroke (group C) (1.14 ± 0.58 and 1.00 ± 0.26 versus 3.14 ± 0.62 $min^{-1}/mU/L \times 10^4$, resp., $P < 0.001$). Also, the results showed significantly lower Si levels in nondiabetics with ATI (group D) and LI (group E) compared to healthy controls (group F) (3.38 ± 0.77 and 3.03 ± 0.72 versus 6.03 ± 1.69 $min^{-1}/mU/L \times 10^4$, resp., $P < 0.001$) (Figure 1). Simultaneously, PI levels were higher in T2D patients, ATI (group A), and LI (group B) than in T2D patients without ischemic stroke (group C) (20.94 ± 4.31 and 20.07 ± 0.88 versus 16.06 ± 0.91 mU/L, respectively, $P < 0.001$) and in nondiabetics with

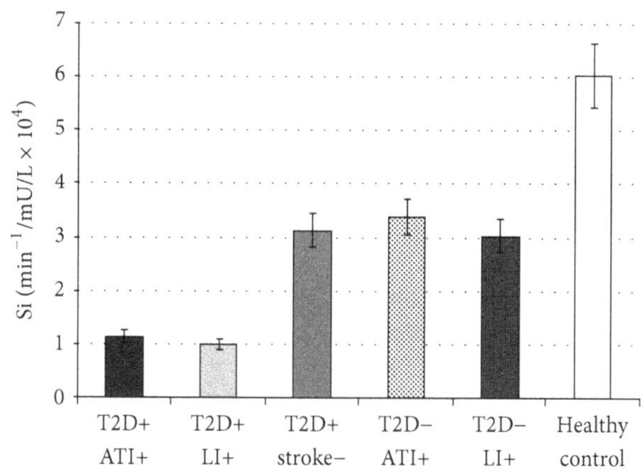

FIGURE 1: Values are expressed as mean ± SE. Bar graphs show the values of insulin sensitivity index (Si) determined by minimal model analysis. Si levels were significantly lower in type 2 diabetic (T2D) patients with different subtypes of ischemic stroke: atherothrombotic infarction (ATI) and lacunar infarction (LI) compared to T2D patients without ischemic stroke, and the same relationship is found in the respective groups in nondiabetics ($P < 0.001$) (ANOVA test).

ATI (group D) or LI (group E) in comparison to healthy controls (group F) (15.57 ± 1.86 and 15.59 ± 1.26 versus 7.54 ± 2.03 mU/L, respectively, $P < 0.001$) (Figure 2).

3.3. Antioxidant Enzyme Activity. When we evaluated antioxidant enzyme activities in T2D patients with ATI (group A) and LI (group B) and without ischemic stroke (group C) and in nondiabetics with ATI (group D) and LI (group E) and healthy controls (group D), we detected the levels

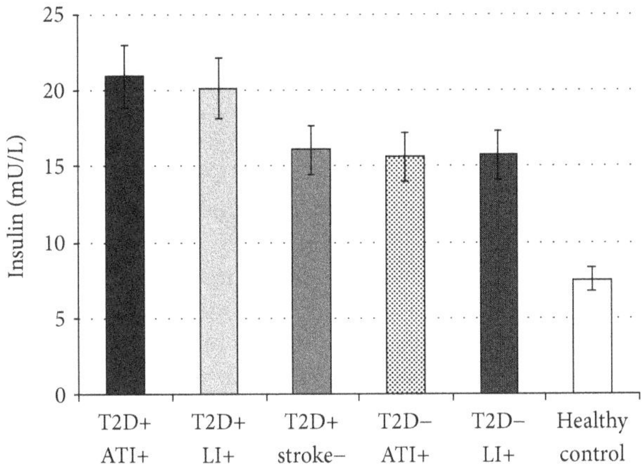

FIGURE 2: Values are expressed as mean ± SE. Bar graphs show the values of basal plasma insulin (PI) level. PI levels were higher in type 2 diabetic (T2D) patients with different subtypes of ischemic stroke: atherothrombotic infarction (ATI) and lacunar infarction (LI) compared to T2D patients without ischemic stroke, and the same relationship is found in the respective groups in nondiabetics ($P < 0.001$) (ANOVA).

TABLE 2: Independent factors related to different subtypes of ischemic stroke in diabetics and nondiabetics in multiple logistic regression analysis.

	Odds ratio (95% CI)	P value
Related to T2D+ ATI+		
Si	0.002 (0.000–0.017)	$P = 0.000$
GR	0.613 (0.422–0.889)	$P = 0.01$
GSH-Px	0.599 (0.332–1.113)	$P = 0.105$
Related to T2D+ LI+		
Si	0.001 (0.0006–0.08)	$P = 0.000$
GR	0.549 (0.369–0.817)	$P = 0.003$
GSH-Px	0.685 (0.362–1.297)	$P = 0.245$
Related to T2D− ATI+		
Si	0.159 (0.056–0.454)	$P = 0.001$
GSH-Px	0.606 (0.428–0.858)	$P = 0.005$
GR	0.795 (0.643–0.982)	$P = 0.033$
Related to T2D− LI+		
Si	0.071 (0.022–0.236)	$P = 0.000$
GSH-Px	0.760 (0.536–1.077)	$P = 0.123$
GR	0.840 (0.680–1.039)	$P = 0.108$

Nagelkerke $R^2 = 0.844$.
Cox and Snell $R^2 = 0.821$.

of the GSH-Px and GR activity being significantly lower in group A and B versus C and in group D and E versus F (GSHPx: A: 21.96 ± 3.56 versus B: 22.51 ± 1.23 versus C: 25.12 ± 1.67 U/gHb, $P < 0.001$; D: 24.75 ± 3.02 versus E: 25.57 ± 1.92 versus F: 28.56 ± 3.91 U/gHb, $P < 0.001$; GR: A: 44.37 ± 3.58 versus B: 43.50 ± 2.39 versus C: 48.58 ± 3.67 U/gHb, $P < 0.001$; D: 24.75 ± 3.02 versus E: 25.57 ± 1.92 versus F: 28.56 ± 3.91 U/gHb, resp., $P < 0.001$) (Figure 3), while the SOD levels did not differ between the investigated groups (A: 769.57 ± 72.36 versus B: 768.97 ± 34.50 versus C: 789.18 ± 60.28, D: 795.23 ± 48.28 versus E: 797.80 ± 69.21 versus F: 813.88 ± 45.80 mU/mgHb, resp., P = NS).

3.4. Multiple Logistic Regression Analysis. This analysis identified that decreased insulin sensitivity Si and the decreases of GR were related to both ATI and LI in T2D patients. Simultaneously, this model identified decreased insulin sensitivity Si and the level of GR and GSH-Px in nondiabetics with ATI, but predominantly decreased insulin sensitivity Si in nondiabetics with LI (Table 2).

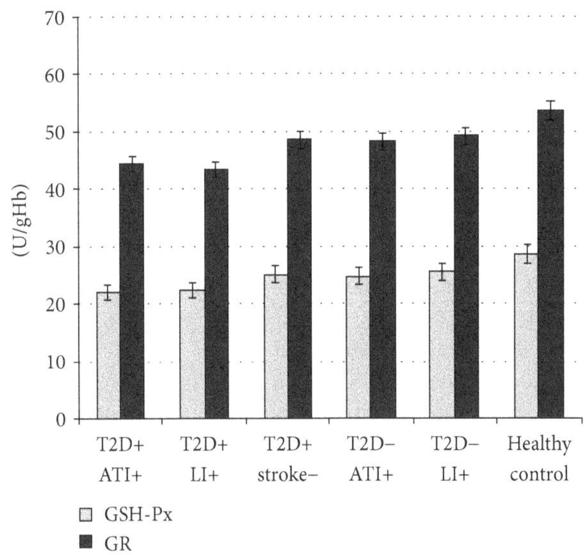

FIGURE 3: Values are expressed as mean ± SE. Bar graphs show the values of antioxidant enzyme glutathione peroxidase (GSH-Px) and glutathione reductase (GR) activity. GSH-Px and GR levels were lower in type 2 diabetes (T2D) patients with different subtypes of ischemic stroke: atherothrombotic infarction (ATI) and lacunar infarction (LI) compared to T2D patients without ischemic stroke, and the same relationship is found in the respective groups in nondiabetics ($P < 0.001$) (ANOVA test).

4. Discussion

In this study, we directly measured the IS level, together with three different types of antioxidant enzyme activities, GSH-Px, SOD, and GR, in T2D patients and nondiabetic individuals with two different subtypes of ischemic stroke in type 2 diabetics.

Our results have shown decreased IS level in T2D patients with two different subtypes of ischemic stroke, ATI and LI, compared to T2D without stroke, while we could not demonstrate the difference between the subtypes, and the same pattern of IS changes was found in the nondiabetics.

To our knowledge, there are scarce data regarding the changes in IS in T2D with ischemic stroke subtypes.

Previous study also suggested that insulin resistance measured using different methodology, the short insulin tolerance test, is independently associated with markers of atherosclerosis detected on carotid arteries in T2D patients [15]. Simultaneously, an association has been documented between insulin resistance and other markers at the large vessels, such as the pulsatility index on cerebral arteries [16].

On the other hand, it has been shown that insulin resistance, evaluated by the homeostasis model assessment (HOMA) index, was higher in diabetic in contrast to nondiabetic patients with LI being a small vessel disease [17]. Additionally, it has been suggested that diabetes, hypertension, and metabolic syndrome which share insulin resistance as a common mechanism, contribute to LI occurrence [18–20]. However, detailed mechanisms of the possible link between the presence of ischemic stroke subtypes and insulin resistance remain to be clarified.

In addition, when we measured the level of insulinemia in these patients, the significantly higher level of insulinemia was detected in both groups of T2D patients, with ATI and LI. The increases in insulin levels might be primarily consequence of the simultaneous presence of insulin resistance in the relevant groups. However, the increases in insulin might contribute to the appearance of the ischemic stroke subtypes. Insulin, as a growth factor, might interfere with the beneficial effects of nitric oxide (NO) on the vasculature [21]. Moreover, insulin infusion during euglycemic insulin clamp was able to suppress endothelium-dependent vasodilation in large arteries, which is reported to be based on increased availability of endothelin-1, leading to downregulation of NAD(P)H oxidase and superoxide anion production [22], and endothelial dysfunction is proposed to play an important role in the pathogenesis of cerebral small vessel disease [23, 24].

Also, our results demonstrated lower values of antioxidant enzymes in T2D patients with ATI or LI than in type 2 diabetics without ischemic stroke. The patients with ATI and LI did not differ regarding the level of antioxidant enzymes. These findings could be explained by the fact that in diabetes there is already reduced capacity of antioxidant protection, which is further significantly disturbed in the acute phase of ischemic stroke [4, 5].

In our data, in patients with ATI and LI, we found the decreases in glutathione-dependent enzymes activity in contrast to other types of antioxidant enzyme activity, for example, SOD. These results imply a prolonged and severe depression of gluthatione dependent antioxidative defense mechanisms irrespective of stroke subtypes.

Since it has been documented that free radicals are extremely difficult to measure directly, antioxidant enzymes have been proposed to represent indirect markers of oxidative stress [5].

Numerous, but mostly experimental, studies provided evidence of an association between ischemic stroke and decreased antioxidant enzyme activity, although this possible association in humans has been less investigated [9, 25]. Moreover, the analyses of treatment with agents in stroke showing an ability to prevent further depression of antioxidant protection and scavenging reactive free radicals were reported to fail to restore GSH-Px and GR activities [26, 27].

Generally, a recently study that aimed to assess total antioxidant capacity and oxidative stress in diabetic and nondiabetic acute stroke patients with 2 different stroke subtypes, large and small vessel disease strokes, concluded that oxidative stress and counterbalancing antioxidant capacity are more pronounced in diabetic acute stroke patients than in nondiabetics [28].

The study provided different data in comparison to the previous investigations showing decreased GSH-Px activity in both diabetic and nondiabetic patients with coronary heart disease when compared to controls [17, 29, 30].

However, the results from our study have shown the diminished activity of both GSH-Px and GR in T2D patients with ATI and LI, which is consistent with previous reports of decreased GSH-Px levels patients with stroke [6, 8, 31, 32].

The levels of SOD are found to exhibit great variations in the previous study in patients with the stroke [6, 8, 26, 29, 31–37]. Our results could not detect the differences in the SOD levels in different groups of patients, and thus they are in line with data showing no changes in respect to SOD level in both diabetics and nondiabetics irrespective of different subtypes of ischemic stroke [33, 34, 37]. The tentative explanation for the inconsistent findings regarding SOD might reflect the predominant role of intracellular versus extracellular fraction of SOD in free radical scavenging [38].

In our study, the detected antioxidant enzyme activities were not affected by other important factors potentially influencing the enzyme levels, for example, by hyperglycemia, aging, duration of diabetes, and presence of macrovascular complications, due to the fact that in all groups of T2D patients had similar levels of metabolic and satisfactory metabolic control and that patients were matched in respect of age, duration of diabetes, and the prevalence of macrovascular complications.

The multiple regression analysis applied to our data has demonstrated that decreased IS together with the decreases in GR are related to both ATI and LI in T2D patients. In nondiabetics, the decreases in Si levels and the diminished GR are found to be related only to ATI. The analysis reveals the potential difference in the mechanisms underlying the onset of the two subtypes of the stroke in T2D patients compared to nondiabetics. The results imply that higher levels of insulin resistance combined with lower levels of GR, detected in T2D patients compared to nondiabetics, were underlying the onset of LI together ATI in T2D in contrast to the findings in nondiabetics. In this context, our results are consistent with the findings that LI represents the most frequent ischemic stroke subtype in T2D. Taken together, our data imply that insulin resistance exerts its pathogenic influence on the level of gluthatione dependent antioxidant enzymes, especially in T2D.

5. Conclusions

In conclusion, our results suggest that the presence of different subtypes of ischemic stroke is associated with insulin resistance and diminished antioxidant enzyme activity in both subtypes of ischemic stroke in T2D. The results also imply that atherogenic influence of decreased IS in the different subtypes of stroke in T2D might be exerted through a significantly reduced glutathione dependent antioxidant enzyme activity, while the mechanisms relating the effects of insulin resistance and decreased antioxidant enzyme activity remain to be clarified.

Conflict of Interests

The authors have no financial interests or other conflict of interests.

Acknowledgment

This work was funded by projects 175097 from the Ministry of Science, Republic of Serbia.

References

[1] T. Ohira, E. Shahar, L. E. Chambless, W. D. Rosamond, T. H. Mosley, and A. R. Folsom, "Risk factors for ischemic stroke subtypes: the atherosclerosis risk in communities study," *Stroke*, vol. 37, no. 10, pp. 2493–2498, 2006.

[2] K. Matsumoto, S. Miyake, M. Yano et al., "Insulin resistance and classic risk factors in type 2 diabetic patients with different subtypes of ischemic stroke," *Diabetes Care*, vol. 22, no. 7, pp. 1191–1195, 1999.

[3] K. Shinozaki, H. Naritomi, T. Shimizu et al., "Role of insulin resistance associated with compensatory hyperinsulinemia in ischemic stroke," *Stroke*, vol. 27, no. 1, pp. 37–43, 1996.

[4] S. Love, "Oxidative stress in brain ischemia," *Brain Pathology*, vol. 9, no. 1, pp. 119–131, 1999.

[5] H. A. Kontos, "Oxygen radicals in cerebral ischemia: the 2001 Willis lecture," *Stroke*, vol. 32, no. 11, pp. 2712–2716, 2001.

[6] C. Zimmermann, K. Winnefeldb, S. Streckb, M. Roskosb, and R. L. Haberla, "Antioxidant status in acute stroke patients and patients at stroke risk," *European Neurology*, vol. 51, pp. 157–161, 2004.

[7] C. Nodin, C. Zhu, K. Blomgren, M. Nilsson, and F. Blomstrand, "Decreased oxidative stress during glycolytic inhibition enables maintenance of ATP production and astrocytic survival," *Neurochemistry International*, vol. 61, no. 3, pp. 291–301, 2012.

[8] M. A. Haidara, H. Z. Yassin, M. Rateb, H. Ammar, and M. A. Zorkani, "Role of oxidative stress in development of cardiovascular complications in diabetes mellitus," *Current Vascular Pharmacology*, vol. 4, no. 3, pp. 215–227, 2006.

[9] G. W. Kim, T. Kondo, N. Noshita, and P. H. Chan, "Manganese superoxide dismutase deficiency exacerbates cerebral infarction after focal cerebral ischemia/reperfusion in mice: implications for the production and role of superoxide radicals," *Stroke*, vol. 33, no. 3, pp. 809–815, 2002.

[10] World Health Organization, "Definition, diagnosis, and classification: diabetes mellitus: report of a WHO study group," Tech. Rep. series 727, World Health Organization, Geneva, Switzerland, 1985.

[11] "Special report from the National Institute of Neurological Disorders and Stroke. Classification of cerebrovascular diseases III," *Stroke*, vol. 21, no. 4, pp. 637–676, 1990.

[12] "World Health Organization-International Society of Hypertension guidelines for the menagment of hypertesion," *Journal of Hypertension*, vol. 17, article 151, 1999.

[13] G. Pacini and R. N. Bergman, "MINMOD: a computer program to calculate insulin sensitivity and pancreatic responsivity from the frequently sampled intravenous glucose tolerance test," *Computer Methods and Programs in Biomedicine*, vol. 23, no. 2, pp. 113–122, 1986.

[14] E. Colak, N. Majkic-Singh, S. Stankovic et al., "Parameters of antioxidative defense in type 2 diabetic patients with cardiovascular complication," *Annals of Medicine*, vol. 37, pp. 613–620, 2005.

[15] S. W. Park, S. K. Kim, Y.-W. Cho et al., "Insulin resistance and carotid atherosclerosis in patients with type 2 diabetes," *Atherosclerosis*, vol. 205, no. 1, pp. 309–313, 2009.

[16] J. S. Park, M. H. Cho, K. Y. Lee et al., "Cerebral arterial pulsatility and insulin resistance in type 2 diabetic patients," *Diabetes Research and Clinical Practice*, vol. 79, no. 2, pp. 237–242, 2008.

[17] T. Rundek, H. Gardener, Q. Xu et al., "Insulin resistance and risk of ischemic stroke among nondiabetic individuals from the northern Manhattan study," *Archives of Neurology*, vol. 67, no. 10, pp. 1195–1200, 2010.

[18] E. López-Cancio, A. Galán, L. Dorado et al., "Biological signatures of asymptomatic extra- and intracranial atherosclerosis: the Barcelona-AsIA (Asymptomatic Intracranial Atherosclerosis) study," *Stroke*, vol. 43, no. 10, pp. 2712–2719, 2012.

[19] A. Tuttolomondo, A. Pinto, G. Salemi et al., "Diabetic and nondiabetic subjects with ischemic stroke: differences, subtype distribution and outcome," *Nutrition, Metabolism and Cardiovascular Diseases*, vol. 18, no. 2, pp. 152–157, 2008.

[20] C. E. Zhang, E. P. M. Van Raak, R. P. W. Rouhl et al., "Metabolic syndrome relates to lacunar stroke without white matter lesions: a study in first-ever lacunar stroke patients," *Cerebrovascular Diseases*, vol. 29, no. 5, pp. 503–507, 2010.

[21] R. W. Stout, "Insulin and atheroma. 20-Yr perspective," *Diabetes Care*, vol. 13, no. 6, pp. 631–654, 1990.

[22] G. Arcaro, A. Cretti, S. Balzano et al., "Insulin causes endothelial dysfunction in humans: sites and mechanisms," *Circulation*, vol. 105, no. 5, pp. 576–582, 2002.

[23] M. Wada, H. Nagasawa, K. Kurita et al., "Microalbuminuria is a risk factor for cerebral small vessel disease in community-based elderly subjects," *Journal of the Neurological Sciences*, vol. 255, no. 1-2, pp. 27–34, 2007.

[24] F. Anan, T. Masaki, H. Kikuchi et al., "Association between plasma high-sensitivity C-reactive protein and insulin resistance and white matter lesions in Japanese type 2 diabetic patients," *Diabetes Research and Clinical Practice*, vol. 87, no. 2, pp. 233–239, 2010.

[25] J. E. Jung, G. S. Kim, H. Chen et al., "Reperfusion and neurovascular dysfunction in stroke: from basic mechanisms to potential strategies for neuroprotection," *Molecular Neurobiology*, vol. 41, no. 2-3, pp. 172–179, 2010.

[26] E. Candelario-Jalil, A. González-Falcón, M. García-Cabrera et al., "Assessment of the relative contribution of COX-1 and COX-2 isoforms to ischemia-induced oxidative damage and neurodegeneration following transient global cerebral ischemia," *Journal of Neurochemistry*, vol. 86, no. 3, pp. 545–555, 2003.

[27] H. Guo, L.-M. Hu, S.-X. Wang et al., "Neuroprotective effects of scutellarin against hypoxic-ischemic-induced cerebral injury via augmentation of antioxidant defense capacity," *Chinese Journal of Physiology*, vol. 54, no. 6, pp. 399–405, 2011.

[28] B. Guldiken, M. Demir, S. Guldiken, N. Turgut, B. Turgut, and A. Tugrul, "Oxidative stress and total antioxidant capacity in diabetic and nondiabetic acute ischemic stroke patients," *Clinical and Applied Thrombosis/Hemostasis*, vol. 15, no. 6, pp. 695–700, 2009.

[29] A. Ceriello and E. Motz, "Is oxidative stress the pathogenic mechanism underlying insulin resistance, diabetes, and cardiovascular disease? The common soil hypothesis revisited,"

Arteriosclerosis, Thrombosis, and Vascular Biology, vol. 24, no. 5, pp. 816–823, 2004.

[30] N. Uzel, A. Sivas, M. Uysal, and H. Oz, "Erythrocyte lipid peroxidation and glutathione peroxidase activities in patients with diabetes mellitus," *Hormone and Metabolic Research*, vol. 19, no. 2, pp. 89–90, 1987.

[31] S. Demirkaya, M. A. Topcuoglu, A. Aydin, U. H. Ulas, A. I. Isimer, and O. Vural, "Malondialdehyde, glutathione peroxidase and superoxide dismutase in peripheral blood erythrocytes of patients with acute cerebral ischemia," *European Journal of Neurology*, vol. 8, no. 1, pp. 43–51, 2001.

[32] Y. Dinçer, Z. Alademir, H. Ilkova, and T. Akçay, "Susceptibility of glutatione and glutathione-related antioxidant activity to hydrogen peroxide in patients with type 2 diabetes: effect of glycemic control," *Clinical Biochemistry*, vol. 35, no. 4, pp. 297–301, 2002.

[33] M. M. Kesavulu, R. Girl, B. Kameswara Rao, and C. H. Apparao, "Lipid peroxidation and antioxidant enzyme levels in type 2 diabetics with microvascular complications," *Diabetes and Metabolism*, vol. 26, no. 5, pp. 387–392, 2000.

[34] A. Cherubini, M. C. Polidori, M. Bregnocchi et al., "Antioxidant profile and early outcome in stroke patients," *Stroke*, vol. 31, no. 10, pp. 2295–2300, 2000.

[35] F. N. Ahmed, F. N. Naqvi, and F. Shafiq, "Lipid peroxidation and serum antioxidant enzymes in patients with type 2 diabetes mellitus," *Annals of the New York Academy of Sciences*, vol. 1084, pp. 481–489, 2006.

[36] H. Tavilani, N. Sheikh, A. Rezaie, A. Vaisi-Raygani, and S. Salimi, "Relationship between estradiol and antioxidant enzymes activity of ischemic stroke," *Journal of Biomedicine and Biotechnology*, vol. 2009, Article ID 841468, 5 pages, 2009.

[37] I. Seghrouchni, J. Drai, E. Bannier et al., "Oxidative stress parameters in type I, type II and insulin-treated type 2 diabetes mellitus; insulin treatment efficiency," *Clinica Chimica Acta*, vol. 321, no. 1-2, pp. 89–96, 2002.

[38] F. Kimura, G. Hasegawa, H. Obayashi et al., "Serum extracellular superoxide dismutase in patients with type 2 diabetes: relationship to the development of micro- and macrovascular complications," *Diabetes Care*, vol. 26, no. 4, pp. 1246–1250, 2003.

16

Raghib Syndrome Presenting as a Cryptogenic Stroke: Role of Cardiac MRI in Accurate Diagnosis

Vistasp J. Daruwalla,[1] Keyur Parekh,[2] Hassan Tahir,[1] Jeremy D. Collins,[2] and James Carr[2]

[1]*Conemaugh Memorial Hospital/Temple University, USA*
[2]*Department of Cardiovascular Radiology, Northwestern University Feinberg School of Medicine, USA*

Correspondence should be addressed to Vistasp J. Daruwalla; vdaruwal@conemaugh.org

Academic Editor: Gianluca Pontone

Raghib Syndrome is a rare developmental complex, which consists of persistence of the left superior vena cava (PLSVC) along with coronary sinus ostial atresia and atrial septal defect. This Raghib complex anomaly has also been associated with other congenital malformations including ventricular septal defects, enlargement of the tricuspid annulus, and pulmonary stenosis. Our case demonstrates an isolated PLSVC draining into the left atrium along with coronary sinus atresia in a young patient presenting with cryptogenic stroke without the atrial septal defect. Majority of the cases reported in the literature were found to have the lesion during the postmortem evaluation or were characterized at angiography and/or echocardiography. We stress the importance of modern day imaging like the computed tomography (CT) angiography and cardiac MRI in diagnosis and surgical management of such rare lesions leading to cryptogenic strokes.

1. Introduction

Persistence of the left superior vena cava (PLSVC) is seen in 0.3%–0.5% of normal subjects [1, 2] and in up to 2.1%–4.3% of patients with congenital heart disease [3]. Coronary sinus ostial atresia with a PLSVC is usually associated with an anomalous connection between the coronary sinus ostium and the left atrium [4, 5]. Atresia of the coronary sinus ostium without this anomalous communication is rare since first described in 1738 [6]. Raghib syndrome is a rare developmental complex, which consists of PLSVC draining in the left atrium, coronary sinus ostial atresia, and atrial septal defect in the posteroinferior angle of the atrial septum. Okumori et al. stated that the atrial septal defect was true and this specific type of atrial septal defect associated with an absent coronary sinus [7]. Cases of an intact atrial septum and with PLSVC into left atrium were noted [8].

Due to the association with cardiac level right to left shunts, Raghib Syndrome has a significant risk of paradoxical embolization and is associated with varied degrees of reduced arterial blood oxygen saturation. Most of the cases reported in the literature were detected during postmortem evaluation or were characterized at angiography and/or echocardiography. We report a case of isolated PLSVC draining into the left atrium along with coronary sinus atresia in a young patient presenting with cryptogenic stroke evaluated with transthoracic echocardiography, computed tomography (CT), angiography and Cardiac MRI.

2. Case Presentation

The patient is a 31-year-old African-American, left handed female who was recently diagnosed with hypertension. She presented with left handed clumsiness, most notably in her left index finger and thumb, she also complains of an episode of slurred speech and left sided facial numbness that lasted for about 30 minutes to 1 hour. The patient was initially seen in a local hospital nearby and was reported to have an abnormal EKG with T wave inversions in leads v2–v4 and left ventricular hypertrophy but the patient refused admission and was admitted to our institution 10 days later. Her symptoms had improved two days after the attack but she

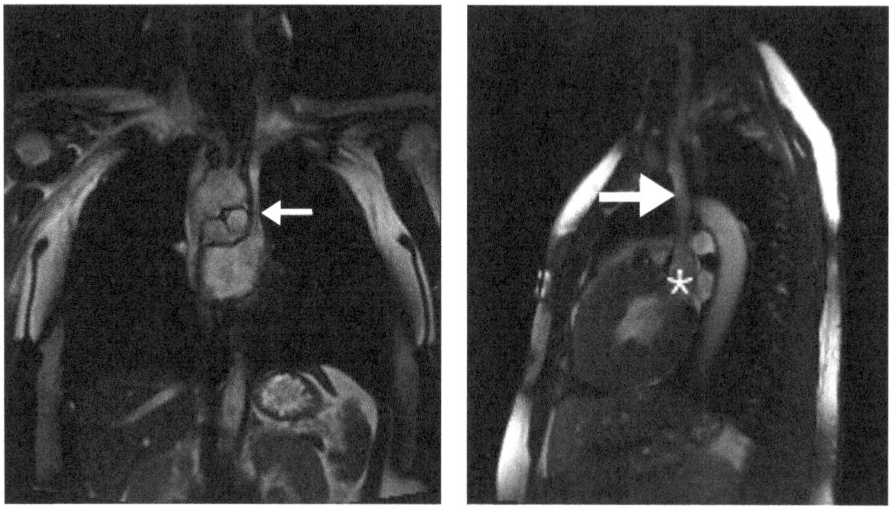

(a) (b)

Figure 1: Coronal and sagittal T2 weighted images show a persistent left superior vena cava (arrow) draining in to the left atrial appendage (star).

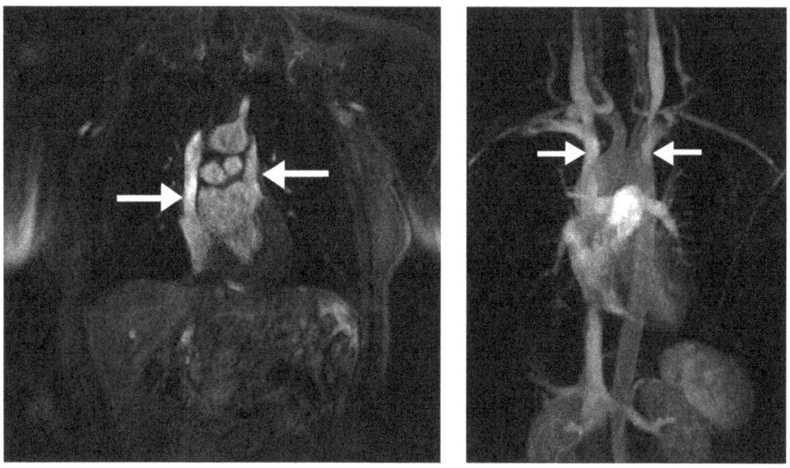

(a) (b)

Figure 2: Static and three-dimensional MR angiography confirms the presence of right and left superior vena cava (arrows) draining in to the corresponding atrial chambers leading to a right-to-left shunt.

still had difficulty with fine motor task like typing. During her stay she maintained a saturation of 95-96%.

Her neurological work-up included an MRI of the brain, which demonstrated a subacute infarct within the right precentral gyrus, involving the region of the hand knob correlating with her left hand weakness (Figure 5).

Transthoracic echocardiography revealed moderate left ventricular hypertrophy without regional wall motion abnormalities. The left atrium was mildly dilated. There was an increased mitral valve E point, ventricular septal separation; the visually estimated ejection fraction was 45–50%. There was no evidence of right to left shunting by agitated saline bubble contrast study performed in the right arm.

Her chest radiography demonstrated abnormal soft tissue densities along the right paratracheal region extending to the right main stem bronchus and along the right cardiomediastinal margin of unclear etiology which was further evaluated with a CT scan. CT imaging demonstrated persistence of the left superior vena cava draining into the left atrium without visualization of a coronary sinus. Cardiac venous drainage is seen directly into the inferior vena cava via the great cardiac vein. Subtle high attenuation contrast extends deep into the interventricular septum. While this may be a myocardial cleft in the same setting of possible left ventricular hypertrophy, the alternate possibility of a sinusoidal VSD is raised as a potential component of Raghib Syndrome. The mass seen in

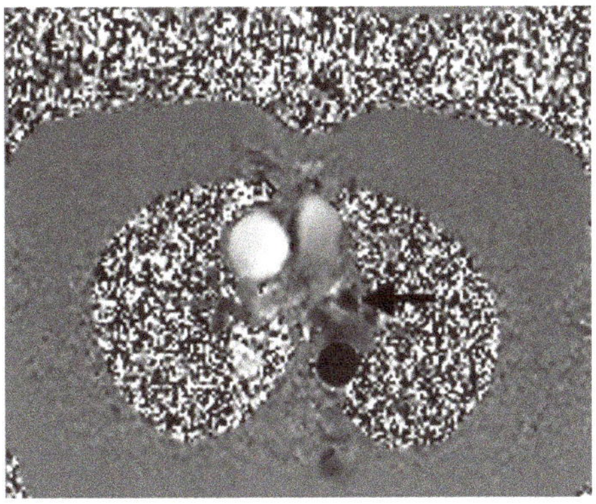

FIGURE 3: Axial 2D phase contrast images in the upper chest show caudally directed flow in the left superior vena cava (arrow).

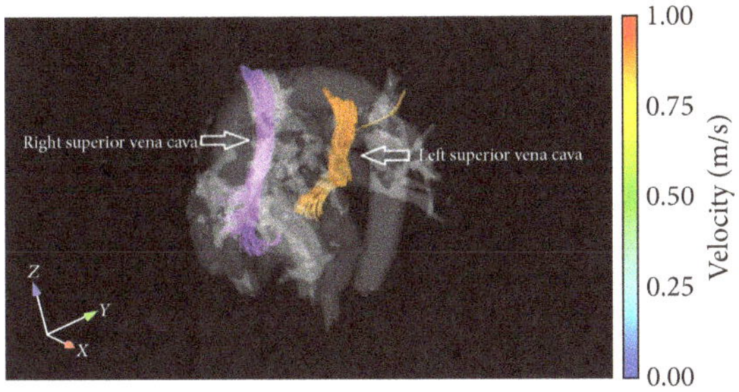

FIGURE 4: Whole heart 4D flow image demonstrating differential flow into the atria. Flow from the right superior vena cava (SVC) to the right atrium and left superior vena cava to the left atrium.

the chest radiograph along the cardiomediastinal margin was correlated to be a 5.4 cm pericardial cyst, and a 1 mm right middle lobe nodule was also noted.

For cryptogenic stroke, the patient underwent upper and lower extremity Doppler ultrasound as well as cardiac MRI. Doppler ultrasound showed no evidence of deep vein thrombosis. Cardiac MR demonstrated concentric hypertrophic cardiomyopathy, with relative sparing of the apical chamber. Left ventricular systolic function was moderately reduced with a calculated ejection fraction of 36%. The persistent left superior vena cava drained into the left atrium resulting in a right to left shunt with a $Qp/Qs = 0.694$ (Figure 1).

The patient's clinical diagnosis was Raghib syndrome with paradoxical embolization causing stroke. Although PLSVC serves as a right to left shunt, our patient during her stay has maintained oxygen saturation of above 90%. The right to left shunt caused by PLSVC is usually small and does not lead to significant oxygen desaturation. Transcatheter treatment is performed in patients with unroofed coronary sinus or an ASD and also seen in a reported case of LSVC which had a bridging with the RSVC by left brachiocephalic vein, such a treatment option was not considered in our patient as she did not have any of the above. She was discharged on aspirin, metoprolol, and a Holter monitor was placed prior to discharge. She will continue to follow up with the hospital for further evaluation 6 months later with a cardiac MRI.

3. Discussion

Raghib Syndrome is a rare cardiac anomaly that was originally described by Raghib et al. in 1965 as a developmental complex consisting of termination of the left superior vena cava in the left atrium, absence of the coronary sinus, and an atrial septal defect commonly located at the posterior-inferior angle of the atrial septum [9]. This complex was considered unique to Raghib Syndrome; however, cases with a normal atrial septum have been reported where the orifice of the unroofed coronary sinus functions as the interatrial communication [10].Our patient demonstrated an isolated persistent left superior vena cava draining into the left atrium along with an absence of the coronary sinus (Figure 6) and absence of ASD (Figure 7). She also has hypertrophic cardiomyopathy leading to ventricular dysfunction; association of this condition with Raghib syndrome has not been reported before.

Embryologically, persistence of the left superior vena cava (PLSVC) occurs due to failure of involution of the left horn of the embryonic sinus venosus and is one the most common venous anomalies of the chest. Drainage of the PLSVC into the left atrium due to congenital defects which prevent the rotation of the sinoatrial region; this in turn causes the left and the right cardinal veins to lie at the same level rather than the usual inferior location of the right cardinal vein, thus blocking the development of the coronary sinus. As a result a PLSVC draining into left atrium is commonly associated with coronary sinus ostial atresia [7]. LSVC may serve as a collateral channel secondary to coronary sinus atresia. This anatomic configuration is vital to recognize at open heart surgery so that the cardiac venous return can be identified and preserved. Retrograde administration of cardioplegia is also relatively contraindicated. The coronary sinus catheter balloon may not be able to occlude the dilated coronary sinus, resulting in failure to ensure retrograde flow of cardioplegia to the myocardium. Also, cardioplegia delivered would largely be distributed to the left internal jugular and left subclavian veins, rather than myocardium [11, 12]. Careful mapping of the coronary venous anatomy and dissection of the coronary sinus are necessary before reanastomoses of the PLSVC into the right atrium is attempted [11].

Precise anatomical detailing and multiresolution image building capacity of cardiac CT scan is of high yield in such cases especially in the plane of the atrioventricular groove in a short axis view. The shunt between the left atrium and the coronary sinus can be easily detected on a cardiac CT scan by insertion of contrast in the left arm vein and noting its presence in the left atrium [13]. MRI on the other hand with its phase contrast cine images may demonstrate turbulent flow from left atrium to coronary sinus, thus providing a distinctive advantage in detecting left to right shunt and estimating the ratio of pulmonary to systemic flow (Figure 3). The 3D images of cardiac CT scan and MRI not only facilitate in diagnosing the anomaly but also play an important role in planning surgical interventions like closure of PLSVC with coils or coronary sinus stent placement (Figure 2) [14, 15]. A novel cardiac MRI 4D flow technique, still under research phase, displays differential flow into the atria (Figure 4).

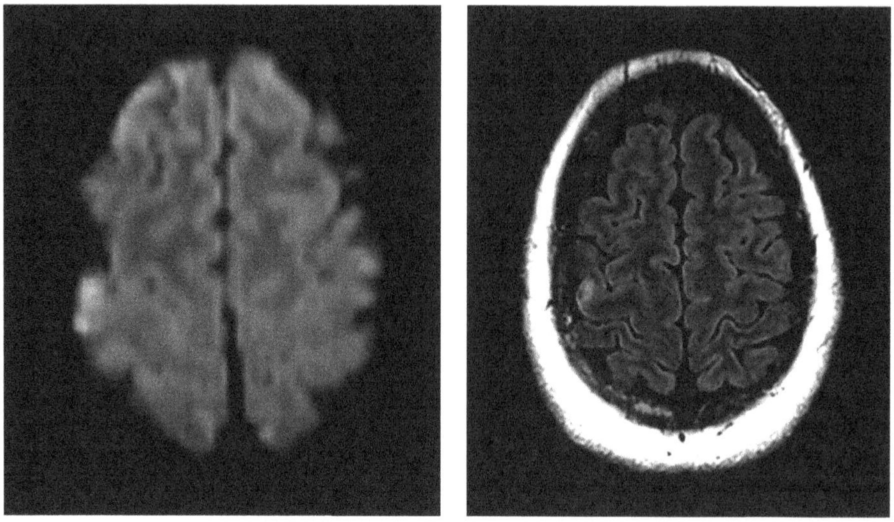

(a) (b)

FIGURE 5: Restricted diffusion on DWI with increase T2 signal on FLAIR and postcontrast enhancement in right frontal lobe is consistent with subacute infarct within the right precentral gyrus.

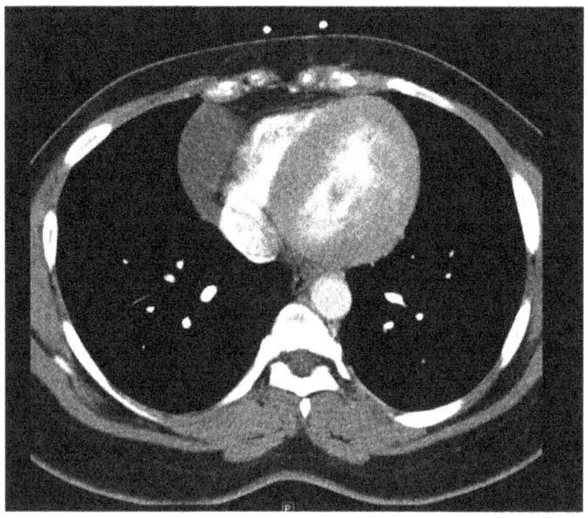

FIGURE 6: Coronary sinus atresia: absence of coronary sinus at the expected location on axial contrast CT chest image.

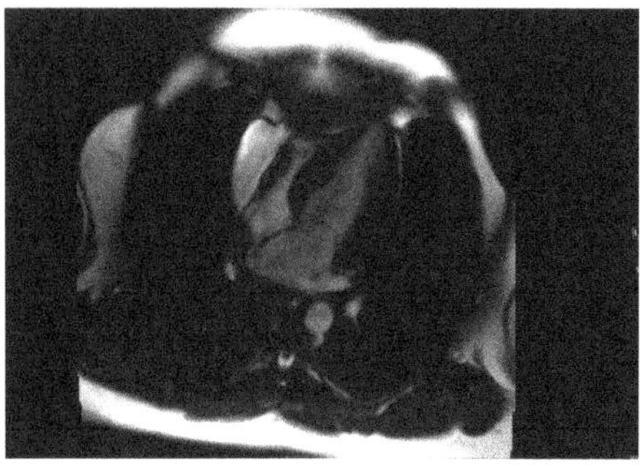

FIGURE 7: Four chamber steady-state free precession imaging shows intact interatrial septum. No ASD noted.

Overall cardiac Ct scan and MRI provide an unparalleled edge in visualization of such rare developmental anomalies and assist in prevention of paradoxical cerebral embolization and abscess formation [16].

4. Conclusion

Raghib Syndrome is considered to be a benign anomaly yet is associated with paradoxical embolization, diminished arterial oxygen saturation, and has implications for cardiac surgery as well as considerations for the location of intravenous access. Cardiac MRI and cardiac CT are useful imaging modalities in the evaluation of anomalies of the systemic venous return, enabling quantification of the flow disturbance and characterization of the anatomy.

Conflict of Interests

The authors declare that there is no conflict of interests regarding the publication of this paper.

References

[1] M. Biffi, G. Boriani, L. Frabetti, G. Bronzetti, and A. Branzi, "Left superior vena cava persistence in patients undergoing pacemaker or cardioverter-defibrillator implantation: a 10-year experience," *Chest*, vol. 120, no. 1, pp. 139–144, 2001.

[2] J. K. Perloff, "Congenital anomalies of vena caval connection," in *The Clinical Recognition of Congenital Heart Disease*, pp. 703–714, WB Saunders, Philadelphia, Pa, USA, 4th edition, 1994.

[3] J. C. Horrow and N. Lingaraju, "Unexpected persistent left superior vena cava: diagnostic clues during monitoring," *Journal of Cardiothoracic Anesthesia*, vol. 3, no. 5, pp. 611–615, 1989.

[4] E. Mantini, C. M. Grondin, C. W. Lillehei, and J. E. Edwards, "Congenital anomalies involving the coronary sinus," *Circulation*, vol. 33, no. 2, pp. 317–327, 1966.

[5] M. R. de Leval, D. G. Ritter, D. C. McGoon, and G. K. Danielson, "Anomalous systemic venous connection: surgical

considerations," *Mayo Clinic Proceedings*, vol. 50, no. 10, pp. 599–610, 1975.

[6] Le Cat, *Histoire de l'Acad Royale des Sciences*, Le Cat, Paris, France, 1738.

[7] M. Okumori, M. Hyuga, S. Ogata, T. Akamatsu, S. Otomi, and S. Ota, "Raghib's syndrome: a report of two cases," *Japanese Journal of Surgery*, vol. 12, no. 5, pp. 356–361, 1982.

[8] D. A. Goor and C. W. Lillehei, *Congenital Malformations of the Heart: Embryology, Anatomy, and Operative Considerations*, Grune & Stratton, New York, NY, USA, 1975.

[9] G. Raghib, H. D. Ruttenberg, R. C. Anderson, K. Amplatz, P. Adams, and J. E. Edwards, "Termination of left superior vena cava in left atrium, atrial septal defect, and absence of coronary sinus," *Circulation*, vol. 31, pp. 906–918, 1965.

[10] H. D. Allen, D. J. Driscoll, R. E. Shaddy, and T. F. Feltes, *Moss and Adam's Heart Disease in Infants, Children and Adolescent*, Lippincott Williams & Wilkins, 2012.

[11] E. N. Nsah, G. W. Moore, and G. M. Hutchins, "Pathogenesis of persistent left superior vena cava with a coronary sinus connection," *Pediatric Pathology*, vol. 11, no. 2, pp. 261–269, 1991.

[12] J. Paval and S. Nayak, "A persistent left superior vena cava," *Singapore Medical Journal*, vol. 48, no. 3, pp. e90–e93, 2007.

[13] G. Brancaccio, F. Miraldi, F. Ventriglia, G. Michielon, R. M. di Donato, and M. de Santis, "Multidetector-row helical computed tomography imaging of unroofed coronary sinus," *International Journal of Cardiology*, vol. 91, no. 2-3, pp. 251–253, 2003.

[14] J. K. Hahm, Y. W. Park, J. K. Lee et al., "Magnetic resonance imaging of unroofed coronary sinus: three cases," *Pediatric Cardiology*, vol. 21, no. 4, pp. 382–387, 2000.

[15] Y. H. Choe, I.-S. Kang, S. W. Park, and H. J. Lee, "MR imaging of congenital heart disease in adolescents and adults," *Korean Journal of Radiology*, vol. 2, no. 3, pp. 121–131, 2001.

[16] E. M. Kim, P. B. Moore, S. P. Singh, and S. G. Lloyd, "Cardiovascular magnetic resonance imaging of the Raghib complex," *Journal of the American College of Cardiology*, vol. 57, no. 8, article e15, 2011.

17

Coexistence of Neurofibromatosis Type-1and MTHFR C677T Gene Mutation in a Young Stroke Patient: A Case Report

Halim Yilmaz,[1] Gulten Erkin,[1] Haluk Gumus,[2] and Lutfiye Nalbant[1]

[1] *The Department of Physical Medicine and Rehabilitation, Konya Education and Research Hospital, 42040 Konya, Turkey*
[2] *The Department of Neurology, Konya Education and Research Hospital, 42040 Konya, Turkey*

Correspondence should be addressed to Halim Yilmaz; drhalimyilmaz@hotmail.com

Academic Editors: Y. Iwasaki, R. Koide, and K. Wessel

In neurofibromatosis type-1 (NF1), cerebrovascular disorders are rarely encountered although vasculopathy is a well-known complication. Several mutations seen in methylenetetrahydrofolate reductase (MTHFR) give rise to the formation of hyperhomocysteinemia and homocystinuria, a considerable risk factor for cardiovascular and cerebrovascular disorders, by leading to enzymatic inactivation. In the paper, a 31-year-old young stroke female patient with the coexistence of neurofibromatosis and MTHFR C677T gene mutation was presented.

1. Introduction

The term "stroke" describes findings of focal neurologic syndromes with sudden onset, developing due to vascular events. Strokes experienced under 45 are called young stroke and go definitely undetected in about half of the cases despite large number of investigations [1, 2]. In spite of the course with "café-au-lait" spots and neurofibromas, NF1 may also influence many organs. Although vasculopathy is a known complication in NF1, cerebrovascular disorders are rarely encountered [3, 4]. Seen in MTHFR gene, various mutations cause the formation of hyperhomocysteinemia and homocystinuria, a significant risk factor for cardiovascular and cerebrovascular disorders, by leading to inactivation of enzymes [5]. We reported a 31-year-old woman with young stroke from the coexistence of neurofibromatosis and MTHFR C677T gene mutation.

2. Case Report

The 31-year-old and 8-year married case was a housewife with a child. In the case applying to a clinic with the complaint of headache nearly 3 months earlier, stroke developed on the same day. No history of systemic disorders such as hypertension, diabetes mellitus and cardiovascular events, drug intake, cigarette smoking and use of alcoholic drinks, spontaneous abortion, and stillbirth was present. Patient's father was determined to have experienced a cerebrovascular event when he was 48. Applying to our clinic with the disability complaints of gait and use of right upper extremity, the patient was admitted with the diagnosis of young stroke. As a result of general and palpable examination on admission, Lisch nodules on both eyes and numerous "café-au-lait" spots and palpable cutaneous neurofibromas which could be seen with naked eyes in lumbar and thoracic regions (Figure 3) were detected. The diagnosis of neurofibromatosis was histopathologically confirmed with biopsy performed with neurofibromas. On neurologic examination, right central facial paralysis, right hemihypoesthesia, and pyramidal findings on right lower and upper extremities were detected. Cranial neurologic examination, except for facial nerves, was within normal limits. Brunstrom's scale was stage II for the right upper extremity, III for the right hand, and V for the right lower extremity. The patient was ambulated for short-distance assisted walking and dependent on routine activities such as feeding, dressing, and gait (functional independence scale score (FIM) = 84). In laboratory tests, whole blood count, lipid levels, electrolytes, tests for liver and kidney functions, coagulation screen, and blood glucose level were within normal limits. Electrocardiography displayed sinus

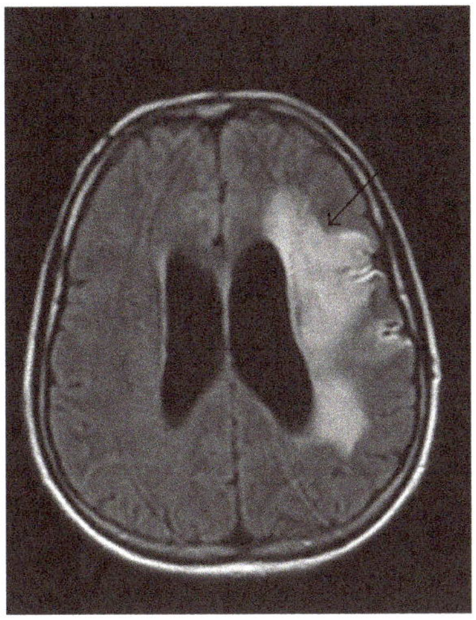

Figure 1: Infarct region compatible with large-size MCA infarct in left frontotemporoparietal lobes on cerebral MRI.

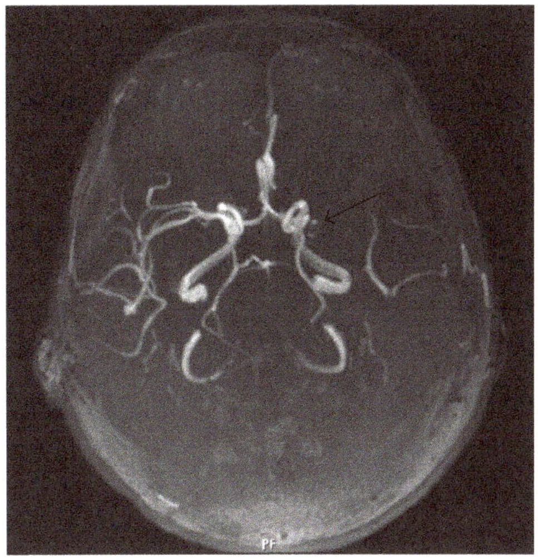

Figure 2: Occlusion from origin of left middle cerebral artery on MRI angiography.

rhythm, and echocardiography and chest X-ray showed no abnormality. In cerebral magnetic resonance imaging (MRI), an infarct region consistent with large-size middle cerebral artery (MCA) infarct extending cortical-subcortical white-matter in left frontotemporoparietal lobes (Figure 1) and, in MRI angiography, an occluded spectrum from the level of left middle cerebral artery origin (Figure 2) were determined. Cranial venous MRI angiography was within normal limits, and scanning showed no abnormality as to vascular occlusive disease. In investigations performed for thrombophilia, heterozygote MTHFR C677T mutation was determined. Homocystein, protein-S, protein-C, antithrombin-III, lipoprotein-a, and factor-5 were within normal limits. Due to the existence of Lisch nodules, "café-au-lait" spots, and cutaneous neurofibromas (Figure 3), NF1 was considered, and with the help of biopsy from cutaneous neurofibromas, the diagnosis of NF1 was supported. Upon investigating the association between NF1 and young stroke cases, a part of patients with NF1 were found to be accompanied by pheochromocytoma, considering that pheochromocytoma may lead to young stroke due to paroxysmal hypertension. Levels of metanephrine and normetanephrine measured in 24 h urine because of pheochromocytoma showed no abnormal results.

As a result, NF1 and heterozygote MTHFR gene mutation were diagnosed in our case with young stroke, and aspirin (300 mg/day) and clopidogrel (75 mg/day) were administered. Due to stroke, the case was started to be rehabilitated in a program (neurophysiologic exercises, neuromuscular electrical stimulation, and gait training). With 4-week intensive rehabilitation program, the case commenced to walk without assistance, and FIM score was 96.

3. Discussion

NF1 is an autosomal, dominantly inherited syndrome and encountered about one out of 3000 individuals. NF1 gene is present on chromosome 17 and provides the synthesis of a protein called neurofibromin, functioning as a tumor suppressor [6]. When a mutation is formed in gene on chromosome 17, optic glioma, tumor formations like neurofibromas, pigmented lesions, and typical skeletal lesions may be observed [7]. With the existence of two and more of the criteria by the National Institution of Health, NF1 cases are diagnosed [6, 8]. The case was diagnosed with NF1 due to the determination of numerous neurofibromas and about 20 "café-au-lait" spots in size of 0.5 cm and over in lumbar and thoracic regions and Lisch nodules in both eyes.

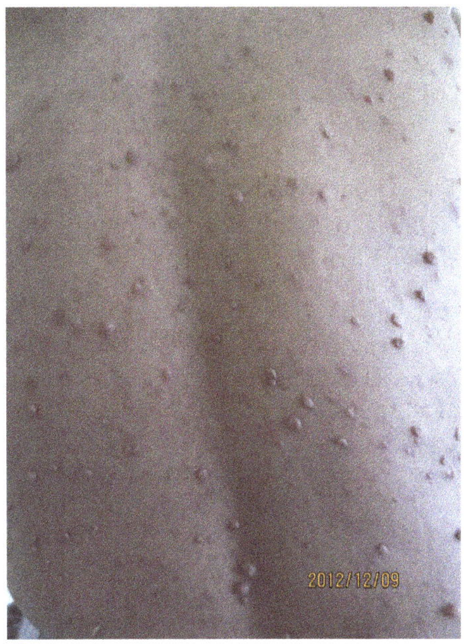

Figure 3: Common neurofibromas and "café-au-lait" spots on thoracolumbar region.

The cause of stroke in young adults is different from that in the elderly. Cerebral vascular abnormalities similar to vascular ectasia were reported to be one of the main reasons of young stroke [9]. The prevalence of cerebrovascular dysplasia is 2–5% in patients NF1 [10]. Most of such disorders are composed of occlusion or stenosis in intracranial arteries, aneurysm at a lesser degree, arteriovenous malformations, and moya-moya disease. Our case was also demonstrated to experience left middle cerebral arterial occlusion through MRI. Due to such vascular disorders, cerebral ischemia, hemorrhage and increase of intracranial pressure could be encountered [11], and the mechanism of vascular abnormalities in NF1 still remains unclear. Occurring due to phenotypical expression of NF1 gene, protein of defective neurofibromin is believed to be responsible for the formation of abnormal vascular smooth muscles. The condition results in vascular ectatic alterations and aneurysmal stenosis in blood vessels [12]. Cases related to vascular abnormalities due to NF1 leading to stroke in young adults are present in literature. In a study, Krishnaswami and Vahidassr reported a 43-year-old young stroke patient with pontine infarct due to vascular ectasia associated with NF1 [2]. In another study, a young woman with stroke accompanied by NF1 was reported by Tang et al. [4].

The association between stroke and MTHFR is a known condition. MTHFR plays a key role in the cycle of pholate and contributes to the metabolism of homocystein amino acid [13]. Such clinical features as peripheral neuropathy, growth retardation, hypotonia, stroke, and thrombosis are encountered in severe deficiency of MTHFR where hyperhomocysteinemia and homocystinuria develop [14, 15]. Conditions where MTHFR deficiency is mild are frequently encountered in general population, and the deficiency is suggested to be a risk factor, especially in the development of arterial disorders [14]. It was notably emphasized in a study that an association is present between two common polymorphisms of MTHFR gene (MTHFR C677T and A1298C), and cerebrovascular disorders and venous thrombosis [13]. Also, in a study performed by Morita et al. with 256 stroke patients and 325 controls, a strong association was suggested to be present between MTHFR C677TT genotype and stroke [16]. In our report, left middle cerebral arterial occlusion and mutation of heterozygote MTHFR C677T gene accompanied by NF1 were reported to lead to stroke in a 31-year-old woman patient. Because of giving rise to stroke in young adults, vascular abnormalities stemming from NF1 should meticulously be taken into account in such patients.

Our case may be the first in literature to determine the coexistence of NF1, the cause of young stroke, and accompanying cerebral artery occlusion and mutation of heterozygote MTHFR C677T gene. Therefore, although the association between stroke and NF1 is rarely encountered in daily practice in young patients applying to clinics with the complaint of stroke, diagnosis of NF1 should be taken into account, and the existence of NF1 should be investigated via a careful dermatologic examination. In addition, in young patients with the complaint of stroke, MTHFR C677T gene mutation should be considered as etiologic reason, and the mutation should be kept in mind to be accompanied by NF1. Young patients diagnosed with NF1 may be suggested to be closely followed up as to neurologic symptoms and complications, and stroke risks in future should be evaluated via cerebral vascular imaging in such patients.

References

[1] U. Utku, "Stroke: definition, etiology, classification and risk factors," *Turkish Journal of Physical Medicine and Rehabilitation*, vol. 53, no. 1, pp. 1–3, 2007.

[2] V. Krishnaswami and D. Vahidassr, "Young stroke due to vascular anomaly from neurofibromatosis type 1," *British Medical Journal Case Reports*, 2012.

[3] E. J. Piovesan, R. H. Scola, L. C. Werneck et al., "Neurofibromatosis, stroke and basilar impression: case report," *Arquivos de Neuro-Psiquiatria*, vol. 57, no. 2 B, pp. 484–488, 1999.

[4] S. C. Tang, M. J. Lee, J. S. Jeng, and P. K. Yip, "Novel mutation of neurofibromatosis type 1 in a patient with cerebral vasculopathy and fatal ischemic stroke," *Journal of the Neurological Sciences*, vol. 243, no. 1-2, pp. 53–55, 2006.

[5] L. L. Stern, P. J. Bagley, I. H. Rosenberg, and J. Selhub, "Conversion of 5-formyltetrahydrofolic acid to 5-methyltetrahydrofolic acid is unimpaired in folate-adequate persons homozygous for the C677T mutation in the methylenetetrahydrofolate reductase gene," *Journal of Nutrition*, vol. 130, no. 9, pp. 2238–2242, 2000.

[6] J. I. Harper, "Familial multiple tumour syndrome," in *Textbook of Dermatology*, R. H. Champion, J. L. Burton, D. A. Burns, and S. M. Breathnach, Eds., pp. 378–384, Blackwell Science, Oxford, UK, 6th edition, 1998.

[7] S. Van Es, K. N. North, K. McHugh, and M. De Silva, "MRI findings in children with neurofibromatosis type 1: a prospective study," *Pediatric Radiology*, vol. 26, no. 7, pp. 478–487, 1996.

[8] D. H. Gutmann, "Recent insights into neurofibromatosis type 1: clear genetic progress," *Archives of Neurology*, vol. 55, no. 6, pp. 778–780, 1998.

[9] P. J. Martin, T. P. Enevoldson, and P. R. Humphrey, "Causes of ischaemic stroke in the young," *Postgraduate Medical Journal*, vol. 73, no. 855, pp. 8–16, 1997.

[10] A. G. Cairns and K. N. North, "Cerebrovascular dysplasia in neurofibromatosis type 1," *Journal of Neurology, Neurosurgery and Psychiatry*, vol. 79, no. 10, pp. 1165–1170, 2008.

[11] D. Ilhan, S. Dağli, B. Adapinar, and D. Özbabalik, "Cerebral intratumoral haemorrhage haemorrhage associated with neurofibromatosis type 1 case report," *Journal of Neurological Sciences*, vol. 26, no. 2, pp. 237–241, 2009 (Turkish).

[12] D. Rea, J. F. Brandsema, D. Armstrong et al., "Cerebral arteriopathy in children with neurofibromatosis type 1," *Pediatrics*, vol. 124, no. 3, pp. e476–e483, 2009.

[13] M. Dikmen, "Metilentetrahidrofolat Redüktaz (MTHFR) Enziminin Moleküler Biyolojisi ve Hastalıklarla İlişkisi. Molecular Biology of Methylenetetrahydrofolate Reductase (MTHFR) Enzyme and Its Association with Diseases. Kocatepe Tıp Dergisi," *The Medical Journal of Kocatepe*, vol. 5, pp. 9–16, 2004.

[14] P. Goyette, A. Pai, R. Milos et al., "Gene structure of human and mouse methylenetetrahydrofolate reductase (MTHFR)," *Mammalian Genome*, vol. 9, no. 8, pp. 652–656, 1998.

[15] P. L. Rady, S. K. Tyring, S. D. Hudnall et al., "Methylenetetrahydrofolate reductase (MTHFR): the incidence of mutations C677T and A1298C in the Ashkenazi Jewish population," *American Journal of Medical Genetics*, vol. 86, no. 4, pp. 380–384, 1999.

[16] H. Morita, H. Kurihara, S. I. Tsubaki et al., "Methylenetetrahydrofolate reductase gene polymorphism and ischemic stroke in Japanese," *Arteriosclerosis, Thrombosis, and Vascular Biology*, vol. 18, no. 9, pp. 1465–1469, 1998.

18

Recovery of Dysphagia in Lateral Medullary Stroke

Hitesh Gupta and Alakananda Banerjee

Max Healthcare, Saket, New Delhi 110017, India

Correspondence should be addressed to Hitesh Gupta; hitesh_gg01@yahoo.com

Academic Editor: Massimiliano Filosto

Lateral medullary stroke is typically associated with increased likelihood of occurrence of dysphagia and exhibits the most severe and persistent form. Worldwide little research exists on dysphagia in brainstem stroke. An estimated 15% of all patients admitted to stroke rehabilitation units experience a brainstem stroke out of which about 47% suffer from dysphagia. In India, a study showed that 22.3% of posterior circulation stroke patients develop dysphagia. Dearth of literature on dysphagia and its outcome in brainstem stroke particularly lateral medullary stroke motivated the author to present an actual case study of a patient who had dysphagia following a lateral medullary infarct. This paper documents the severity and management approach of dysphagia in brainstem stroke, with traditional dysphagia therapy and VitalStim therapy. Despite being diagnosed with a severe form of dysphagia followed by late treatment intervention, the patient had complete recovery of the swallowing function.

1. Introduction

Swallowing mechanism is a sequential event of oral, pharyngeal, and esophageal phases that transports saliva, ingested solids, and fluid from mouth to the stomach and protects the airways during swallowing. Pharyngeal function involves numerous interacting control mechanisms that ultimately link pharyngeal contraction patterns to the adjacent oral cavity and esophagus.

Dysphagia (difficulty in eating and swallowing) is extremely common following a brainstem stroke. About 15% of all patients admitted to stroke rehabilitation units experience a brainstem stroke out of which about 40%–47% of the patients suffer from dysphagia [1]. Dysphagia following brainstem stroke is characteristically associated with a greater likelihood of occurrence, showing signs of most severe form of dysphagia, compared to hemispheric strokes [2]. Worldwide little research exists on dysphagia in brainstem stroke.

Dysphagia has been associated with respiratory complications, increased risk of aspiration pneumonia, nutritional compromise, and dehydration. It is also socially penalizing and affects the patient's quality of life.

A brainstem stroke affects the swallowing function as the major swallowing centers of the nucleus tractus solitarius (NTS), nucleus ambiguus (NA), and the reticular formation are situated in the dorsolateral medulla oblongata [3]. As a result, dysphagia following a lateral medullary stroke (LMS) is often more severe and spontaneous recovery may not completely restore the swallowing function. It may persist for life time or may take months or years to resolve [2]. Factors, such as lesion size and actual stroke location, as detected and correlated with brainstem MRI, can play a significant role in determining dysphagia morbidity. However, MRI results can demonstrate only the area of the infarct and not the swallowing-related structures and, therefore, cannot clarify the variation of swallowing disorders among patients with LMS [3].

Treatment for dysphagia involves traditional therapy [4, 5] (diet modification, exercises to strengthen the oropharyngeal musculature, compensatory maneuvers to facilitate laryngeal elevation and closure during swallowing, and techniques to stimulate and strengthen the swallowing reflex) and advanced VitalStim therapy.

VitalStim therapy is a special form of neuromuscular electrical stimulation (NMES) device, which has received FDA clearance to be used for treatment of pharyngeal dysphagia. It can only be administered under the direction of certified healthcare professionals (speech language pathologists and occupational therapists) [6]. On direct electrical stimulation, contraction of swallowing muscles occurs, which is due to the depolarization of peripheral motor nerve after acetylcholine is released at the end plates.

VitalStim is a dual-channel electrotherapy system, which uses small calibrated electrical current delivered by specially designed electrodes to stimulate the muscles responsible for swallowing. At the same time, trained specialists help patients "reeducate" their muscles through rehabilitation therapy.

Electrodes are simultaneously activated over the submental and laryngeal regions on the throat with the aim of producing a simultaneous contraction of the mylohyoid muscle in the submental region (to elevate the hyoid bone) and the thyrohyoid muscle in the neck (to elevate larynx to the hyoid bone). In VitalStim therapy, electrode placement varies if there is

(i) insufficient length of the neck;
(ii) fresh surgical incision (no direct placement);
(iii) presence of indwelling foreign materials like tracheostomy, staples, sutures, and so forth (avoid placement over them).

VitalStim therapy is contraindicated if patient is not conscious, uncooperative, has behavioral issues, or has any implants like pacemaker and so forth [6].

VitalStim therapy has been used to reeducate patients to utilize their pharyngeal muscles in the throat for patterned activity to commence or reestablish swallowing [4]. It has been theorized that this small electrical stimulation may aid swallowing either by augmenting hyolaryngeal elevation or by escalating sensory input into the central nervous system. The current stimulates motor nerves in the throat instigating the muscles responsible for swallowing to contract. The quality of the swallowing function improves and with repetition muscles may be reeducated. This case study aims to document the severity and the advanced technological management of dysphagia in lateral medullary infarct.

2. Case Study

The patient, a 29-year-old male, came to the Department of Physiotherapy and Rehabilitation, Max Super Speciality Hospital, Saket, New Delhi, with the complaint of inability to swallow. He had to spit out saliva frequently as he was unable to swallow it. The patient had a history of right medullary stroke (infarction) 1 year back. He was treated in a local hospital in Punjab. During the course of his hospitalization, he acquired severe pneumonia due to aspiration while he was feeding orally. Therefore, a nasogastric tube (NGT) was placed for nutritional support. The length of stay in the hospital was two months where all of his functions recovered except swallowing. The patient was discharged with the NGT. He was sent to a neurologist for examination. Clinical dysphagia evaluation [5] was done by a dysphagia therapist, which included a detailed history of the subjective complaints and medical status, cranial nerve testing, and an examination of the phases of swallowing. Cervical auscultation and respiratory status examination were also done [7]. Food trial was not done as the patient could not swallow. It was observed that the patient could not swallow his saliva.

The dysphagia assessment revealed that the patient had good oral motor functions and was able to chew and propel bolus from the mouth but was unable to swallow. The impairment was found in the pharyngeal phase. No hyolaryngeal movement was elicited in an attempt to swallow voluntarily or on stimulating swallowing reflex indicating a complete loss of pharyngeal swallowing phase. This can be explained as follows: when mediated by the swallowing center in the medulla, as any stimulus reaches the pharynx, it causes the food to be pushed further back into pharynx and esophagus by rhythmic but involuntary contractions of several muscles in the back of the mouth, pharynx, and esophagus. Laryngeal elevation is essential for airway protection during the pharyngeal phase of swallowing. It aids opposition of the arytenoids to the base of epiglottis for laryngeal vestibule closure and helps shape the aryepiglottic sinuses to divert the bolus laterally around the vestibule. Anterior movement of the hyoid in conjunction with laryngeal elevation helps to pull open the flexed upper esophageal sphincter so that food or liquid may be propelled through it and into the esophagus [6].

During phonation, soft palate movement was reduced, but protective reflexes like gag, cough, and the ability to clear throat were good. Among the lower cranial nerves, glossopharyngeal (IX nerve) and vagus (X nerve) nerves were found to be relatively more impaired. Disuse atrophy made his chance of recovery even worse as it is believed that, after 72 hours of stroke, disuse atrophy starts if any particular muscle does not work [8–10]. In this case his pharyngeal muscles were not in use for more than a year.

American Speech-Language-Hearing Association (ASHA) National Outcome Measurement System (NOMS) swallowing level scale was used as a parameter for evaluating the swallowing function on which the patient was rated level 1. The ASHA level is a measurement of both the level of supervision required and the diet level that intuitively reflects a patient's functional status [11]. A FEES (fibreoptic endoscopy evaluation of swallowing) was not done.

3. Course of Treatment Planning and Recovery

After detailed assessment and counseling of the patient, a treatment program of traditional therapy combined with VitalStim therapy was planned in the outpatient department of physiotherapy and rehabilitation to be followed five days a week. Studies have shown the effectiveness of combined traditional therapy and VitalStim therapy in stroke patients [6, 12]. The treatment was started and, for convenience, the management was divided into two phases.

4. Phase One

The initial goal was to elicit swallowing reflex to initiate hyolaryngeal movement. Documented laryngeal elevation in normal adults is approximately 0–2.50 cm or 20 mm [13, 14]. Therapy commenced after familiarizing the patient with the treatment protocol and VitalStim device.

The sensory threshold of the patient was identified as the lowest current level at which he reported a "tingling sensation" on the skin. Following this, the current intensity was raised to the level reported as "grabbing sensation" by the patient, which in our case ranged between 12 and 14 mA.

Each VitalStim therapy session lasted for 60 minutes and five sessions were taken per week. In conjunction with VitalStim therapy, traditional therapy was provided which involved sensory stimulatory activities to elicit swallowing reflex with the use of lemon drops, salt, honey, and ice under the supervision of the dysphagia therapist. Sensory input from the gut has a major influence on the activity of brainstem swallowing centers and cortical sensory and motor areas [15].

A flicker in the hyolaryngeal excursion on stimulating swallowing reflex was noticed on clinical palpations after completion of 34 sessions of VitalStim therapy. Subjectively the patient was sensitive to voluntary swallowing attempts, though after every attempt, it was seen that there were clinical laryngeal penetration signs like coughing and wet and gurgling voice which required throat clearing followed by spitting of saliva. Pharyngeal strengthening exercises like Shaker exercise, Mendelssohn's maneuver, effortful swallow, and Masako exercise were also incorporated [5, 16].

5. Phase Two

After 12 weeks, approximately more than 50% of hyolaryngeal excursion, not functional (MMT) [14], was observed on clinical palpation. Food trials were introduced along with VitalStim therapy. Among the eight types of consistencies of food groups [5], initially group 4 (pudding thick consistency) foods like ice cream, curd, and jelly were given as they have minimal risk of aspiration. Patients with neurogenic dysphagia experience more difficulty with fluids than with thicker or solid consistencies [17].

The patient experienced weakness of pharyngeal peristalsis while swallowing, resulting in food residue in the pharyngeal pockets followed by throat clearing and coughing. The patient had coughs during food trials but was gradually able to swallow the food bolus partially along with the saliva by attempting to swallow repeatedly after throat clearing instead of spitting out. The quantity and frequency of spitting reduced significantly. Chewable food was introduced to reinforce the physiological oropharyngeal coordination of swallowing. The patient was advised a home regime of pharyngeal exercises and practice of swallowing with recommended safe consistencies of food, like groups 4 (pudding thick) and 5 (mechanical soft chewable), three to four times a day.

After 17 weeks and 76 sessions of VitalStim therapy, hyolaryngeal excursion became approximately 80%, which was functionally weak (MMT) [14], and the patient was able to swallow foods of groups 3 (honey thick liquids), 4 (pudding thick), 5 (mechanical soft chewable), and 6 (chewy food) slowly and comfortably without any signs of laryngeal penetration. On completion of 79 sessions of treatment in a period of 18 weeks, the patient attained fully functional (MMT) [14] hyolaryngeal excursion and started swallowing foods of groups 1 (thin liquids), 2 (nectar thick liquids), 7 (food that falls apart), and 8 (mixed textures) without any clinical signs and symptoms of laryngeal penetration and aspiration.

It was noted that the patient was able to swallow all consistencies (groups 1 to 8) in a safe manner and rated level 7 on ASHA scale. He was suggested to continue Shaker and Mendelssohn's maneuver for pharyngeal strengthening as well as follow the general aspiration precautions. The NGT was subsequently removed. The patient had a followup in the department of physiotherapy and rehabilitation after 6 months. Reassessment showed no deficit in swallowing function.

6. Discussion

Evidence of combined traditional therapy and VitalStim therapy to treat dysphagia due to stroke is documented [6, 12]. Numerous researches exist on dysphagia management in patients with cerebral stroke, but less work has been reported worldwide on the management of dysphagia in brainstem stroke, especially in cases of lateral medullary infarct. One of the case studies on dysphagia following lateral medullary infarct reported resolution of dysphagia 18 months after stroke [2]. The peculiarity of this case was that the patient did not receive any kind of attention to swallowing or intervention until after a year. Also, it signifies that the chances of spontaneous recovery of dysphagia followed by lateral medullary infarct are less compared to dysphagia following a hemispheric stroke [1]. After almost 16 months of dysphagia, the patient started intensive swallow rehabilitation therapy under the guidance of a dysphagia therapist at Max Healthcare, Saket, New Delhi, India, and, in only four months, regardless of severe dysphagia and late intervention, the patient recovered and achieved complete ability to swallow, eat, and drink by mouth.

Technologic advances like VitalStim therapy, transcranial magnetic stimulation (TMS), and functional magnetic stimulation (FMS) have enhanced the assessment and treatment of patients with dysphagia by permitting better quantification of impairment and treatment effectiveness [18]. Dysphagia due to brainstem stroke can be managed efficiently and early intervention may help in reducing recovery period and dysphagia related complications. An important aspect in patient care is improving the recognition and management of dysphagia or the difficulty or inability to swallow.

Fiberoptic endoscopic evaluation of swallowing (FEES) is a useful tool in the assessment of swallowing. The purpose of the examination is to determine if there is aspiration (food or liquid going into the airway) during or after swallowing, or if the food or liquid remains in the throat after the swallowing. It provides information regarding the structure and functions of the pharyngeal phase of swallowing and swallowing safety [19].

The patient's refusal for undergoing fiberoptic endoscopic evaluation of swallowing (FEES) has been the limitation of this study.

Future study is needed in a larger population of patients with lateral medullary stroke to understand the recovery pattern and effectiveness of combined traditional therapy and VitalStim therapy for improving swallowing function.

Conflict of Interests

The authors declare that there is no conflict of interests regarding the publication of this paper.

References

[1] E. Kruger, R. Teasell, K. Salter, N. Foley, and C. Hellings, "The rehabilitation of patients recovering from brainstem strokes: case studies and clinical considerations," *Topics in Stroke Rehabilitation*, vol. 14, no. 5, pp. 56–64, 2007.

[2] H. M. Finestone, R. W. Teasell, and J. Heitzner, "Case study of dysphagia and aspiration following a brain stem stroke," *Topics in Stroke Rehabilitation*, vol. 6, no. 3, pp. 41–45, 1999.

[3] I. Aydogdu, C. Ertekin, S. Tarlaci, B. Turman, N. Kiylioglu, and Y. Secil, "Dysphagia in lateral medullary infarction (Wallenberg's Syndrome): an acute disconnection syndrome in premotor neurons related to swallowing activity?" *Stroke*, vol. 32, no. 9, pp. 2081–2087, 2001.

[4] M. Bülow, R. Speyer, L. Baijens, V. Woisard, and O. Ekberg, "Neuromuscular electrical stimulation (NMES) in stroke patients with oral and pharyngeal dysfunction," *Dysphagia*, vol. 23, no. 3, pp. 302–309, 2008.

[5] *Occupational Therapy Dysphagia Training Information*, Physical Medicine and Rehabilitation Department Mayo Clinic, Rochester, NY, USA, 2006.

[6] M. Freed and Y. Wijting, *Training Manual for Patients Assessment, Treatment Using Vitalstim Electrical Stimulation*, Chattanooga Group, Hixson, Tenn, USA, 2006.

[7] P. M. Zenner, D. S. Losinski, and R. H. Mills, "Using cervical auscultation in the clinical dysphagia examination in long-term care," *Dysphagia*, vol. 10, no. 1, pp. 27–31, 1995.

[8] L. M. Burkhead, C. M. Sapienza, and J. C. Rosenbek, "Strength-training exercise in dysphagia rehabilitation: principles, procedures, and directions for future research," *Dysphagia*, vol. 22, no. 3, pp. 251–265, 2007.

[9] M. L. Urso, P. M. Clarkson, and T. B. Price, "Immobilization effects in young and older adults," *European Journal of Applied Physiology*, vol. 96, no. 5, pp. 564–571, 2006.

[10] M. A. Nicosia, J. A. Hind, E. B. Roecker et al., "Age effects on the temporal evolution of isometric and swallowing pressure," *Journals of Gerontology A—Biological Sciences and Medical Sciences*, vol. 55, no. 11, pp. M634–M640, 2000.

[11] National Outcomes Measurements System (NOMS). American Speech-Language Hearing Association, *Adult Speech-Language Pathology Training Manual*, American Speech-Language Hearing Association, Rockville, Md, USA, 1998.

[12] W. Xia, C. Zheng, Q. Lei et al., "Treatment of post-stroke dysphagia by vitalstim therapy coupled with conventional swallowing training," *Journal of Huazhong University of Science and Technology—Medical Science*, vol. 31, no. 1, pp. 73–76, 2011.

[13] O. Bretan and M. A. A. Henry, "Laryngeal mobility and dysphagia," *Arquivos de Gastroenterologia*, vol. 34, no. 3, pp. 134–138, 1997.

[14] H. J. Hislop and J. Montgomery, "8. Assessment of muscles innervated by cranial nerves," in *Daniels and Worthingham's: Techniques of Manual Examination*, p. 335, 2007.

[15] S. Hamdy, J. C. Rothwell, Q. Aziz, and D. G. Thompson, "Organization and reorganization of human swallowing motor cortex: implications for recovery after stroke," *Clinical Science*, vol. 99, no. 2, pp. 151–157, 2000.

[16] P. W. Duncan, R. Zorowitz, B. Bates et al., "Management of adult stroke rehabilitation care: a clinical practice guideline," *Stroke*, vol. 36, no. 9, pp. e100–143, 2005.

[17] A. M. O. Bakheit, "Management of neurogenic dysphagia," *Postgraduate Medical Journal*, vol. 77, no. 913, pp. 694–699, 2001.

[18] R. Momosaki, M. Abo, S. Watanabe, W. Kakuda, N. Yamada, and K. Mochio, "Functional magnetic stimulation using a parabolic coil for dysphagia after stroke," *Neuromodulation*, 2013.

[19] S. E. Langmore, K. Schatz, and N. Olsen, "Fiberoptic endoscopic examination of swallowing safety: a new procedure," *Dysphagia*, vol. 2, no. 4, pp. 216–219, 1988.

19

Left Atrial Appendage Closure for Stroke Prevention in Patients with Atrial Fibrillation and Hereditary Hemorrhagic Telangiectasia

Sebastiaan Velthuis,[1] Martin J. Swaans,[1] Johannes J. Mager,[2] Benno J. W. M. Rensing,[1] Lucas V. A. Boersma,[1] and Martijn C. Post[1]

[1] *Department of Cardiology, St. Antonius Hospital, 3435 CM Nieuwegein, The Netherlands*
[2] *Department of Pulmonology, St. Antonius Hospital, 3435 CM Nieuwegein, The Netherlands*

Correspondence should be addressed to Sebastiaan Velthuis, s.velthuis1@antoniusziekenhuis.nl

Academic Editors: C. D. Barrett, C. Firschke, A. J. Mansur, and K. Roberts-Thomson

Atrial fibrillation (AF) is the most common cardiac arrhythmia, affecting millions of individuals worldwide, and a major risk factor for disabling cerebral embolic stroke. Hereditary hemorrhagic telangiectasia (HHT) is an autosomal dominant inherited disorder, characterized by vascular abnormalities with high-bleeding tendency and therefore intolerance for oral anticoagulation. We report a case of percutaneous closure of the left atrial appendage, which might be a good alternative strategy instead of chronic oral anticoagulation to protect patients with high-risk AF and HHT from cerebral embolic strokes.

1. Introduction

Atrial fibrillation (AF) is the most common cardiac arrhythmia and a major risk factor for cerebral embolic stroke. Although oral anticoagulation (OAC) is highly effective in stroke prevention, a substantial number of patients is unable to sustain chronic OAC because of high-bleeding risks. Among these are patients with hereditary hemorrhagic telangiectasia (HHT), who frequently encounter inconvenient epistaxis, gastrointestinal bleedings, or life-threatening bleedings from cerebral or pulmonary arteriovenous malformations. Since most thromboembolic complications in patients with AF arise from the left atrial appendage (LAA), a percutaneous transcatheter LAA closure device was recently developed.

This is the first paper about the feasibility of percutaneous LAA closure in patients with high-risk AF and HHT, which can be a promising strategy to protect these patients against embolic stroke, while avoiding the need for long-term OAC.

2. Case Presentation

We present a 79-year-old man who had been previously diagnosed with HHT, based on the clinical Curaçao criteria [1]; his family history revealed numerous first-degree relatives with HHT, physical examination demonstrated several telangiectasia on hands, face, lips, and ears, and he suffered from recurrent epistaxis. DNA analysis confirmed the clinical diagnosis with an ALK-1 gene mutation on chromosome 12. Visceral AVMs in the brain, lungs, liver, or gastro-intestinal tract were excluded with magnetic resonance imaging, echocardiography, computed-tomography, and endoscopy. In addition to HHT, the patient was known with arterial hypertension, a recent cerebral ischemic stroke, and permanent AF. His $CHADS_2$-score of four indicated a high risk of recurrent stroke (8.5%/year) [2]. Since visceral sources of life-threatening hemorrhages were ruled out, a trial of OAC (warfarin) was started. This resulted in extensive epistaxis, requiring repeated blood transfusions despite treatment with iron supplements and nasal cauterizations.

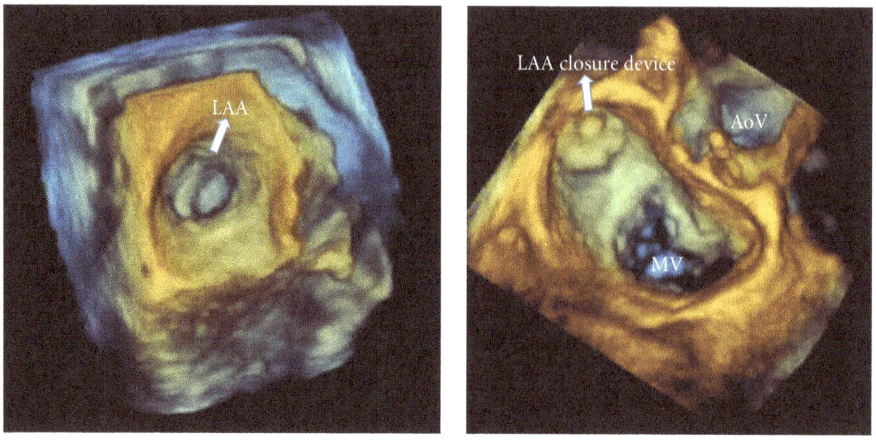

(a) (b)

Figure 1: Real-time three-dimensional transoesophageal echocardiographic imaging of the left atrial appendage as seen from the left atrial perspective. (a) Preprocedural view of LAA. (b) LAA closure device deployed. (LAA: left atrial appendage; AoV; aortic valve; MV; mitral valve).

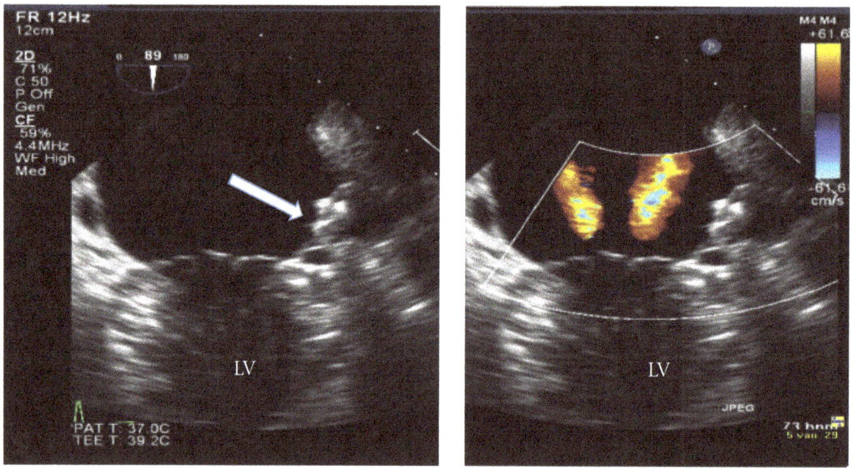

(a) (b)

Figure 2: Two-dimensional transoesophageal echocardiographic imaging of the left atrium at 45-days followup. (a) Successful occlusion of the LAA without thrombus formation on the atrial surface of the device despite the limited use of anticoagulation therapy (aspirin only). (b) No residual flow around the device. LV: left ventricle.

Because of this clinical dilemma, the patient was referred to our HHT-specialized cardiology department and was accepted for percutaneous LAA closure to protect against recurrent stroke, while avoiding the need for long-term OAC. A 27 mm Watchman LAA Occlusion Device (Atritech Inc., Plymouth, Minnesota) was implanted in the LAA using biplane fluoroscopy and 3D-transoesophageal echocardiography (TEE) guidance, according to the recent literature (Figure 1) [3]. Because of the patient's high-bleeding risk, postprocedural anticoagulation was limited to aspirin for at least six weeks to allow for device endothelialization and to prevent thrombotic complications. Control TEE at 45 days demonstrated successful closure of the LAA without thrombus formation on the atrial surface of the device (Figure 2), and aspirin was discontinued. During one-year followup, no thromboembolic complications or severe HHT-related bleedings occurred.

3. Discussion

This is the first paper about the feasibility of a percutaneous LAA closure device in patients with high-risk AF and HHT. Percutaneous closure of the LAA might be a new strategy to protect this population against cerebral embolic stroke without the need for chronic OAC and subsequent high-bleeding risks.

HHT-related gene mutations result in abnormal angiogenesis and fragile vessels with increased bleeding tendency [4]. Recurrent epistaxis is the most common symptom of

HHT, affecting 78–96% of patients [5]. Epistaxis often leads to iron-deficiency anemia and is an important factor reducing quality of life [6]. Gastro-intestinal (GI) telangiectasia is present in 80% of HHT patients, from which 30% will develop GI-bleedings and causes increased morbidity and mortality [7]. Approximately 23% of HHT patients have cerebral AVMs. The bleeding risk from cerebral AVMs in HHT is estimated around 0.5% per year [8], which may have devastating consequences. Pulmonary AVMs are present in up to 58% of HHT patients [9] and carry the risk of hemoptysis or hemothorax, which is caused by a ruptured endobronchial or subpleural AVM and reported in up to 8% [10].

Because of this inconvenient and sometimes life-threatening bleeding tendency, the decision to start OAC in patients with high-risk AF and HHT should be based on a careful individual risk assessment of both thromboembolic and hemorrhagic complications.

Previous studies demonstrated that the LAA is the source of thrombi in more than 90% of patients with nonvalvular AF [11], which led to the development of the Watchman left atrial appendage occlusion device. This percutaneous transcatheter device excludes the LAA from the systemic circulation and protects against embolic stroke, without the need for long-term OAC. The Watchman device was investigated in the PROTECT-AF trial, which demonstrated that percutaneous closure of the LAA was noninferior to chronic OAC therapy [3]. After device implantation, all patients in the PROTECT-AF trial were treated with warfarin for 45 days, clopidogrel and aspirin for six months, and then aspirin lifelong. Therefore, the exact safety and efficacy of percutaneous LAA device closure in patients with high-bleeding risks and intolerance for short-term OAC remains unknown. At our institution, HHT patients must be eligible for at least 6 weeks of aspirin therapy, which is tested before device implantation using a nosebleed diary. A careful risk-benefit assessment is made prior to LAA device implantation for every individual with HHT, in order to arrange a tailor-made postprocedural anticoagulation treatment. We underscore that the optimum strategy to prevent device-related thromboembolic complications without raising the risk of bleeding in patients with contraindications for OAC has to be established in future studies. At present, percutaneous LAA occlusion may be an acceptable option in selected HHT patients with high-risk AF who are not candidates for long-term OAC.

4. Conclusion

Percutaneous closure of the LAA might provide an alternative strategy to chronic anticoagulation therapy for stroke prevention in patients with high-risk AF and HHT.

Acknowledgment

The Cardiology Department receives proctoring fees from Boston Scientific for Training and Educational Services.

References

[1] C. L. Shovlin, A. E. Guttmacher, E. Buscarini et al., "Diagnostic criteria for hereditary hemorrhagic telangiectasia (Rendu-Osler-Weber syndrome)," *American Journal of Medical Genetics*, vol. 91, no. 1, pp. 66–67, 2000.

[2] A. J. Camm, P. Kirchhof, G. Y. Lip et al., "Guidelines for the management of atrial fibrillation: the Task Force for the Management of Atrial Fibrillation of the European Society of Cardiology (ESC)," *European Heart Journal*, vol. 31, pp. 2369–2429, 2010.

[3] D. R. Holmes, V. Y. Reddy, Z. G. Turi et al., "Percutaneous closure of the left atrial appendage versus warfarin therapy for prevention of stroke in patients with atrial fibrillation: a randomised non-inferiority trial," *The Lancet*, vol. 374, no. 9689, pp. 534–542, 2009.

[4] A. Fernandez-L, F. Sanz-Rodriguez, R. Zarrabeitia et al., "Blood outgrowth endothelial cells from Hereditary Haemorrhagic Telangiectasia patients reveal abnormalities compatible with vascular lesions," *Cardiovascular Research*, vol. 68, no. 2, pp. 235–248, 2005.

[5] H. Plauchu, J. P. de Chadarevian, A. Bideau, and J. M. Robert, "Age-related clinical profile of heredity hemorrhagic telangiectasia in an epidemiologically recruited population," *American Journal of Medical Genetics*, vol. 32, no. 3, pp. 291–297, 1989.

[6] G. Pasculli, F. Resta, E. Guastamacchia, L. di Gennaro, P. Suppressa, and C. Sabbà, "Health-related quality of life in a rare disease: hereditary hemorrhagic telangiectasia (HHT) or Rendu-Osler-Weber Disease," *Quality of Life Research*, vol. 13, no. 10, pp. 1715–1723, 2004.

[7] A. V. Longacre, C. P. Gross, M. Gallitelli, K. J. Henderson, R. I. J. White, and D. D. Proctor, "Diagnosis and management of gastrointestinal bleeding in patients with hereditary hemorrhagic telangiectasia," *American Journal of Gastroenterology*, vol. 98, no. 1, pp. 59–65, 2003.

[8] R. B. Willemse, J. J. Mager, C. J. J. Westermann, T. T. C. Overtoom, H. Mauser, and J. G. Wolbers, "Bleeding risk of cerebrovascular malformations in hereditary hemorrhagic telangiectasia," *Journal of Neurosurgery*, vol. 92, no. 5, pp. 779–784, 2000.

[9] M. W. F. van Gent, M. C. Post, R. J. Snijder, C. J. J. Westermann, H. W. M. Plokker, and J. J. Mager, "Real prevalence of pulmonary right-to-left shunt according to genotype in patients with hereditary hemorrhagic telangiectasia: a transthoracic contrast echocardiography study," *Chest*, vol. 138, no. 4, pp. 833–839, 2010.

[10] B. A. Ference, T. M. Shannon, R. I. J. White, M. Zawin, and C. M. Burdge, "Life-threatening pulmonary hemorrhage with pulmonary arteriovenous malformations and hereditary hemorrhagic telangiectasia," *Chest*, vol. 106, no. 5, pp. 1387–1390, 1994.

[11] J. L. Blackshear and J. A. Odell, "Appendage obliteration to reduce stroke in cardiac surgical patients with atrial fibrillation," *Annals of Thoracic Surgery*, vol. 61, no. 2, pp. 755–759, 1996.

20

Epidermoid Causing Ischemic Stroke in the Brainstem

Raghvendra Ramdasi,[1] Amit Mahore,[1] Abhijeet Kulkarni,[1] Vithal Rangarajan,[1] Manoj Patil,[1] and Juhi Kawale[2]

[1]*Department of Neurosurgery, King Edward Memorial Hospital and Seth Gordhandas Sunderdas Medical College, Parel, Mumbai 400012, India*
[2]*Department of Medicine, King Edward Memorial Hospital and Seth Gordhandas Sunderdas Medical College, Parel, Mumbai 400012, India*

Correspondence should be addressed to Raghvendra Ramdasi; drraghavr@gmail.com

Academic Editor: José Luis González-Gutiérrez

Intracranial tumors may rarely cause stroke. We report an epidermoid cyst causing stroke in a pediatric patient. We have also reviewed the literature and pathogenesis of stroke caused by intracranial tumors.

1. Introduction

Stroke as a presenting symptom of intracranial tumors is extremely rare. Epidermoids referred to as "an ordered disorder" usually produce symptoms of slowly progressive mass lesion [1]. We report a pediatric case of brainstem infarct caused by this "well mannered" epidermoid tumor in cerebellopontine angle. This phenomenon was only once reported in adults [2].

2. Case Presentation

A 12-year-old boy was brought by parents into a rural hospital with complaint of headache for the last 6 months. Computed tomography (CT) scan of brain revealed a hypodense lesion in right cerebellopontine angle and basal cistern (Figure 1(a)). The provisional diagnoses were arachnoid cyst and epidermoid cyst. The patient was referred to tertiary care centre for further management as neurosurgical and magnetic resonance imaging (MRI) facilities were not available at the rural hospital. However, the parents did not follow the medical advice. He was brought to our emergency department after 5 months when he developed altered sensorium and left hemiparesis of sudden onset. On examination, the patient was drowsy and not obeying commands. The patient had good spontaneous activity of right sided limbs without any spontaneous movements of left sided limbs. There was definite paucity of movements of left sided limbs to the central painful stimuli as compared to those of the right sided limbs. The exact assessment of weakness was not possible due to the drowsy state. The right pupil was larger as compared to the left pupil and was not reacting to light. The left sided limbs had hyperreflexia. The left plantar reflex showed extensor response. The rest of the findings were unremarkable.

Magnetic resonance imaging (MRI) of the brain was done within one hour of arrival of the patient and approximately 12 hours after the onset of symptoms. It revealed the lesion with isointensity on T1 weighted imaging and hyperintensity on T2 weighted imaging in right cerebellopontine angle extending to basal cistern (Figures 1(b) and 1(c)). There was another lesion in right half of midbrain with hyperintensity on T1, T2, and FLAIR images (Figures 1(d), 1(e), 1(f), and 1(g)), restricting diffusion on diffusion weighted image (DWI) like the first lesion (Figure 1(h)). The lesion showed low signal on apparent diffusion coefficient (ADC) map ruling out T2 shine-through effect. These findings were suggestive of right cerebellopontine angle epidermoid with right midbrain infarct. The restriction of diffusion on DWI ruled out the possibility of arachnoid cyst. His other investigations including coagulation profile and electrolytes were normal.

The patient was operated on, on emergency basis via right retrosigmoid approach, and near-complete excision

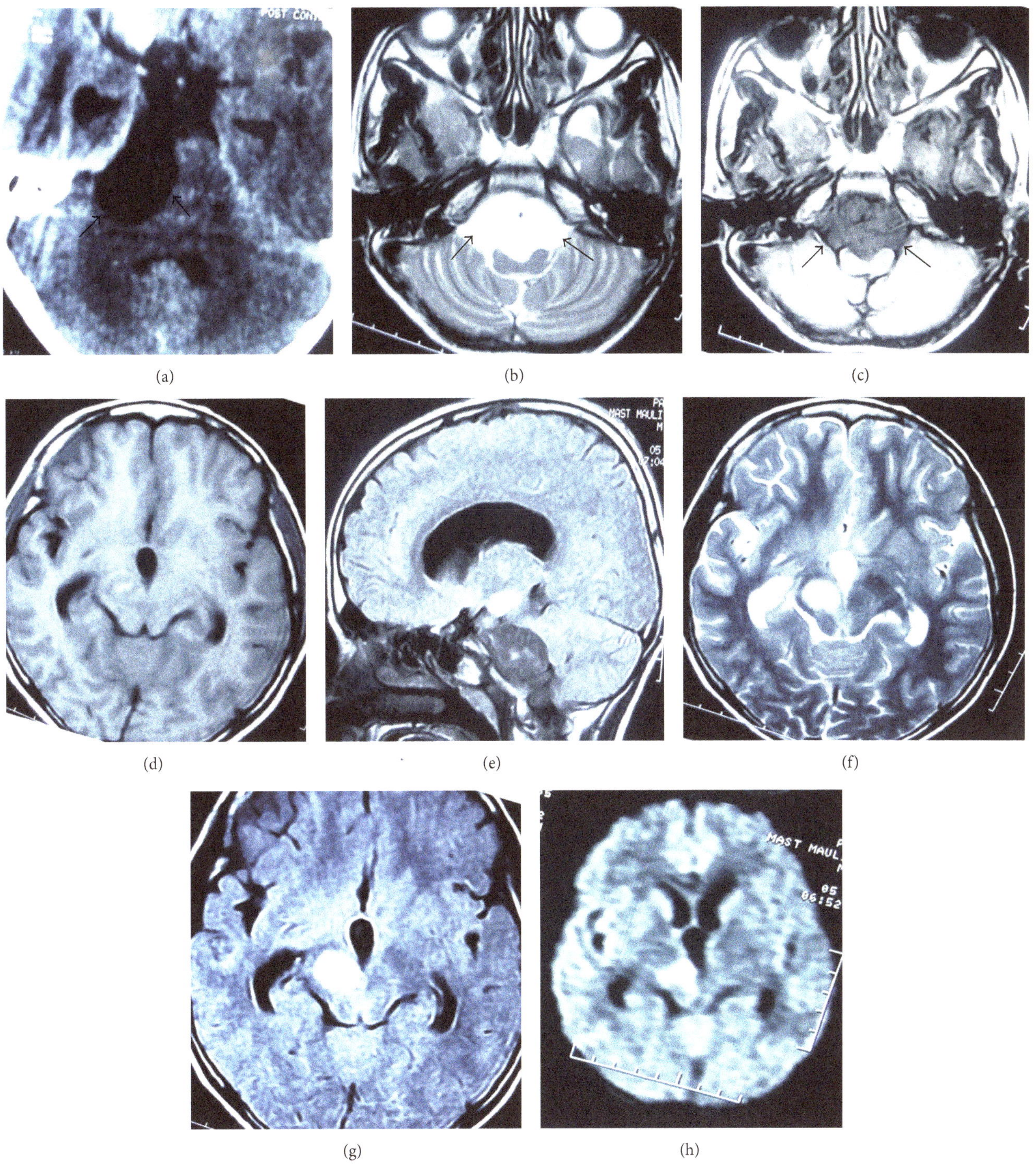

FIGURE 1: (a) Axial image of plain computed tomography (CT) showing hypodense lesion in right cerebellopontine angle and prepontine cistern with compression of the brainstem. Axial T2 (b) and T1 (c) weighted MR images showing the lesion to be hypointense on T1 and hyperintense on T2 sequence (black arrows outline the tumour). (d) and (e) are T1 weighted axial and sagittal images. (f), (g), and (h) are axial T2, FLAIR, and diffusion weighted images, respectively, revealing another lesion of hyperintensity and restricted diffusion in right half of midbrain.

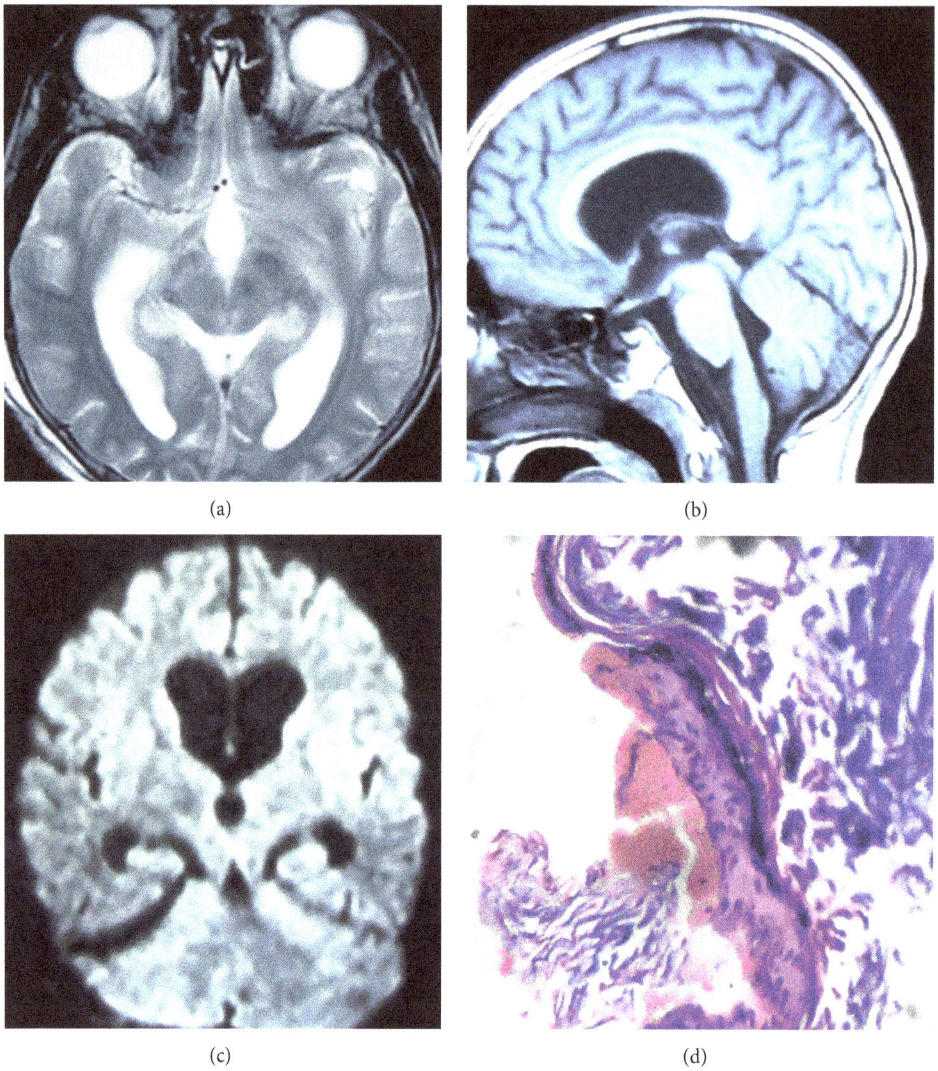

Figure 2: (a) Axial T2, sagittal T1 (b), and diffusion weighted postoperative image (c) showing complete excision of the lesion and resolution of the infarct. (d) The photomicrograph of the lesion (H&E, 100x) showing stratified squamous lining epithelium with lamellated keratin.

of epidermoid cyst was done leaving behind the capsular fragments densely adherent to vessels and nerves.

The patient improved in sensorium with partial improvement of hemiparesis after the surgery. Magnetic resonance imaging (MRI), done one month after the surgery, was suggestive of complete resolution of the infarct (Figures 2(a), 2(b), and 2(c)). Histopathological examination revealed the lesion lined by stratified squamous epithelium with lamellated keratinconsistent with epidermoid cyst (Figure 2(d)). At follow-up of 1 year after the surgery he was completely normal.

3. Discussion

Schnitker and Lehnert in 1952 described middle cerebral artery infarct in a case of pituitary apoplexy [3]. There are few cases of intracranial tumors causing infarct, the mechanisms of which differ from each other [2]. Pituitary adenoma is the most common benign tumor causing infarct. These encase the vessels and compress them subsequently. Infrequently these may cause vasospasm [2, 4]. Meningiomas cause infarct by compression of the vessels [5]. Malignant gliomas cause infarct by invasion of vessels [6–8]. Ruptured dermoid cyst results in vasospasm and infarct [9, 10]. One case of ruptured craniopharyngeal cyst causing infarct is reported and vasospasm is the implicated mechanism [11].

Epidermoids account for approximately 1% of all intracranial tumors. Although these lesions are congenital, patients are usually symptomatic in their third to fifth decade [12]. Two cases of epidermoid causing brainstem infarct were reported where stretching of the vessel was the postulated mechanism [2]. It is likely that the tumor in our case stretched one or more branches of the basilar artery leading to the infarct.

In all the cases reviewed, we found only one pediatric case described by Pozzati et al. [13]. Our case is the second paediatric case of tumors causing infarct and the youngest one. It is the first pediatric case and the third case of epidermoid causing infarct.

T1 hyperintensity with no blooming on gradient echo as in our case may represent incomplete stroke as described by Baheti et al. and warrant urgent intervention [14].

The two cases described before were treated medically for two weeks and the postoperative improvement in their deficits is not mentioned [2]. In our case we operated on the patient within 16 hours of the ictus and he improved remarkably in his deficits. We did not give antiplatelet treatment to our patient because surgery was anticipated in our case. The use of antiplatelets is known to increase the incidence of hematoma in major neurosurgical procedures.

4. Conclusion

Epidermoids may cause acute symptoms as brainstem infarct. The exact mechanism is unknown, but the stretching of the vessels may play an important role. Early surgery instead of medical treatment can reverse the insult. When primary cause of stroke is tumor or tumor-like lesion, the early surgery rather than antiplatelet treatment should be considered.

Conflict of Interests

The authors declare that there is no conflict of interests regarding the publication of this paper.

Authors' Contribution

Each author has contributed in management of patient, review of literature, and/or preparation of the paper.

References

[1] M. Kothari and A. Goel, "The heuristics of craniospinal epidermoid tumors," *Neurology India*, vol. 54, no. 2, p. 143, 2006.

[2] S. Yilmazlar, H. Kocaeli, and T. Cordan, "Brain stem stroke associated with epidermoid tumours: report of two cases," *Journal of Neurology, Neurosurgery and Psychiatry*, vol. 75, no. 9, pp. 1340–1342, 2004.

[3] M. T. Schnitker and H. B. Lehnert, "Apoplexy in a pituitary chromophobe adenoma producing the syndrome of middle cerebral artery thrombosis; case report," *Journal of Neurosurgery*, vol. 9, no. 2, pp. 210–213, 1952.

[4] S. Mohindra, P. Kovai, and R. Chhabra, "Fatal bilateral ACA territory infarcts after pituitary apoplexy: a case report and literature review," *Skull Base*, vol. 20, no. 4, pp. 285–288, 2010.

[5] S. Mathis, B. Bataille, S. Boucebci et al., "A rare cause of stroke in young adults: occlusion of the middle cerebral artery by a meningioma postpartum," *Case Reports in Neurological Medicine*, vol. 8, pp. 652–653, 2013.

[6] P. E. Kaplan, R. Santana, J. Cohen, and J. Leestma, "Glioblastoma multiforme presenting as stroke: an electrophysiological and clinicopathological case report," *Archives of Physical Medicine and Rehabilitation*, vol. 60, no. 2, pp. 74–77, 1979.

[7] E. Auff and K. Vass, "Cerebellar glioblastoma presenting clinically as Wallenberg's syndrome," *Archiv für Psychiatrie und Nervenkrankheiten*, vol. 230, no. 4, pp. 361–364, 1981.

[8] H. Chen, H. Cebula, R. Schott, J.-L. Dietemann, and S. Froelich, "Glioblastoma multiforme presenting with ischemic stroke: case report and review of the literature," *Journal of Neuroradiology*, vol. 38, no. 5, pp. 304–307, 2011.

[9] M. G. Kang, K. J. Kim, J. I. Seok, and D. K. Lee, "Intracranial dermoid cyst rupture with midbrain and thalamic infarction.," *Neurology*, vol. 72, no. 8, p. 769, 2009.

[10] J. M. Ramírez-Moreno, M. Ortega-Martínez, M. A. Fernández-Gil et al., "Isolated mesencephalic stroke related to a ruptured intracranial dermoid cyst," *Neurocirugia*, vol. 20, no. 3, pp. 272–277, 2009.

[11] N. Shida, N. Nakasato, K. Mizoi, M. Kanaki, and T. Yosimot, "Symptomatic vessel narrowing caused by spontaneous rupture of craniopharyngioma cyst—case report," *Neurologia Medico-Chirurgica*, vol. 38, no. 10, pp. 666–668, 1998.

[12] N. Oulali, F. Moufid, M. R. Ghailan, and B. Hosni, "Epidermoid cyst of the cisterna magna and fourth ventricle," *Pan African Medical Journal*, vol. 13, article 19, 2012.

[13] E. Pozzati, G. Frank, M. T. Nasi, and G. Giuliani, "Pituitary apoplexy, bilateral carotid vasospasm, and cerebral infarction in a 15-year-old boy," *Neurosurgery*, vol. 20, no. 1, pp. 56–59, 1987.

[14] N. N. Baheti, A. Cherian, W. P. R. C. Kesavadas, and B. Thomas, "Ischemic hyperintensities on T1-weighted magnetic resonance imaging of patients with stroke: New insights from susceptibility weighted imaging," *Neurology India*, vol. 58, no. 1, pp. 90–94, 2010.

21

Lower Body Positive Pressure Application with an Antigravity Suit in Acute Carotid Occlusion

Karine Berthet,[1] Anne Claire Lukaszewicz,[2] Marie-Germaine Bousser,[1] and Didier Payen[2]

[1] *Department of Neurology, Lariboisière Hospital, Assistance Publique Hôpitaux de Paris and University Paris 7 Diderot, 2 rue Ambroise Paré, 75475 Paris Cedex 10, France*
[2] *Department of Anesthesiology & Critical Care Medicine, Lariboisière Hospital, Assistance Publique Hôpitaux de Paris and University Paris 7 Diderot, 2 rue Ambroise Paré, 75475 Paris Cedex 10, France*

Correspondence should be addressed to Didier Payen, dpayen1234@aol.com

Academic Editor: David S. Liebeskind

The challenge in acute stroke is still to reperfuse as early as possible the ischemic territory. Since fibrinolytic therapies have a limited window with potential risk of bleeding, having a nonpharmacologic mean to recruit vessels in area surrounding necrosis might be useful. We propose here to use antigravity suit inflated at "venous" pressure levels to shift blood towards thoracic and brain territories. We report two cases of spectacular clinical recovery after acute carotid occlusion.

1. Introduction

We report two cases where an anti-gravity suit (also named MAST: Medical Antishock Trousers [1, 2]) was applied with a low gradient of pressure during the acute phase of symptomatic carotid occlusion to amplify the blood volume shift towards the craniothoracic territory [3, 4], improving cerebral haemodynamic conditions and neurological symptoms. The impact of anti-gravity suit application on cerebral vascularisation was measured by transcranial Doppler.

2. Case 1

A 28-year-old woman was seen 2 hours after the sudden onset of total right brachial monoplegia, right facial palsy, and mutism (NIH Stroke Scale: 17) due to a left middle cerebral artery (MCA) infarct. She received intravenous recombinant tissue plasminogen activator (rt-PA) 2.5 hours after stroke onset, without subsequent improvement. Cerebral MRI diffusion-weighted images and T2 flair-weighted images performed 24 hours later showed increased signal in the whole superficial left MCA territory (Figures 2(a) and 3(a)). The MR Angiography (MRA) showed a proximal left internal carotid artery (ICA) occlusion, a tight stenosis on the distal right ICA, no signal in the right siphon and right MCA, while there was a weak signal in the left MCA (Figure 4). T1-FAT-SAT-weighted images showed bilateral ICA dissection (Figure 5). Doppler study showed a high resistance to flow in both common carotid arteries and low bilateral MCA flow with low systolic and diastolic velocities. Intravenous heparin treatment was started 24 hours after rt-PA administration and the patient was lying in a strict −20 degrees head down tilt [5].

Two days after stroke onset, there was no clinical improvement and the patient developed bradycardia (40 pulses/min) and hypotension (100/70 mmHg). Lower body positive pressure (LBPP) was applied using an anti-gravity suit (Trauma Air Pants; Life Support Products Inc., St Louis, Missouri, USA) for 150 minutes. The anti-gravity suit included three independent bladders connected to three pneumatic extremities with manometers providing instantaneous pressure values. The garment was applied from ankle to costal margin and the bladder pressures were set at 20 mmHg on the lower limbs and 10 mmHg on the abdominal area, to keep a positive pressure gradient [3, 4]. During the procedure the patient was lying in a supine position. The following parameters were recorded at baseline, after intravenous infusion of 500 mL of fluid load (colloid), 15 minutes and 150 minutes during LBPP application and 10 minutes after gravity suit deflation: right arm mobility, blood

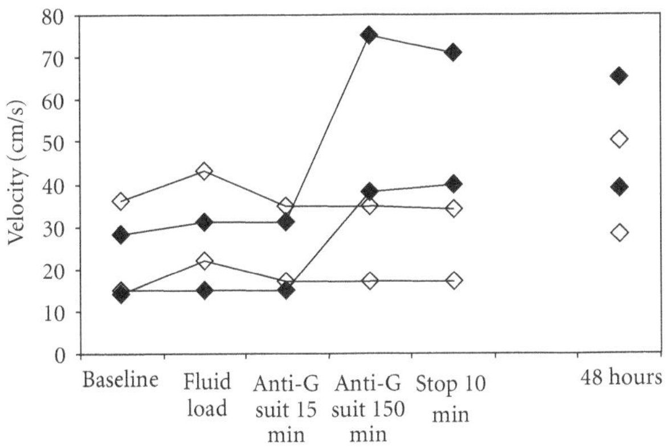

(a)

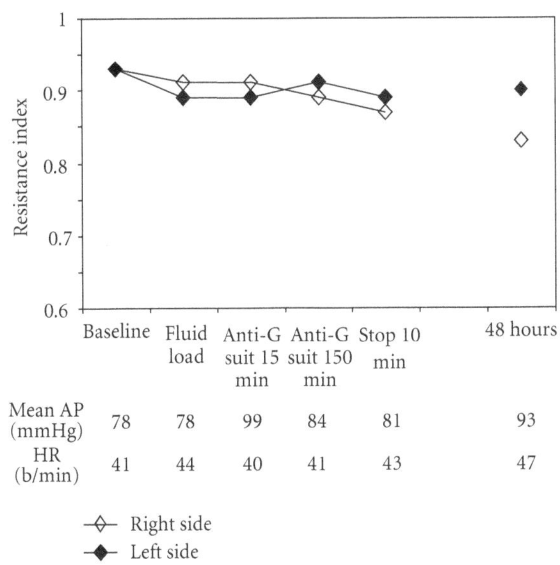

(b)

FIGURE 1: (a) Patterns of intracranial MCA blood flow velocities with time in both the right and left sides, before, during, and after (10 minutes and 48 hours) LBPP application. Note the left side improvement in systolic and diastolic blood flow velocity induced by LBPP, which was sustained for at least 2 days. (b) Vascular resistance index (RI) evolution (method for computation: systolic V/diastolic V). A clear difference between right and left RI occurred only after 48 hours of LBPP application. Corresponding mean arterial pressure (mean AP) and heart rate (HR) at each time.

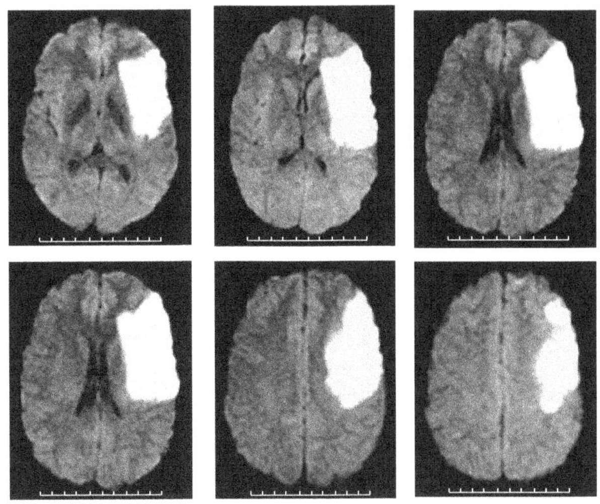

(a)

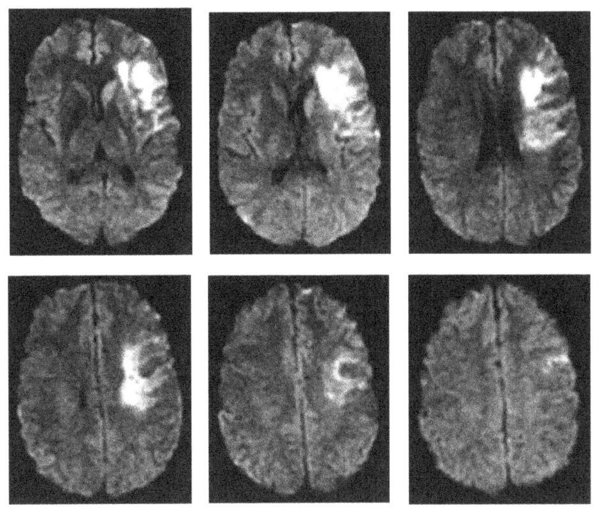

(b)

FIGURE 2: MRI diffusion-weighted images showing left superficial MCA infarct. (a) 24 hours after stroke onset, (b) 5 days after stroke onset.

pressure, heart rate, systolic and diastolic velocities recorded on both MCAs and resistance index (RI) recorded on both common carotids arteries (CCAs).

During LBPP application and up to 48 hours later, there was a 50% increase in systolic and diastolic MCA velocities (Figure 1). The RI decreased on both CCAs from 0.93 to 0.86 and continued to decrease on the right side after the procedure. Heart rate and blood pressure remained stable during LBPP application and during the proceeding days.

Three days after LBPP application the patient started to recover her right hand mobility and her facial palsy started to improve. One week after LBPP application she had completely recovered her right arm and facial mobility. She finally went back home 3 weeks after hospitalisation.

On MRI performed 5 days after stroke onset, diffusion-weighted images showed reduced diffusion abnormalities and reduced infarct size on T2 flair-weighted images (Figures 2(b) and 3(b)). The MRA showed recanalisation of the right ICA with good visualisation of siphon and MCA but a persistent left ICA occlusion (Figure 6).

3. Case 2

A 61-year-old. man was admitted in our stroke unit after 2 reversible episodes of left monocular blindness associated with a total right distal upper limb paralysis. His medical past history was hypertension, hypercholesterolemia, and tobacco use. At the admission the clinical examination showed a total right wrist extension paresis, the so-called "pseudoradial

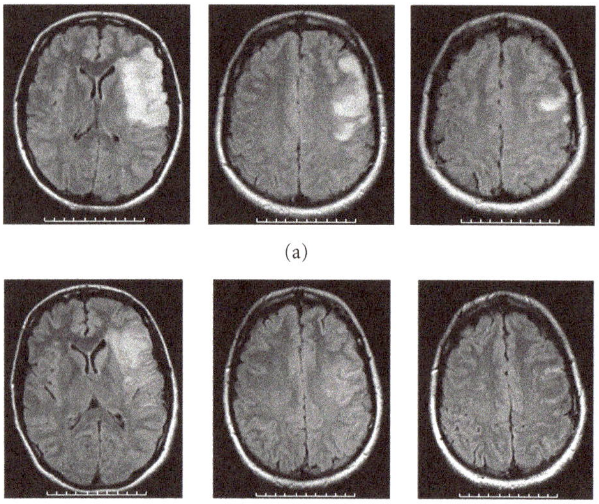

(a)

(b)

FIGURE 3: MRI T2 flair-weighted images showing left superficial MCA infarct. (a) 24 hours after stroke onset, (b) 5 days after stroke onset.

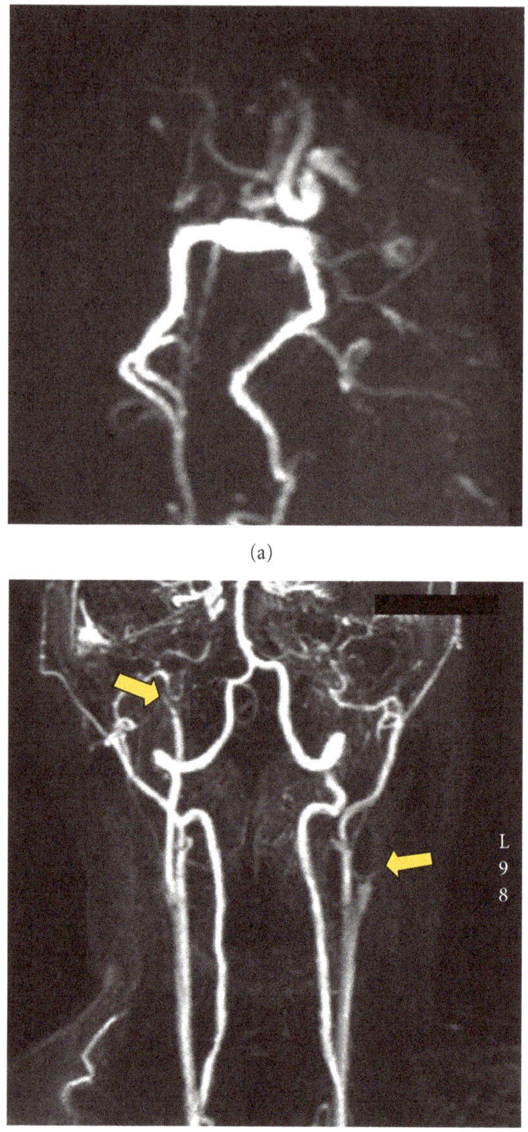

(a)

(b)

FIGURE 4: (a) Intracranial MRA of Willis circle: right siphon, right and left MCAs were not visible. Posterior communicating arteries were also not visible, with visible posterior cerebral arteries. (b) Cervical MRA showing proximal left internal carotid artery occlusion and distal right internal carotid artery tight stenosis (arrows).

paresis" related to a small left frontal infarction visible on MRI (DWI). The MR angiography (MRA) and the duplex scanning showed an occlusion of the left internal carotid artery due to atherosclerosis and a negative flow in the ophthalmic artery downstream. The intracranial MRA showed poor collateral supply by anterior communicating artery and an apparent nonfunctional posterior communicating artery. We decided to apply LBPP process for 2 reasons: (1) the worsening of the right hand deficit (See the movie in Supplementary Materials available online at doi:10.4061/2010/950524), (2) this worsening was not related to a fall in systemic blood pressure (167/84 mmHg). The LBPP was applied once during 90 minutes following the same procedure than in case one. The repeated measurements of blood pressure and heart rate did not show any significant changes along the procedure. The transcranial Doppler showed a decreased of the left MCA resistance to flow index ([systolic velocity-diastolic velocity]/systolic velocity, 0.5 at baseline to 0.4 at the end of the procedure) while there was slight changes on the MCA velocities (64/32 to 75/45 cm/sec). The left ophthalmic artery flow remained negative during and after LBPP application. Heart rate and blood pressure remained stable during LBPP application. The clinical improvement was sustained after anti-G suit deflation (as presented on the movie) consisting in the recovery of the pseudoradial palsy with persisting ataxia lasting few days. The total recovery was obtained before discharge.

4. Discussion

We report two patients with symptomatic carotid artery occlusion in whom LBPP was applied with an anti-gravity suit during the acute phase of stroke. The patients made a remarkable recovery in parallel with significant cerebral hemodynamic improvement not related to global systemic hemodynamic changes.

LBPP is known to shift blood from the lower body compartment towards the upper part of the body, which improves cardiac preload and output [4, 6, 7] and potentially cerebral perfusion [8]. The addition of an abdominal compression to lower limbs was supposed to be more efficient to push more blood to the brain than compression of lower limb only [6].

Several mechanisms might be discussed for neurological improvement: (1) recanalization of carotid occlusion, (2) development of collaterals, and (3) recruitment of smaller

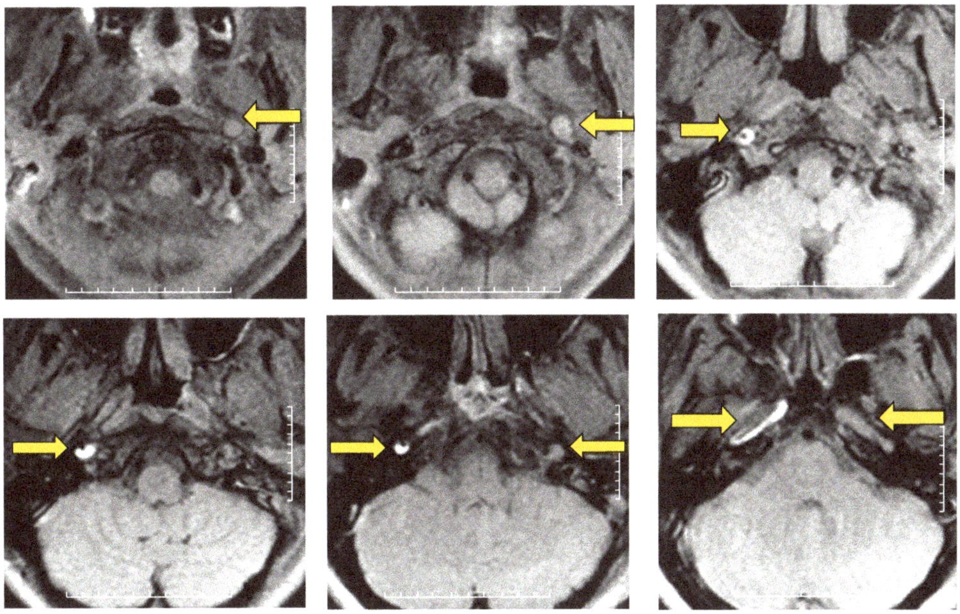

FIGURE 5: MRI T1-FAT-SAT-weighted images showing the dissecting process visible as a hypersignal in the wall of both ICAs as well as an enhancement of ICA diameter (arrows).

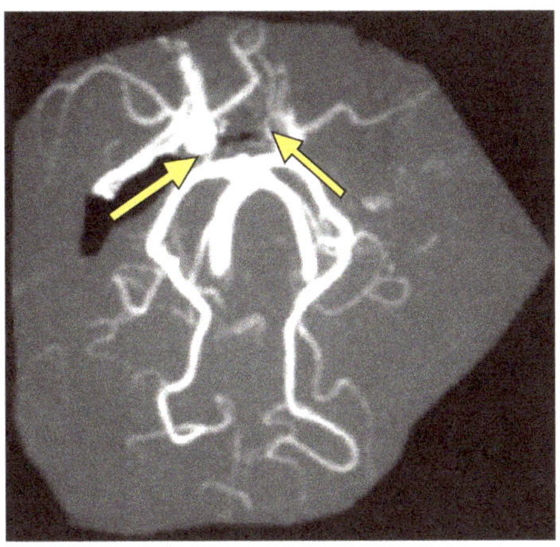

FIGURE 6: Intracranial MRA showing recanalisation of the right ICA; the right and left MCAs are visible as well as both posterior communicating arteries (arrows).

vessels in watershed fields. For the first patient, it is unlikely that rt-PA administration played a major role in this dramatic improvement since there was no improvement 24 hours after treatment, which decreases the likelihood of a favourable outcome to 20% [9, 10], and the efficacy of rt-PA in carotid occlusions is debatable [11, 12].

The reopening of the carotid artery, which was unusually rapid for the spontaneous evolution of a dissection [13], may have played an important role in case 1 evolution. Whether LBPP application contributed to this reopening, though likely with RI decrease on right CCA, is open to debate and we cannot rule out coincidental recanalization of the ICA occlusion. In case 1, the parallel improvement in the clinical status and flow parameters on transcranial Doppler (TCD) during and after LBPP application suggests a beneficial effect of LBPP application on brain perfusion, particularly through restitution of blood flow in the ischemic left MCA territory. It could be due to the recruitment of collateral pathway through Willis circle explaining the increase of systolic and diastolic velocities recorded on left MCA during LBPP application (case 1, Figure 1), as well as the improvement of anterior cerebral circulation shown by the MRA performed 5 days after stroke onset (right siphon and right MCA were visible and the posterior communicating arteries were functional on Figure 6). The second case reported which showed a clinical improvement (film) during the LBPP application showed a weak improvement in cerebral velocities. The temporal relationship between clinical recovery and LBPP application suggests a benefit.

Another possible beneficial effect could be the recruitment of smaller vessels in watershed fields especially in case 2. The clinical improvement during the LBPP application could be related to the new partition in the frontal region of blood which could play a role in the recruitment of small vessels by an efficient loading or even a reopening.

Two recent reports showed the impact of a mechanical external counter-pulsation on cerebral velocities in healthy volunteers [8] and on functional outcome in patients with stroke [14]. In this study the LBPP application was limited to the lower limbs by the mean of a cyclic external counter-pulsation at diastolic time of heart cycle which is more complex than our classical anti-gravity suit. Furthermore, we can expect that the anti-gravity suit could mobilised a higher blood volume in respect of the abdominal compartment implication.

Even if this paper is limited to two patients, without control group, the remarkable recovery observed in these two patients together with the improvement in hemodynamic parameters on TCD might be related to LBPP application through improvement of cerebral perfusion. We need definitively, further investigation during the acute phase of ischemic stroke to conclude on the beneficial effect of this noninvasive tool.

Acknowledgment

This work was supported in part by the Plan quadriennal EA 322 2002-2006.

References

[1] L. R. Frank, "Is MAST in the past? The pros and cons of MAST usage in the field," *Journal of Emergency Medical Services*, vol. 25, no. 2, pp. 38–41, 44–45, 2000.

[2] N. McSwain, "Pneumatic anti-shock garment in the '90s," *Emergency*, vol. 26, no. 4, pp. 53–56, 1994.

[3] D. M. Payen, C. J. L. Brun-Buisson, P. A. Carli, et al., "Hemodynamic, gas exchange, and hormonal consequences of LBPP during PEEP ventilation," *Journal of Applied Physiology*, vol. 62, no. 1, pp. 61–70, 1987.

[4] D. M. Payen, P. A. Carli, C. J. L. Brun-Buisson, et al., "Lower body positive pressure vs. dopamine during PEEP in humans," *Journal of Applied Physiology*, vol. 58, no. 1, pp. 77–82, 1985.

[5] A. W. Wojner-Alexandrov, Z. Garami, O. Y. Chernyshev, and A. V. Alexandrov, "Heads down: flat positioning improves blood flow velocity in acute ischemic stroke," *Neurology*, vol. 64, no. 8, pp. 1354–1357, 2005.

[6] S. Bondurant and J. B. Hickam, "Circulatory and pulmonary effects of acute central vascular engorgement in normal subjects," *Diseases of the Chest*, vol. 35, no. 1, pp. 83–87, 1959.

[7] S. Bondurant, J. B. Hickam, and J. K. Isley, "Pulmonary and circulatory effects of acute pulmonary vascular engorgement in normal subjects," *The Journal of Clinical Investigation*, vol. 36, no. 1, pp. 59–66, 1957.

[8] A. W. Alexandrov, M. Ribo, K. S. Wong, et al., "Perfusion augmentation in acute stroke using mechanical counterpulsation-phase IIa: effect of external counterpulsation on middle cerebral artery mean flow velocity in five healthy subjects," *Stroke*, vol. 39, no. 10, pp. 2760–2764, 2008.

[9] D. L. Brown, K. C. Johnston, D. P. Wagner, and E. C. Haley Jr., "Predicting major neurological improvement with intravenous recombinant tissue plasminogen activator treatment of stroke," *Stroke*, vol. 35, no. 1, pp. 147–150, 2004.

[10] G. Saposnik, S. Di Legge, F. Webster, and V. Hachinski, "Predictors of major neurologic improvement after thrombolysis in acute stroke," *Neurology*, vol. 65, no. 8, pp. 1169–1174, 2005.

[11] D. Georgiadis, O. Lanczik, S. Schwab, et al., "IV thrombolysis in patients with acute stroke due to spontaneous carotid dissection," *Neurology*, vol. 64, no. 9, pp. 1612–1614, 2005.

[12] I. Linfante, R. H. Llinas, M. Selim, et al., "Clinical and vascular outcome in internal carotid artery versus middle cerebral artery occlusions after intravenous tissue plasminogen activator," *Stroke*, vol. 33, no. 8, pp. 2066–2071, 2002.

[13] B. Guillon, V. Biousse, C. Tzourio, and M. G. Bousser, "Cervical artery dissection: recent data and pathophysiological hypothesis," *Revue de Medecine Interne*, vol. 20, no. 5, pp. 412–420, 1999.

[14] J. H. Han, T. W. Leung, W. W. Lam, et al., "Preliminary findings of external counterpulsation for ischemic stroke patient with large artery occlusive disease," *Stroke*, vol. 39, no. 4, pp. 1340–1343, 2008.

22

Impaired Emotion Recognition after Left Hemispheric Stroke: A Case Report and Brief Review of the Literature

Hugo P. Aben,[1,2] Yael D. Reijmer,[2] Johanna M. A. Visser-Meily,[3] Jacoba M. Spikman,[4] Geert Jan Biessels,[2] Paul L. M. de Kort,[1] and PROCRAS Study Group[1,2,3,4]

[1]*Department of Neurology, Elisabeth Tweesteden Hospital, Tilburg, Netherlands*
[2]*Department of Neurology, Brain Center Rudolf Magnus, University Medical Center Utrecht, Utrecht, Netherlands*
[3]*Department of Rehabilitation Medicine, Brain Center Rudolf Magnus, University Medical Center Utrecht, Utrecht, Netherlands*
[4]*Department of Clinical and Experimental Neuropsychology, University of Groningen, Groningen, Netherlands*

Correspondence should be addressed to Hugo P. Aben; h.aben@etz.nl

Academic Editor: Majaz Moonis

Impaired recognition of emotion after stroke can have important implications for social competency, social participation, and consequently quality of life. We describe a case of left hemispheric ischemic stroke with impaired recognition of specifically faces expressing fear. Three months later, the patient's spouse reports that the patient was irritable and slow in communication, which may be caused by the impaired emotion recognition. The case is discussed in relation to the literature concerning emotion recognition and its neural correlates. Our case supports the notion that emotion recognition, including fear recognition, is regulated by a network of interconnected brain regions located in both hemispheres. We conclude that impaired emotion recognition is not uncommon after stroke and can be caused by dysfunction of this emotion-network.

1. Introduction

Social cognition concerns the psychological processes by which we perceive, process, and interpret social information [1]. Nowadays, neurologists are increasingly aware of the importance of screening for deficits in social cognition [2]. For example, screening for impaired social cognition has become more common in patients with traumatic brain injury [2, 3]. After stroke, impaired social cognition is prevalent, with a reported prevalence rate of 49% [4]. Despite the high prevalence, deficits in social cognition after stroke are often overlooked by the neurologist, and it is generally not spontaneously mentioned by the patient or his caregiver.

After stroke, impaired social cognition is partly reflected by worse emotion recognition in studies that compared patients to healthy controls in tasks examining facial, prosodic, and lexical emotional stimuli [5, 6]. These studies show that impaired emotion recognition after stroke is not limited to one modality: a stroke affects general processing of emotion for different modalities.

Impaired emotion recognition after stroke has a negative influence on social participation, and it can have important implications for a patient's quality of life [7]. Moreover, it can affect social competence [8], it predicts social behavior disorders [9], and it is negatively correlated with maintenance of personal and professional relations [10, 11].

We present a case with a profound difficulty in the recognition of faces expressing fear after insular stroke. Furthermore, the case is discussed in relation to the literature concerning emotion recognition and its neural correlates.

2. Case Description

A sixty-five-year-old, right-handed man, who had just retired from his work as a detective, presented with global aphasia, agitation, and a mild paresis of his right arm, which started acutely 5 hours before admission. He had no known vascular risk factors, and he had a degree in higher vocational education. The admission CT scan of his brain revealed no signs of ischemia or hemorrhage. One day after admission, the total

Table 1: The patient's results for the "Ekman 60 Faces Test."

Emotion	Nr correct answers	Mean scores reference sample (SD)	Cutoff values
Anger	8/10	7.33 (1.90)	4
Disgust	6/10	9.00 (1.62)	6
Fear	1/10*	6.47 (2.03)	3
Happiness	10/10	9.93 (0.42)	9
Sadness	5/10	8.03 (1.66)	5
Surprise	5/10*	8.66 (1.44)	6
Total	35/60*	49.41 (4.88)	41

The mean scores, standard deviations. and cutoff values for the reference sample (aged 61–70) are derived from the FEEST manual. This sample consisted of 58 healthy participants with an IQ > 90. Cutoff values have been calculated by using the nearest integer value to a z-value of 1.65 below average [12]. *Scores below the cutoff value.

Table 2: Neuropsychological assessment of the patient.

Domain	T-score	Tests	T-scores
Attention and processing speed	46.6	Reaction Time Test, Vienna Test System, S1, S2	50.5
		Symbol Digit Modalities Test	44.2
		Trail Making Test A	41.0
(Working) memory and learning	39.2	WAIS Digit Span Forward and Backward	41.7
		The Rey Auditory Verbal Learning Test	38.0
Frontal-Executive functions	39.8	Controlled Oral Word Association Test	30.0*
		Hayling Test	40.0
		Reaction time test, Vienna Test System, S3	47.0
		Trail Making Test B	44.0
Language	31.6*	Boston Naming Test	23.1*
		Semantic fluency	40.0
Visuospatial function	NA	Bells Test, no T-score available, 1 omission	NA

This table shows the T-scores of the patient for each of the tested domains in the neuropsychological assessment. *Scores below 1.5 standard deviations.

score on the Montreal Cognitive Assessment (MoCA) was 20 out of a maximum of 30 points, mainly failing the subdomains language (0/3), delayed recall (2/5), and visuospatial function (2/5). The patient correctly copied the cube and made no mistake in the contour of the clock. However, he did not add numbers to the clock and placed the hands at ten to eleven, instead of ten past eleven. Two days after admission, the patient did not report any complaints. The aphasia, paresis, and agitation had resolved quickly, and the patient was discharged home. As part of an observational study, the PROCRAS study, see Additional Points for more information, the patient underwent a detailed neuropsychological assessment and MRI scan of his brain 4 weeks after the stroke. Apart from complaining of being tired more quickly, he had no other complaints at that point. As part of the neuropsychological assessment, the "Ekman 60 Faces Test," part of the Facial Expressions of Emotion: Stimuli and Tests (FEEST), was performed [12]. Interestingly, out of 10 presented fearful faces, he recognized only 1 facial expression correctly. For his performance on other emotions, see Table 1. His total score on the FEEST was nearly 3 standard deviations below the norm. There were no symptoms of depression or anxiety on the Hospital Anxiety and Depression Scale (HADS). Moreover, there were no signs of prosopagnosia, and the Bells Test revealed no visuospatial dysfunction. Further extensive neuropsychological testing revealed problems with naming objects on the Boston Naming Test but no impaired performance on the verbal fluency test. In Table 2, the T-scores for each domain and the subtests that constitute these domains are presented. The MRI showed a lesion of the posterior part of the left insula but also of a part of the left temporal cortex and the left parietal cortex as can be seen in Figure 1. In order to investigate potential impairments in brain connectivity, the brain network of the patient was reconstructed from the diffusion weighted MR images as described in Reijmer et al. [13]. The mean fractional anisotropy of the white matter tracts connected to each of the 90 cortical and subcortical brain regions was calculated. The brain networks of 25 age-matched healthy control participants served as a reference group. Results showed that the connectivity strength of the patient was markedly reduced (>1.5 SD lower compared to the reference sample) in several parietal, temporal, and subcortical regions, primarily in the left hemisphere (Figure 2), indicating disconnection of a network of brain regions.

Three months after the stroke, the patient felt no restrictions in his ability to perform hobbies such as gardening and reading, and he experienced no difficulties in social

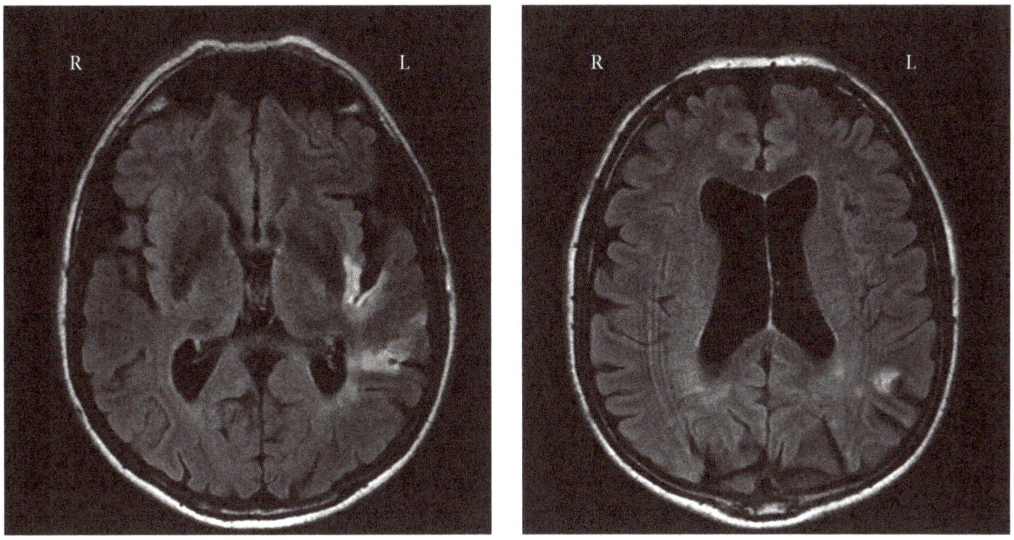

Figure 1: Transversal fluid attenuated inversion recovery (FLAIR) images of the patient, revealing a lesion to the posterior part of the insula and part of the left temporal cortex and left parietal cortex.

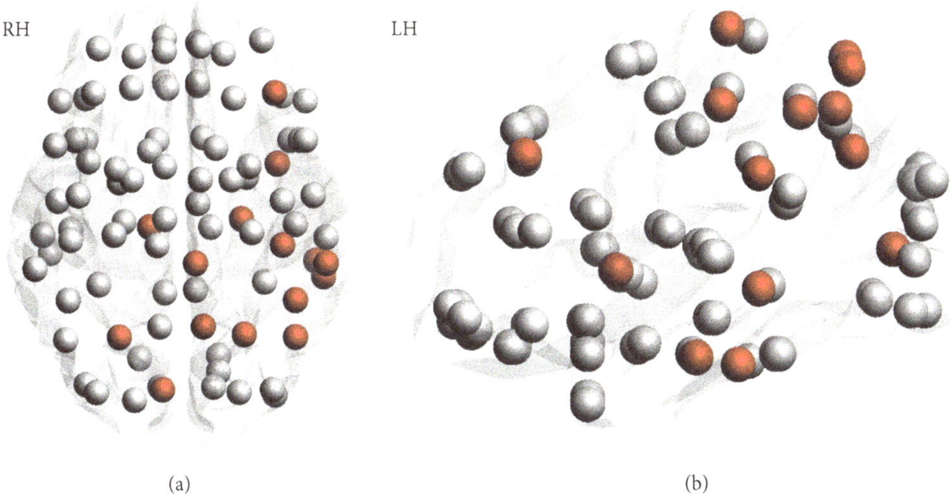

Figure 2: Axial (a) and lateral (b) view of the disconnectivity profile of the patient (obtained from analyzing the DTI-MRI data). Nodes represent 90 cortical and subcortical brain regions [38]. The red nodes indicate regions with more than 1.5 standard deviations of decreased connectivity strength compared to 25 age-matched healthy controls. Note that nodes surrounding the ischemic zone are affected. In addition, however, nodes in the contralesional hemisphere and a frontal node are affected. This suggests that the stroke affected a network of brain regions.

contact. However, his wife reported that he has been slower in communication and manifests slight irritability ever since the stroke.

3. Discussion

In this article, we present a case with a profound deficit in the recognition of facial emotions expressing fear after enduring a stroke of the posterior part of the left insula and parts of the left temporal and parietal cortex. There was no evidence of depressive or anxious symptoms on follow-up, suggesting that the difficulty in recognition of fearful faces was not caused by a depressive or anxiety disorder. It has not been ruled out that visuospatial dysfunction caused the impaired recognition of facial emotions. However, the score of 2/5 for the MoCA's visuospatial subdomain might have been caused by a language disorder rather than a visuospatial disorder. Moreover, the Bells Test revealed no abnormalities at the neuropsychological examination 4 weeks after stroke, making a neglect very unlikely. It was not clear whether our patient had difficulties in emotion recognition before the stroke, for example, due to an autism spectrum disorder or traumatic brain injury in the past. However, we think that his higher education level and his work as a detective require at least adequate social cognitive skills. Therefore, it is plausible to attribute the profound deficit in fear recognition to the stroke. This case stood out because of two reasons. First, the stroke involved the left hemisphere, while emotion recognition is generally attributed to the right hemisphere [5]. Secondly, the deficit in recognition of fearful faces after ischemia of the posterior part of the insula seems to contradict earlier findings in the literature [14–16]. Recognition of fear has been strongly linked to activity in the amygdala [16], whereas the insula is thought to be specifically engaged in the recognition of disgust [14, 15]. We will discuss the literature in relation to the case and these two findings.

3.1. Laterality in Emotion Recognition. Researchers have still not reached consensus on the specific contribution of the right and left hemisphere to emotion recognition. A recent review of many studies examining emotion recognition after stroke found more support for the hypothesis that emotion recognition seems to be largely lateralized to the right hemisphere, independent of valence [5, 17]. Several studies report that left hemispheric stroke patients perform as good as healthy controls in the recognition of emotions [18–21]. However, other studies do reveal differences in emotion recognition between patients with a left hemispheric stroke and healthy controls [22–24]. The left hemispheric stroke of our patient is in line with these studies and adds to the theory that the left hemisphere also contributes to the process of emotion recognition. According to the motoric direction theory, the left hemisphere is specialized in "approach" emotions (i.e., happiness, anger, and surprise), whereas the right hemisphere is responsible for recognizing "withdrawal" emotions (i.e., sadness, fear, and disgust) [25]. The patient had relative ease in recognizing anger and happiness, although he scored below the cutoff score for surprise. He scored relatively low for the withdrawal emotions: fear, sadness, and disgust. Although the patient does partly fit the pattern of this hypothesis, the location of the stroke would suggest that the specialization of both hemispheres is just the opposite of what the motoric direction theory suggests. Possibly, disconnectivity between both hemispheres (Figure 2) could explain this mismatch.

3.2. Neural Correlates of Emotion Recognition. Several brain structures have been suggested to be involved in emotion recognition. For example, lesions to left or right temporal cortex lead to impaired emotion recognition [26]. However, lesions to the basal ganglia [27, 28], the cerebellum [29], the thalamus [30], the right inferior parietal cortex, and the anterior infracalcarine cortex [18] can have the same consequence. It is well known that activity in the amygdala has been strongly linked to recognition of fear [16], and a lesion of the amygdala causes an impairment in fear recognition [31–33]. However, this does not imply that lesions of the amygdala are the unique cause of impaired fear recognition. For example, a study reported that a lesion to the right infracalcarine cortex also seems to lead to a specific impairment in the recognition of fear [18]. This suggests that even the recognition of one single emotion, in this case the emotion fear, is a process that involves, like all cognitive functions [34], a network of brain structures.

A meta-analysis of fMRI and PET studies [16] in healthy controls concluded that the neural network involved in recognition of emotion consists of three important structures. The first is the medial prefrontal cortex (MPFC), which has a general role in emotional processing. The other two are the anterior cingulate cortex (ACC) and the insula, which are more specifically involved in emotion recognition, especially in more cognitive demanding tasks [16].

3.3. The Insula and Emotion Recognition. Because our patient had a stroke involving, among others, the posterior part of the left insula, this specific lesion might have caused the difficulty in recognition of emotion. In behavioral and imaging studies, the insula is found to be engaged in the recognition of disgust [14, 15]. However, less is known about the consequences of a lesion to the insula. Several case studies describe different responses to an acute lesion of the left insula. In one study, a patient had impairments in global cognitive functioning as reflected by cognitive screening with the MoCA [35], comparable with the case we described. In a double case report, one patient with insular stroke had only slightly slower response times but no impaired emotion recognition [36]. The second case that is described had a subcortical stroke, disconnecting the connections from the insula to the frontal cortex. In this case, an impaired recognition of all negative emotions was found. Another study reported on a patient with behavioral changes after an isolated stroke of the anterior part of the right insula [37]. Although emotion perception was not assessed, an additional SPECT scan showed hypoperfusion in several right anterior brain structures, most of which are thought to be involved in an emotion-network.

3.4. A Matter of (Dis)connection? As stated earlier, the left insula plays a role in a network of structures involved in emotion recognition. This can be supported by a recent study in which direct electrical stimulation was applied to the left insula during awake surgery in thirteen patients causing a decreased recognition of all negative emotions [39]. Another study found that impaired emotion recognition was associated with dysfunction of a bilateral fronto-temporal-limbic network in 180 patients with traumatic brain injury (TBI) [40]. A different study found that damage anywhere to the inferior frontooccipital fasciculus or the inferior longitudinal fasciculus is associated with impaired emotion recognition [41]. The seemingly contradicting evidence of different presentations after insular stroke can be better interpreted as the consequence of disconnection to frontal or a variety of contralateral regions [42]. This implies that the process of emotion recognition is not confined to a specific location, a lesion anywhere in this "emotion-network" may lead to a deficit in emotion recognition [43].

We hypothesize that in our patient the stroke caused damage to the network involved in emotion recognition, which is supported by the analysis of the DTI-MRI data (Figure 2). Although this analysis does not provide direct evidence for emotion recognition being a network-function, it does support this theory by showing disconnection in more brain structures than those directly affected by the stroke. We propose that the profound impairment of recognition of fear can be explained by a disconnection of fibers to this emotion-network.

3.5. Impact of Impaired Emotion Recognition after Stroke. Impaired emotion recognition has been found to negatively impact social participation and quality of life after stroke [44]. For deficits in emotion regulation, the same consequences have been established [45]. The patient's spouse reported that the patient showed slight irritability and slowness in communication after the stroke, although the patient himself stated having no difficulties in social interaction. We hypothesize that the deficit in emotion recognition could partly contribute to these symptoms, and this deficit could consequently lead to restrictions in social participation.

4. Conclusions

Impaired emotion recognition is prevalent after stroke. However, it is not often reported by the patient or the caregiver, it is not easily recognized, and it is not routinely investigated in clinical practice. This is unfortunate, since impaired emotion recognition negatively impacts social participation. Detection of impaired emotion recognition may help in guidance of the patient and his caregiver. In turn, this should help people better reintegrate into daily life and increase quality of life.

Emotion recognition is a complex process involving many neural structures. A lesion anywhere in this emotion-network can lead to dysfunction. Further research on emotion recognition should shift its focus from the specific localization of emotion recognition to identifying the brain regions and the functional and structural connections that form part of this emotion-network.

Additional Points

In the Prediction of Cognitive Recovery After Stroke (PROCRAS) study, we aim to investigate the additional value of measures of structural connectivity derived from diffusion tensor imaging- (DTI-) MRI in the prediction of cognitive recovery after stroke. Patients with the clinical diagnosis of a stroke with a MoCA total score below 26 undergo a neuropsychological assessment and DTI-MRI 3–6 weeks after stroke. One year after stroke the neuropsychological assessment is repeated to assess the primary endpoint.

Conflicts of Interest

The authors declare no conflicts of interest regarding the publication of this paper.

Acknowledgments

The names of the PROCRAS study group are as follows: H. Aben, M.D. (author); P. de Kort MD, Ph.D. (author); G. J. Biessels, M.D., Ph.D. (author); A. Meily-Visser M.D., Ph.D. (author); J. Spikman, Ph.D. (author); Y. Reijmer, Ph.D. (author); J. Smetsers, M.S.; L. Luijten, M.D.; P. van de Sande; J. de Bresser, M.D., Ph.D.; M. de Groot, Ph.D.; B. Jakobs, Ph.D. The PROCRAS study is funded by ZonMW (Grant no. 842003011); Y. Reijmer receives funding from Alzheimer Nederland and ZonMw/Memorabel (Grant no. 733050503).

References

[1] J. D. Henry, W. von Hippel, P. Molenberghs, T. Lee, and P. S. Sachdev, "Clinical assessment of social cognitive function in neurological disorders," *Nature Reviews Neurology*, vol. 12, no. 1, pp. 28–39, 2016.

[2] M. R. Benedictus, J. M. Spikman, and J. Van Der Naalt, "Cognitive and behavioral impairment in traumatic brain injury related to outcome and return to work," *Archives of Physical Medicine and Rehabilitation*, vol. 91, no. 9, pp. 1436–1441, 2010.

[3] J. M. Spikman, M. E. Timmerman, M. V. Milders, W. S. Veenstra, and J. van der Naalt, "Social cognition impairments in relation to general cognitive deficits, injury severity, and prefrontal lesions in traumatic brain injury patients," *Journal of Neurotrauma*, vol. 29, no. 1, pp. 101–111, 2012.

[4] S. E. Starkstein, R. C. Leiguarda, J. P. Federoff, T. R. Price, and R. G. Robinson, "Neuropsychological and neuroradiologic correlates of emotional prosody comprehension," *Neurology*, vol. 44, no. 3, pp. 515–522, 1994.

[5] R. Yuvaraj, M. Murugappan, M. I. Norlinah, K. Sundaraj, and M. Khairiyah, "Review of emotion recognition in stroke patients," *Dementia and Geriatric Cognitive Disorders*, vol. 36, no. 3-4, pp. 179–196, 2013.

[6] J. C. Borod, L. K. Obler, H. M. Erhan et al., "Right hemisphere emotional perception: evidence across multiple channels," *Neuropsychology*, vol. 12, no. 3, pp. 446–458, 1998.

[7] K. Kim, Y. M. Kim, and E. K. Kim, "Correlation between the activities of daily living of stroke patients in a community setting and their quality of life," *Journal of Physical Therapy Science*, vol. 26, no. 3, pp. 417–419, 2014.

[8] S. L. Langer, L. C. Pettigrew, J. F. Wilson, and L. X. Blonder, "Personality and social competency following unilateral stroke," *Journal of the International Neuropsychological Society*, vol. 4, no. 5, pp. 447–455, 1998.

[9] P. Narme, M. Roussel, H. Mouras, P. Krystkowiak, and O. Godefroy, "Does impaired socioemotional functioning account for behavioral dysexecutive disorders? Evidence from a transnosological study," *Aging, Neuropsychology, and Cognition*, pp. 1–14, 2016.

[10] G. Yeates, M. Rowberry, S. Dunne et al., "Social cognition and executive functioning predictors of supervisors' appraisal of interpersonal behaviour in the workplace following acquired brain injury," *NeuroRehabilitation*, vol. 38, no. 3, pp. 299–310, 2016.

[11] L. X. Blonder, L. C. Pettigrew, and R. J. Kryscio, "Emotion recognition and marital satisfaction in stroke," *Journal of Clinical and Experimental Neuropsychology*, vol. 34, no. 6, pp. 634–642, 2012.

[12] A. Young, D. Perrett, A. Calder, R. Sprengelmeyer, and P. Ekman, *Facial Expressions of Emotion—Stimuli and Tests (FEEST)*, v.1.0, Thames Valley Test Company, v.1.0 edition, 2002.

[13] Y. D. Reijmer, A. Leemans, K. Caeyenberghs, S. M. Heringa, H. L. Koek, and G. J. Biessels, "Disruption of cerebral networks and cognitive impairment in Alzheimer disease," *Neurology*, vol. 80, no. 15, pp. 1370–1377, 2013.

[14] P. Krolak-Salmon, M.-A. Hénaff, J. Isnard et al., "An attention modulated response to disgust in human ventral anterior insula," *Annals of Neurology*, vol. 53, no. 4, pp. 446–453, 2003.

[15] R. Adolphs, D. Tranel, and A. R. Damasio, "Dissociable neural systems for recognizing emotions," *Brain and Cognition*, vol. 52, no. 1, pp. 61–69, 2003.

[16] K. L. Phan, T. Wager, S. F. Taylor, and I. Liberzon, "Functional neuroanatomy of emotion: a meta-analysis of emotion activation studies in PET and fMRI," *NeuroImage*, vol. 16, no. 2, pp. 331–348, 2002.

[17] J. C. Borod, "Interhemispheric and intrahemispheric control of emotion: a focus on unilateral brain damage," *Journal of Consulting and Clinical Psychology*, vol. 60, no. 3, pp. 339–348, 1992.

[18] R. Adolphs, H. Damasio, D. Tranel, and A. R. Damasio, "Cortical systems for the recognition of emotion in facial expressions," *Journal of Neuroscience*, vol. 16, no. 23, pp. 7678–7687, 1996.

[19] D. Bowers, R. M. Bauer, H. B. Coslett, and K. M. Heilman, "Processing of faces by patients with unilateral hemisphere lesions. I. Dissociation between judgments of facial affect and facial identity," *Brain and Cognition*, vol. 4, no. 3, pp. 258–272, 1985.

[20] S. Charbonneau, B. P. Scherzer, D. Aspirot, and H. Cohen, "Perception and production of facial and prosodic emotions by chronic CVA patients," *Neuropsychologia*, vol. 41, no. 5, pp. 605–613, 2003.

[21] J. J. Schmitt, W. Hartje, and K. Willmes, "Hemispheric asymmetry in the recognition of emotional attitude conveyed by facial expression, prosody and propositional speech," *Cortex*, vol. 33, no. 1, pp. 65–81, 1997.

[22] K. Kucharska-Pietura, M. L. Phillips, W. Gernand, and A. S. David, "Perception of emotions from faces and voices following unilateral brain damage," *Neuropsychologia*, vol. 41, no. 8, pp. 1082–1090, 2003.

[23] M. K. Mandal, J. C. Borod, H. S. Asthana, A. Mohanty, S. Mohanty, and E. Koff, "Effects of lesion variables and emotion type on the perception of facial emotion," *Journal of Nervous and Mental Disease*, vol. 187, no. 10, pp. 603–609, 1999.

[24] M. Peper and E. Irle, "The decoding of emotional concepts in patients with focal cerebral lesions," *Brain and Cognition*, vol. 34, no. 3, pp. 360–387, 1997.

[25] R. J. Davidson, P. Ekman, C. D. Saron, J. A. Senulis, and W. V. Friesen, "Approach-withdrawal and cerebral asymmetry: emotional expression and brain physiology I," *Journal of Personality and Social Psychology*, vol. 58, no. 2, pp. 330–341, 1990.

[26] C. Xi, Y. Zhu, C. Zhu, D. Song, Y. Wang, and K. Wang, "Deficit of theory of mind after temporal lobe cerebral infarction," *Behavioral and Brain Functions*, vol. 9, no. 1, article 15, 2013.

[27] J. Kemp, M.-C. Berthel, A. Dufour et al., "Caudate nucleus and social cognition: neuropsychological and SPECT evidence from a patient with focal caudate lesion," *Cortex*, vol. 49, no. 2, pp. 559–571, 2013.

[28] C. C. Y. Cheung, T. M. C. Lee, J. T. H. Yip, K. E. King, and L. S. W. Li, "The differential effects of thalamus and basal ganglia on facial emotion recognition," *Brain and Cognition*, vol. 61, no. 3, pp. 262–268, 2006.

[29] M. Adamaszek, K. C. Kirkby, F. Dagata et al., "Neural correlates of impaired emotional face recognition in cerebellar lesions," *Brain Research*, vol. 1613, pp. 1–12, 2015.

[30] E. Wilkos, T. J. B. Brown, K. Slawinska, and K. Akucharska, "Social cognitive and neurocognitive deficits in inpatients with unilateral thalamic lesions—pilot study," *Neuropsychiatric Disease and Treatment*, vol. 11, pp. 1031–1038, 2015.

[31] R. Adolphs, F. Gosselin, T. W. Buchanan, D. Tranel, P. Schyns, and A. R. Damasio, "A mechanism for impaired fear recognition after amygdala damage," *Nature*, vol. 433, no. 7021, pp. 68–72, 2005.

[32] D. R. Bach, R. Hurlemann, and R. J. Dolan, "Impaired threat prioritisation after selective bilateral amygdala lesions," *Cortex*, vol. 63, pp. 206–213, 2015.

[33] D. Dellacherie, D. Hasboun, M. Baulac, P. Belin, and S. Samson, "Impaired recognition of fear in voices and reduced anxiety after unilateral temporal lobe resection," *Neuropsychologia*, vol. 49, no. 4, pp. 618–629, 2011.

[34] H.-J. Park and K. Friston, "Structural and functional brain networks: from connections to cognition," *Science*, vol. 342, no. 6158, Article ID 1238411, 2013.

[35] P. Julayanont, D. Ruthirago, and J. C. DeToledo, "Isolated left posterior insular infarction and convergent roles in verbal fluency, language, memory, and executive function," *Proceedings (Baylor University Medical Center)*, vol. 29, no. 3, pp. 295–297, 2016.

[36] B. Couto, L. Sedeño, L. A. Sposato et al., "Insular networks for emotional processing and social cognition: comparison of two case reports with either cortical or subcortical involvement," *Cortex*, vol. 49, no. 5, pp. 1420–1434, 2013.

[37] H.-J. Cho, S.-J. Kim, S. J. Hwang et al., "Social-emotional dysfunction after isolated right anterior insular infarction," *Journal of Neurology*, vol. 259, no. 4, pp. 764–767, 2012.

[38] N. Tzourio-Mazoyer, B. Landeau, D. Papathanassiou et al., "Automated anatomical labeling of activations in SPM using a macroscopic anatomical parcellation of the MNI MRI single-subject brain," *NeuroImage*, vol. 15, no. 1, pp. 273–289, 2002.

[39] C. Papagno, A. Pisoni, G. Mattavelli et al., "Specific disgust processing in the left insula: new evidence from direct electrical stimulation," *Neuropsychologia*, vol. 84, pp. 29–35, 2016.

[40] O. Dal Monte, F. Krueger, J. M. Solomon et al., "A voxel-based lesion study on facial emotion recognition after penetrating brain injury," *Social Cognitive and Affective Neuroscience*, vol. 8, no. 6, pp. 632–639, 2013.

[41] C. L. Philippi, S. Mehta, T. Grabowski, R. Adolphs, and D. Rudrauf, "Damage to association fiber tracts impairs recognition of the facial expression of emotion," *Journal of Neuroscience*, vol. 29, no. 48, pp. 15089–15099, 2009.

[42] R. Limongi, A. Tomio, and A. Ibanez, "Dynamical predictions of insular hubs for social cognition and their application to stroke," *Frontiers in Behavioral Neuroscience*, vol. 8, article 380, 2014.

[43] D. P. Kennedy and R. Adolphs, "The social brain in psychiatric and neurological disorders," *Trends in Cognitive Sciences*, vol. 16, no. 11, pp. 559–572, 2012.

[44] C. L. Cooper, L. H. Phillips, M. Johnston, B. Radlak, S. Hamilton, and M. J. McLeod, "Links between emotion perception and social participation restriction following stroke," *Brain Injury*, vol. 28, no. 1, pp. 122–126, 2014.

[45] C. L. Cooper, L. H. Phillips, M. Johnston, M. Whyte, and M. J. Macleod, "The role of emotion regulation on social participation following stroke," *British Journal of Clinical Psychology*, vol. 54, no. 2, pp. 181–199, 2015.

23

Cardiac Fibroelastoma versus Thrombus: Echocardiographic Evidence can be Misleading

John P. O'Laughlin,[1] Gautam Verma,[1] and Iosif Gulkarov[2,3]

[1]*Department of Internal Medicine, New York Methodist Hospital, 506 6th Street, Brooklyn, NY 11215, USA*
[2]*Department of Cardiothoracic Surgery, New York Methodist Hospital, 263 7th Avenue, Brooklyn, NY 11215, USA*
[3]*Department of Cardiothoracic Surgery, Weill Cornell Medicine, 68th Street M404, New York, NY 10021, USA*

Correspondence should be addressed to Iosif Gulkarov; gulkai01@yahoo.com

Academic Editor: Saadeh Al-Jureidini

We present a case of a young female with stroke symptoms who underwent valve sparing resection of a presumed fibroelastoma based on echocardiographic findings. After confirming embolic stroke, she underwent excision of the lesion, which on pathology revealed a nonbacterial thrombus. Ultimately, this led to a more extensive work-up leading to the discovery of a papillary serous ovarian carcinoma, the underlying cause of her hypercoagulable state. The initial echocardiographic findings painted the clear picture of a papillary tumor on the aortic valve which was likely the source of the emboli resulting in ischemic stroke. This unique case presentation illustrates that imaging, including echocardiography, may not always coincide with the clinical diagnosis. Thus, understanding the differential diagnoses of cardiac masses is of vital clinical significance. The distinction of fibroelastoma versus the much less common finding of aortic thrombus may lead to early diagnosis of malignancy and prevention of life threatening events due to stroke or undiagnosed disease.

1. Introduction

The incidence of primary cardiac tumors is rare with the top three most common tumors consisting of myxomas, lipomas, and fibroelastomas (in order of respective occurrence) [1–3]. Fibroelastomas are described as having a papillary structure and may be found throughout the endocardial tissues, with an affinity for valvular structures [4]. Clinical presentation of this tumor can vary with most patients presenting asymptomatic with incidental finding on echocardiography. Location of the tumor can impact clinical presentation. Tumors on the right side of the heart are commonly asymptomatic or patients may present with pulmonary emboli [5], whereas left sided tumors can result in life threatening embolic phenomena [5]. This is a result of the fragile nature of the tumor's composition and their high affinity for platelet aggregation [5].

Echocardiography remains the cornerstone for identification of cardiac tumors, but the diagnosis based on imaging is not always definitive. Cardiac masses have variations in shape and size making it difficult to diagnose a tumor versus a thrombus based on imaging findings and clinical presentation. The sensitivity and specificity have been estimated to be near 90% when using transthoracic echocardiography in diagnosis of papillary fibroelastoma if tumor size is greater than 2 mm [5]. However, there is still room for an alternative diagnosis. We present a unique case of a presumed aortic valve fibroelastoma that after valve sparing excision turned out to be a nonbacterial thrombus.

2. Case

A 26-year-old previously healthy female presented to emergency department with complaints of headaches for two weeks associated with right sided numbness, weakness, diplopia, facial droop, dysarthria, and ataxia. The patient underwent work-up for a cerebral vascular accident. MRI confirmed the diagnosis of acute stroke involving the left posterior cerebral artery territory with smaller foci of ischemia in

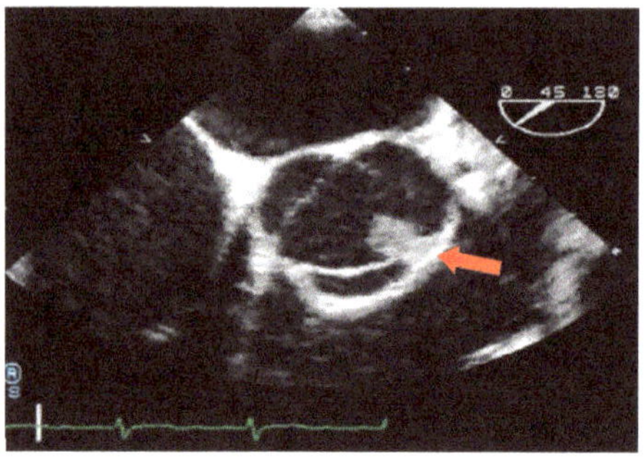

FIGURE 1: Transesophageal echocardiograph illustrating large, papillary, solid, fixed mass, measuring 7 × 7 mm on the left coronary cusp, on the left ventricular aspect of the aortic valve.

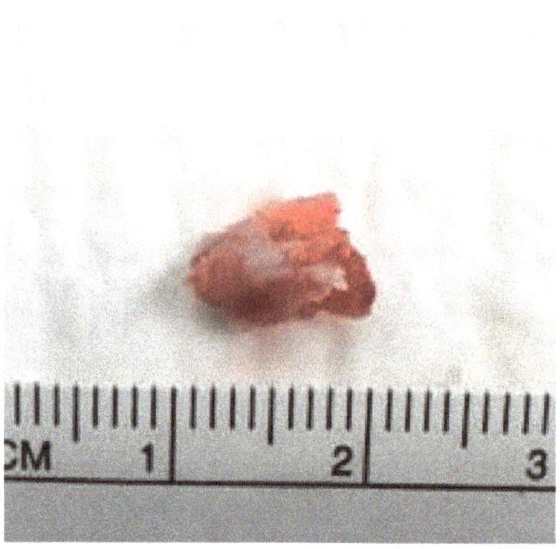

FIGURE 2: Mass surgically excised from left coronary cusp of aortic valve, approximately 9 × 5 mm. Pathology consistent with thrombus.

various cerebral territories, consistent with embolic phenomena. Transesophageal echocardiography revealed a large, papillary, solid, fixed mass, measuring 7 × 7 mm on the left coronary cusp (Figure 1) of the aortic valve that was suspected to be an aortic fibroelastoma due to its papillary structure and size. She underwent valve sparing excision of the fibroelastoma (Figure 2). Pathology later returned consistent with thrombus. The patient was recommended to have a hypercoagulable work-up as an outpatient but was lost to follow-up.

Four months after the initial surgery she presented with complaints of left lower quadrant abdominal pain, described as sharp and stabbing in nature. CT scan of the abdomen and pelvis revealed massive ascites. Recommended correlation study with transvaginal ultrasound was conducted and revealed a complex mass of mixed echogenicity with mildly increased vascularity measuring 7.6 × 7.2 × 9.0 cm, located posterior to the uterus and extending to the right adnexa. Biopsy of the lesion revealed adenocarcinoma. She went on to undergo bilateral salpingooophorectomy, omentectomy, lysis of adhesions, and peritoneal biopsies confirming a final diagnosis of papillary serous ovarian carcinoma, Stage IIc.

3. Discussion

Stroke-like symptoms in otherwise healthy young adults can be very alarming. Initial assessment involves multiple brain imaging modalities before a suspected diagnosis is made, as strokes can be ischemic or hemorrhagic in nature. Cardiac emboli are a common source of ischemic stroke and may be the result of bacterial or nonbacterial thrombi, or cardiac tumors. Due to the vast differential of cardiac masses, assessment and diagnosis pose a challenging task for physicians, especially cardiac tumors. Nonneoplastic processes such as thrombus and valvular vegetations can mimic tumors; therefore physicians should consider them as part of the differential diagnosis.

Cardiac tumors can be categorized into primary cardiac neoplasms or metastatic deposits from other remote primary neoplasms; most commonly breast, lung, lymphomas, melanomas, and renal tumors [6]. Primary cardiac neoplasms can be either benign or malignant. The most common malignant tumors include angiosarcoma and rhabdomyosarcoma. Benign lesions include myxomas, lipomas, and fibroelastomas and represent the most frequent type of intracardiac lesions [1–3]. Myxomas are the most common benign primary cardiac tumor seen in patients 30–60 years of age with increased incidence in women [7]. Myxomas are solitary tumors which arise from the interatrial septum normally within the left atrium [8, 9]. Lipomas are the second most common tumor, occurring in middle to late adulthood, composed of adipocytes, and occur in all chambers within the heart [10, 11]. Fibroelastomas are the third most common tumor, also presenting in middle to late adulthood [11]. They are commonly described as having a papillary structure and can arise from any endocardial surface, but most are found on the aortic or mitral valves [4, 11].

The occurrence of primary cardiac neoplasms is rare and diagnosed in about 0.001–0.03% of echocardiographic studies, reported by Sutsch et al., 1991, based an analysis of 20,305 echocardiographs [12]. Transthoracic or transesophageal echocardiography is the primary imaging modality in initial work-up of cardiac tumors. Transthoracic echocardiography (TTE) is a convenient imaging modality as it is cost effective, noninvasive, and provides efficient results. Within minutes clinicians have vital information regarding the shape, size, mobility, and precise location of masses within the heart [13]. Transesophageal echocardiography (TEE), though similar to TTE, provides clinicians with superior imaging when compared to TTE due to better acoustic windows resulting from lack of signal loss from penetration through adjacent thoracic wall and lung structures [14]. As a result, better visualization helps to identify morphology of smaller cardiac tumors, less than 5 mm, that may otherwise be missed on TTE [14]. TEE is more invasive and requires mild anesthesia. TEE is usually only warranted if there is a high clinical suspicion for a cardiac mass not seen on TTE or lack of identifiable characteristics of a mass on TTE due to poor acoustic windows [6]. Enhancement of masses during echocardiography with the use of a contrast medium may help to further elucidate whether a cardiac mass is a tumor or thrombus [6, 15]. However, this is only beneficial if the tumor is of malignant origin as these tumors are highly vascularized and will enhance on imaging [6, 15, 16]. The use of contrast echocardiography in distinguishing between benign cardiac tumors and thrombi provides no clinical benefit and is unreliable due to their lack of vascularity and enhancement [6, 16].

Treatment of cardiac masses normally depends on the clinical presentation and type of tumor. There is no defined protocol nor evidence based approach to treating these patients; thus clinical judgement in coordination with imagery must be utilized. Benign tumors, including papillary fibroelastomas, are commonly surgically excised due to the high risk of embolic phenomena [17]. On the other hand, malignant tumors typically have poor outcomes despite surgical intervention due to metastatic disease and high rates of recurrence [6, 18].

Our patient presented with stroke due to thromboembolic disease from aortic valve vegetation that was believed to be a papillary fibroelastoma due to its papillary structure on echocardiography and patient's lack of clinical evidence of bacterial endocarditis. TTE and TEE studies revealed findings consistent with a large papillary lesion. Due to the acute risk of further embolic phenomena valve sparing excision was performed revealing a nonbacterial thrombus. Even with the use of contrast echocardiography or cardiac MRI, we would not have been able to differentiate between thrombus and papillary fibroelastoma [19]. Therefore, the benefits of pursuing excision outweighed the risk of surgery as the patient was at high risk for potentially fatal stroke events.

4. Conclusion

Echocardiographic imaging can only provide limited information on the characteristic morphology of cardiac masses, with further contribution to pathologic etiology improved with use of contrast echocardiography or cardiac MRI (limited availability at most institutions). Despite clinical objective evidence supporting benign cardiac tumor etiology (i.e., TEE study consistent with papillary fibroelastoma), one must take the entire clinical picture into account before pursuing invasive surgical procedures. This unique case provides an example that medicine and surgery is not always "textbook" in nature. Even though the echocardiographic evidence supported our clinical suspicion, pathologic analysis did not coincide. Further investigative research must be done to help clinicians and surgeons diagnostically differentiate benign cardiac tumors (myxomas, papillary fibroelastomas, and lipomas) from the less commonly occurring native aortic thrombus. We also recommend that when aortic thrombi are suspected or discovered on imaging, an age-appropriate malignancy work-up should be performed as approximately 15% of cancer patients may have thromboembolic events throughout their disease process [20].

Abbreviations

TTE: Transthoracic echocardiograph
TEE: Transesophageal echocardiograph
MRI: Magnetic Resonance Imaging.

Competing Interests

The authors declare that there are no competing interests regarding the publication of this paper.

References

[1] F. H. Edwards, D. Hale, A. Cohen, L. Thompson, A. T. Pezzella, and R. Virmani, "Primary cardiac valve tumors," *The Annals of Thoracic Surgery*, vol. 52, no. 5, pp. 1127–1131, 1991.

[2] S. Moustafa, C. Sauvé, P. Pagé, and K. Serri, "Incidental finding of a papillary fibroelastoma of the mitral valve chordae," *European Journal of Echocardiography*, vol. 9, no. 5, pp. 745–746, 2008.

[3] A. Al-Mohammad, H. Pambakian, and C. Young, "Fibroelastoma: case report and review of the literature," *Heart*, vol. 79, no. 3, pp. 301–304, 1998.

[4] R. M. Gowda, I. A. Khan, C. K. Nair, N. J. Mehta, B. C. Vasavada, and T. J. Sacchi, "Cardiac papillary fibroelastoma: a comprehensive analysis of 725 cases," *American Heart Journal*, vol. 146, no. 3, pp. 404–410, 2003.

[5] N. Bouhzam, B. Kurtz, F. Doguet, H. Eltchaninoff, and F. Bauer, "Incidental Papillary fibroelastoma: multimodal imaging and surgical decisions in 2 patients," *Texas Heart Institute Journal*, vol. 39, no. 5, pp. 731–735, 2012.

[6] I. A. Paraskevaidis, C. A. Michalakeas, C. H. Papadopoulos, and M. Anastasiou-Nana, "Cardiac tumors," *ISRN Oncology*, vol. 2011, Article ID 208929, 5 pages, 2011.

[7] P. A. Araoz, S. L. Mulvagh, H. D. Tazelaar, P. R. Julsrud, and J. F. Breen, "CT and MR imaging of benign primary cardiac neoplasms with echocardiographic correlation," *Radiographics*, vol. 20, no. 5, pp. 1303–1319, 2000.

[8] A. Burke and R. Virmani, "Tumors of the heart and great vessels," in *Atlas of Tumor Pathology*, Armed Forces Institute of Pathology, Washington, DC, USA, 3rd edition, 1996.

[9] K. Reynen, "Cardiac myxomas," *The New England Journal of Medicine*, vol. 333, no. 24, pp. 1610–1617, 1995.

[10] D. H. O'Donnell, S. Abbara, V. Chaithiraphan et al., "Cardiac tumors: optimal cardiac MR sequences and spectrum of imaging appearances," *American Journal of Roentgenology*, vol. 193, no. 2, pp. 377–387, 2009.

[11] D. Kassop, M. S. Donovan, M. K. Cheezum et al., "Cardiac masses on cardiac CT: a review," *Current Cardiovascular Imaging Reports*, vol. 7, no. 8, article 9281, 2014.

[12] G. Sutsch, R. Jenni, L. von Segesser, and J. Schneider, "Heart tumors: incidence, distribution, diagnosis. Exemplified by 20,305 echocardiographies," *Schweizerische Medizinische Wochenschrift*, vol. 121, no. 17, pp. 621–629, 1991.

[13] G. Gulati, S. Sharma, S. S. Kothari, R. Juneja, A. Saxena, and K. K. Talwar, "Comparison of echo and MRI in the imaging evaluation of intracardiac masses," *CardioVascular and Interventional Radiology*, vol. 27, no. 5, pp. 459–469, 2004.

[14] H. P. Kühl and P. Hanrath, "The impact of transesophageal echocardiography on daily clinical practice," *European Journal of Echocardiography*, vol. 5, no. 6, pp. 455–468, 2004.

[15] S. L. Mulvagh, H. Rakowski, M. A. Vannan et al., "American society of echocardiography consensus statement on the clinical applications of ultrasonic contrast agents in echocardiography," *Journal of the American Society of Echocardiography*, vol. 21, no. 11, pp. 1179–1201, 2008.

[16] J. N. Kirkpatrick, T. Wong, J. E. Bednarz et al., "Differential diagnosis of cardiac masses using contrast echocardiographic perfusion imaging," *Journal of the American College of Cardiology*, vol. 43, no. 8, pp. 1412–1419, 2004.

[17] N. K. Jha, M. Khouri, D. M. Murphy et al., "Papillary fibroelastoma of the aortic valve—a case report and literature review," *Journal of Cardiothoracic Surgery*, vol. 5, article 84, 2010.

[18] M. Hirota, N. Ishikawa, M. Oi, and T. Tedoriya, "Large primary cardiac sarcoma on the left ventricular free wall: is total excision contraindicated?" *Interactive Cardiovascular and Thoracic Surgery*, vol. 11, no. 5, pp. 670–672, 2010.

[19] J. Barkhausen, P. Hunold, H. Eggebrecht et al., "Detection and characterization of intracardiac thrombi on MR imaging," *American Journal of Roentgenology*, vol. 179, no. 6, pp. 1539–1544, 2002.

[20] S. R. Deitcher, "Cancer and thrombosis: mechanisms and treatment," *Journal of Thrombosis and Thrombolysis*, vol. 16, no. 1-2, pp. 21–31, 2003.

24

Giant Left Ventricular Thrombus in a Patient with Acute Ischemic Stroke: A Case Report and Minireview

Fan Ye,[1,2] Burton V. Silverstein,[3] Matheen A. Khuddus,[3] Christopher L. Bray,[1,2] and Arthur C. Lee[3]

[1]*College of Medicine, University of Central Florida, Orlando, FL 32827, USA*
[2]*Department of Medicine and Graduate Medical Education, North Florida Regional Medical Center, Gainesville, FL 32605, USA*
[3]*North Florida Regional Medical Center, The Cardiac and Vascular Institute, Gainesville, FL 32605, USA*

Correspondence should be addressed to Fan Ye; fan.ye@ucf.edu

Academic Editor: Tayfun Sahin

A 56-year-old healthy male with no obvious risk factors or significant past medical history was admitted to the emergency room with acute ischemic stroke. On his transthoracic echocardiography (TTE), an extremely large thrombus was detected at the apex involving the distal anterior wall. The thrombus was predominantly adherent but with a mobile tip. The patient was subsequently managed with dual antiplatelet therapy. In this report, we present an interesting case of an acute ischemic stroke secondary to a giant left ventricular thrombus in a patient with no past significant cardiac or neurologic medical history.

1. Introduction

Left ventricular thrombus was one of the most feared complications in patients with severe ischemic heart disease including myocardial infarction (MI) or left ventricular (LV) aneurysm [1]. Protrusion and mobility of thrombus carry a high risk for recurrent embolic strokes. The majority of reported cases of left ventricular thrombus were complications of acute MI, though it is a relatively rare complication in this day and age of expeditious revascularization but can be devastating if not diagnosed early on. However, the data on patients with large LV thrombus but without cardiac or thrombotic history are deficient.

2. Case Presentation

A 56-year-old Caucasian male patient with no past significant medical history or thrombotic medication use presented to the hospital with right arm weakness, slurred speech, and vertigo continuing for less than 24 hours. He had never been a smoker or illicit drug user. He was physically active and only drank socially. He had no family history of cardiovascular, pulmonary, or hypercoagulable diseases.

In his initial evaluation, brain computer tomography (CT) showed acute/subacute infarct of the right posterior frontal region, brain magnetic resonance imaging (MRI) confirmed acute infarct in the left inferior frontal/suprasylvian region, and head/neck CT angiography (CTA) scan revealed no evidence for large vessel occlusion or visualized intraluminal clot. He was admitted to the neurological unit with a diagnosis of ischemic stroke and was treated with dual antiplatelet therapy using aspirin and clopidogrel. The ECG revealed sinus rhythm with frequent premature ventricular complexes and low-voltage QRS (Figure 1). The lipid panel was normal as well as kidney and liver function. Transthoracic echocardiography (TTE) detected anterior and apical wall akinesias with an LV ejection fraction (EF) of 25–30%, structurally normal valves, and an extremely large thrombus (10 cm × 12 cm) invading the apex and distal anterior wall which was predominantly adherent but with a mobile tip (Figure 2). Troponin × 3 was negative, and coagulability workup was within normal range. Subsequent myocardial perfusion imaging revealed severe hypokinesis involving the mid and apical anterior, mid anteroseptal, basal and mid inferoseptal, and basal, mid, and apical inferior wall of the left ventricle, consistent with infarction in the distribution of multiple vessels, with partial viability.

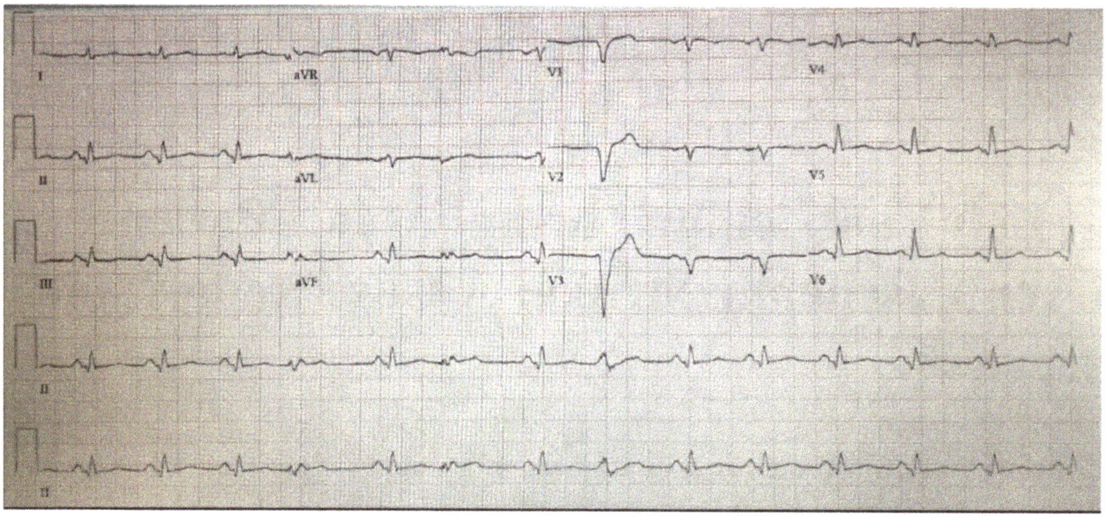

Figure 1: EKG at admission showing sinus rhythm with frequent premature ventricular complexes and low-voltage QRS.

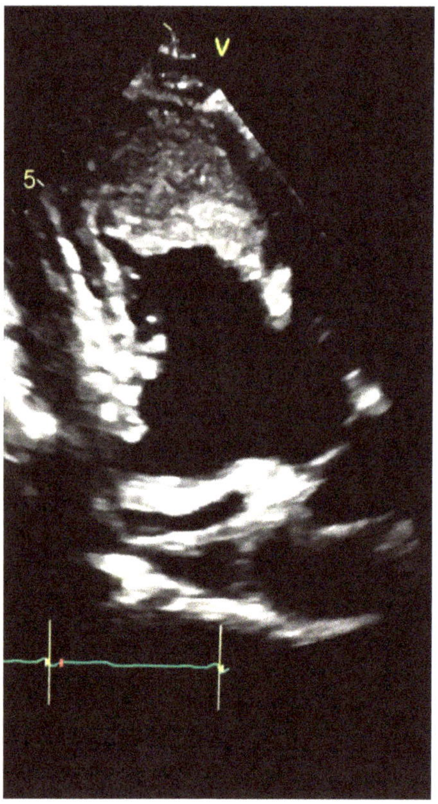

Figure 2: Transthoracic echocardiogram showing the left ventricle filled with thrombus.

Both the cardiovascular surgeon and cardiologist agreed that the majority of the thrombus appeared densely adherent with only a small portion being somewhat mobile on echocardiography and determined the risk of myocardial resection with surgery outweighed the benefits. As a result, the patient was managed medically with aspirin 325 mg daily, clopidogrel 75 mg daily, and apixaban 5 mg bid. In addition, carvedilol 6.25 mg bid and lisinopril 10 mg daily were initiated for treatment of the ischemic cardiomyopathy. The patient was discharged three days later without any medicine side effects. We recommended a renal profile, complete blood count in three days, and TTE monthly.

3. Discussion

In our patient, no particular features were encountered to suggest cardiac or vascular etiology to the stroke, yet a large thrombus was detected.

The rare incidence of left ventricular thrombus has been reported in other diseases, including takotsubo cardiomyopathy [2], heparin-induced thrombocytopenia [3], Behçet disease [4], and disseminated intravascular coagulation [5]. There are limited data as to the exact frequency of LV thrombus in patients with ischemic stroke, but it has been reported to be about 2.4% in symptomatic patients by transesophageal echocardiography [6]. However, most of these studies were retrospective, nonserial, or autopsy reports. Although our patient had no significant past medical history, we speculate that his LV thrombus was secondary to his ischemic cardiomyopathy. The thrombus became firmly attached to the left ventricle, enhancing the underlying myocardial scar, limiting potential infarct expansion, and partially protecting against LV rupture. As a consequence, the patient had no symptoms until the tip of the thrombus became mobile and occluded his CNS perfusion.

Thrombi in the heart occur predominantly in males and are accompanied with ischemic or nonischemic cardiomyopathy including valvular abnormalities, arrhythmias, thromboembolism, pericarditis, and myocarditis [7]. We have recently reported that the lack of mobility is one of the key factors in most risk assessment models of thromboembolism [8]. In our patient, potential underlying myocardial ischemia caused subendothelial injury with inflammatory changes, and left ventricle regional wall akinesia resulted in blood stasis. This combination contributed to the in vivo thrombus formation [9].

The optimal management of large and pedunculated left ventricular thrombus is still controversial, especially those with low LVEF. The management is particularly challenging in patients with high bleeding risk. New oral anticoagulants (dabigatran, rivaroxaban, apixaban, etc.) have been reported in successfully treating left venous thrombus, without having limitations of vitamin K antagonists which include slow onset of action, regular monitoring, and need for dose adjustments [10]. Further evidence demonstrated that new oral anticoagulants were found to be noninferior or superior compared to warfarin in prevention of thromboembolism in patients with nonvalvular atrial fibrillation [11]. Surgical removal is generally recommended for mobile thrombi due to a significant increase in embolization risk. However, deterioration of LV function, introduction of ventricular arrhythmia, and potential dissection of the left ventricle are all serious complications related to surgery [12–14].

4. Conclusion

Although the reported incidence of LV thrombus which is most often seen in patients with MI has reduced significantly in the past decade with the advancement of new medications or intracardiac devices, early detection and treatment of LV thrombus in patients without past cardiac or thrombotic medical history may cause substantial variation in the reported mortality rates. Our patient had a giant LV thrombus, and his future potential risk for another systemic embolization was thought to be high. Therefore, prompt recognition and appropriate treatment of LV thrombus formation are essential to avoid deterioration of LV function and other severe complications in non-MI patients.

Consent

Informed consent was obtained from the patient.

Conflicts of Interest

The authors report no conflicts of interest regarding the content herein.

Acknowledgments

The authors thank Ms. Marquez Megan and Dr. Hale Toklu for their assistance in proofreading the manuscript.

References

[1] J. V. Nixon, "Left ventricular mural thrombus," *Archives of Internal Medicine*, vol. 143, no. 8, pp. 1567–1571, 1983.

[2] H. Herath, S. Pahalagamage, L. C. Lindsay et al., "Takotsubo cardiomyopathy complicated with apical thrombus formation on first day of the illness: a case report and literature review," *BMC Cardiovascular Disorders*, vol. 17, no. 1, p. 176, 2017.

[3] G. T. Stavridis, M. Vasili, H. Ashrafian, T. Athanasiou, E. Melissari, and A. Manginas, "Trans-aortic endoscopic ventricular thrombectomy in a patient with HIT and concomitant aortic and ventricular thromboses," *General Thoracic and Cardiovascular Surgery*, vol. 64, no. 10, pp. 621–624, 2016.

[4] T. Lisitsyna, Z. Alekberova, P. Ovcharov, A. Volkov, J. Korsakova, and E. Nasonov, "Left ventricular intracardiac thrombus in a patient with Behçet disease successfully treated with immunosuppressive agents without anticoagulation: a case report and review of the literature," *Rheumatology International*, vol. 35, no. 11, pp. 1931–1935, 2015.

[5] D. Belov, R. Lyubarova, S. Fein, and M. Torosoff, "Disseminated intravascular coagulation with congestive heart failure and left ventricular thrombus: a case report with literature review of 7 cases," *American Journal of Case Reports*, vol. 16, p. 53, 2015.

[6] R. P. Ward, C. W. Don, K. T. Furlong, and R. M. Lang, "Predictors of long-term mortality in patients with ischemic stroke referred for transesophageal echocardiography," *Stroke*, vol. 37, no. 1, pp. 204–208, 2006.

[7] J. M. Lee, J. J. Park, H. W. Jung et al., "Left ventricular thrombus and subsequent thromboembolism, comparison of anticoagulation, surgical removal, and antiplatelet agents," *Journal of Atherosclerosis and Thrombosis*, vol. 20, no. 1, pp. 73–93, 2013.

[8] F. Ye, C. Stalvey, M. A. Khuddus et al., "A systematic review of mobility/immobility in thromboembolism risk assessment models for hospitalized patients," *Journal of Thrombosis and Thrombolysis*, vol. 44, no. 1, pp. 94–103, 2017.

[9] L. Chi, S. Rebello, and B. Lucchesi, "In vivo models of thrombosis," in *Antithrombotics*, pp. 101–127, Springer-Verlag, Heidelberg, Berlin, Germany, 1999.

[10] E. Yildirim, K. Kalkan, E. Ipek, S. Demirelli, and E. Ermiş, "Successful resolution of left ventricular thrombus with apixaban treatment," *International Journal of the Cardiovascular Academy*, vol. 2, no. 2, pp. 57-58, 2016.

[11] C. January, L. Wann, J. Alpert et al., "AHA/ACC/HRS guideline for the management of patients with atrial fibrillation: a report of the American College of Cardiology/American Heart Association Task Force on Practice Guidelines and the Heart Rhythm Society," *Circulation*, vol. 114, no. 7, pp. e257–e354, 2014.

[12] M. Nili, E. Deviri, R. Jortner, B. Strasberg, and M. J. Levy, "Surgical removal of a mobile, pedunculated left ventricular thrombus: report of 4 cases," *Annals of Thoracic Surgery*, vol. 46, no. 4, pp. 396–400, 1988.

[13] J. H. Kuh and Y. Seo, "Transatrial resection of a left ventricular thrombus after acute myocarditis," *Heart and Vessels*, vol. 20, no. 5, pp. 230–232, 2005.

[14] I. L. Mazza, J. P. Jacobs, A. Aldousany, A. C. Chang, and R. P. Burke, "Video-assisted cardioscopy for left ventricular thrombectomy in a child," *Annals of Thoracic Surgery*, vol. 66, no. 1, pp. 248–250, 1996.

25

Case of Stroke from Cerebral Vasculitis following Carfilzomib, Lenalidomide, and Dexamethasone Therapy in a Patient with Relapsing Multiple Myeloma

Deborah Osafehinti and Kaveh Zivari

Department of Internal Medicine, Maimonides Medical Center, Brooklyn, NY, USA

Correspondence should be addressed to Deborah Osafehinti; dosafehinti@maimonidesmed.org

Academic Editor: Sergio Storti

Lenalidomide, a synthetic derivation of thalidomide, in recent years, has been the backbone of multiple myeloma treatment leading to improved survival. Common adverse effects from lenalidomide-based regimens include hypertension, heart disease, and venous thromboembolism. Hence, thromboprophylaxis is recommended to reduce the risk of stroke. We report a case of stroke from cerebral vasculitis in a patient receiving carfilzomib, lenalidomide, and dexamethasone for relapsing multiple myeloma, not previously published. Medical oncologists should be aware of other causes of stroke among multiple myeloma patients receiving a lenalidomide-based regimen to prevent its occurrence.

1. Introduction

Multiple myeloma (MM) is a hematological malignancy characterized by the neoplastic proliferation of plasma cells leading to monoclonal immunoglobulin production [1–3]. It accounts for 10 to 15% of all hematological malignancies [2, 4], and in the United States, there are more than 20,000 new cases of multiple myeloma every year [4]. Treatment choice is mainly dependent on the functional status of the patient and the aggressiveness of the disease. These include autologous stem cell transplant (for those who are transplant eligible) and chemotherapy [3, 4]. The overall survival rates and treatment response have improved over the past decade following the introduction of novel targeted therapies such as the immunomodulatory agents (IMiD), thalidomide, and proteasome inhibitors (PI), bortezomib [5, 6]. However, MM remains an incurable disease, and many patients will relapse despite receiving appropriate treatment.

The US FDA recently approved the combination of carfilzomib (Kyprolis), a proteasome inhibitor, lenalidomide (Revlimid), a synthetic derivative of thalidomide [7], and dexamethasone for patients with relapsed/refractory multiple myeloma after reports showed better survival outcomes compared to earlier regimens [8, 9]. In the ASPIRE trial, patients treated with the carfilzomib (Kyprolis), lenalidomide (Revlimid), and dexamethasone regimen (i.e., KRd regimen) resulted in a progression-free survival median of 26.3 months compared to 17.6 months in patients treated with lenalidomide and dexamethasone (Rd) regimen [9]. However, grade≥3 adverse effects and serious effects were higher in the KRd arm than the Rd arm, some of which include hypertension, ischemic heart disease, heart failure, and venous thromboembolism [9, 10]. Specifically, by substituting an amino group in the phthaloyl ring, lenalidomide has less adverse side effects compared to thalidomide [11]. The same change in the phthaloyl ring of lenalidomide results in a complex immune modulation effect that is responsible for its activity. However, this complex can lead to lenalidomide toxicity. Most cases of lenalidomide toxicity include skin lesions [11–14], urticaria [15], but rarely vasculitis [13]. We report a case of a patient on the KRd regimen who presented with stroke caused by cerebral vasculitis.

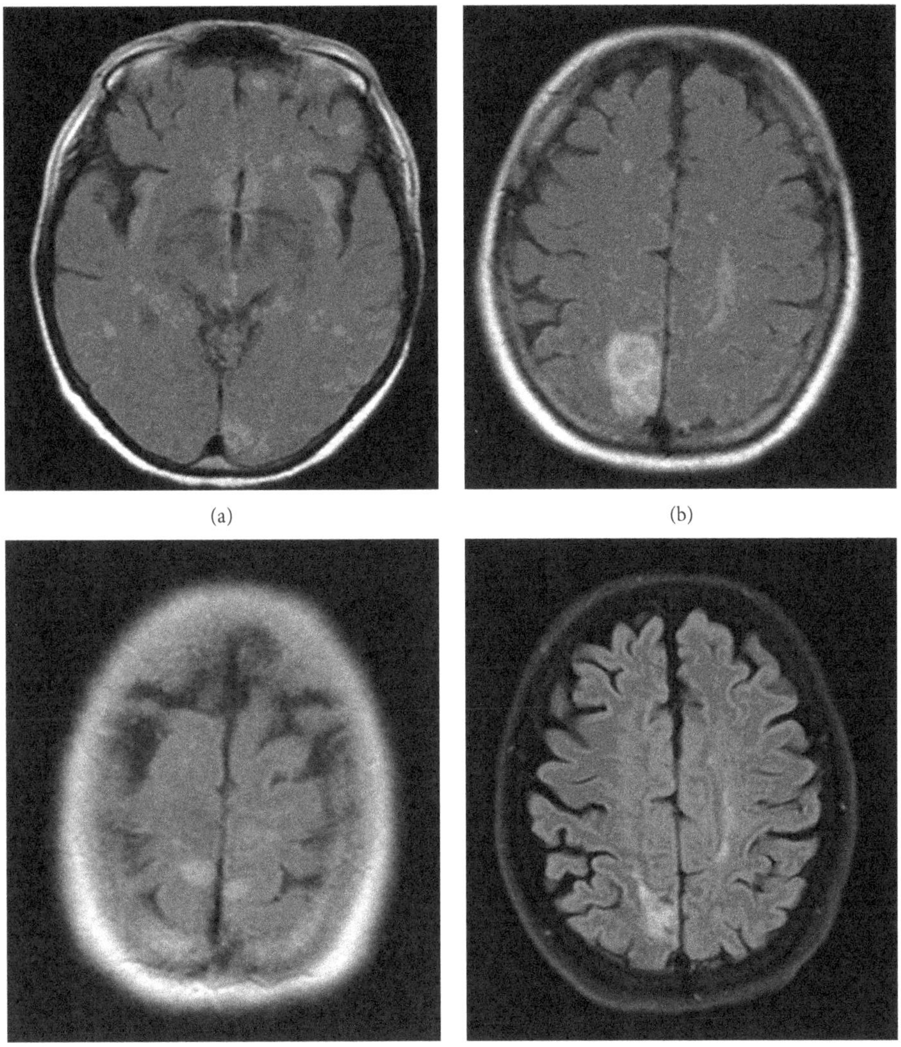

(a) (b) (c) (d)

Figure 1: MRI brain showing acute ischemic regions. (a-b) Acute infarcts in the posterior circulation involving bilateral cerebellar hemispheres, medial bilateral occipital and parietal lobes, and the posterior watershed region at the vertex with small amount of hemorrhagic conversion within the right parietal parasagittal lesion. (c-d) MRI image of infarct in the medial occipital lobe and parietal lobes bilaterally.

2. Case

We present a 59-year-old female with a history of multiple myeloma diagnosis in 2015. Laboratory results at the time of diagnosis had shown hemoglobin of 6.4 g/dl, platelet of 43,000/Ul, and creatinine of 1.2 mg/dl increased from her baseline of 0.7 mg/dl. Serum protein electrophoresis showed an immunoglobulin A level of 9680 mg/dl with low immunoglobulin G and M levels. She had induction chemotherapy with cyclophosphamide, bortezomib, and dexamethasone (CyBorD) regimen, received autologous bone marrow transplantation in 2016, and subsequently went into remission. Unfortunately, she relapsed in 2017 and then started a salvage regimen with carfilzomib, lenalidomide, and dexamethasone every two weeks to 1 month as well as daily low-dose aspirin.

In February 2019, she was admitted to our hospital with complaints of increased lethargy, multiple falls, and worsening headaches for 4 to 5 days. Physical examination showed mild left facial droop. Aside from being a current everyday smoker (about five cigarette sticks per day) with COPD and a former heroin abuser on a methadone maintenance program, she had no history of diabetes, hypertension, or previous strokes. CT of the head revealed a mass-like structure in the right precentral region measuring approximately 1.5 cm by 0.9 cm surrounded by a large area of vasogenic edema without midline shift and a small age-indeterminate infarct in the left posterior paramedian parietal lobe. MRI of the brain (Figure 1) revealed non-enhancing acute infarcts in the posterior circulation involving bilateral cerebellar hemispheres, medial bilateral occipital and parietal lobes, and the posterior watershed region at the vertex with small amount of hemorrhagic

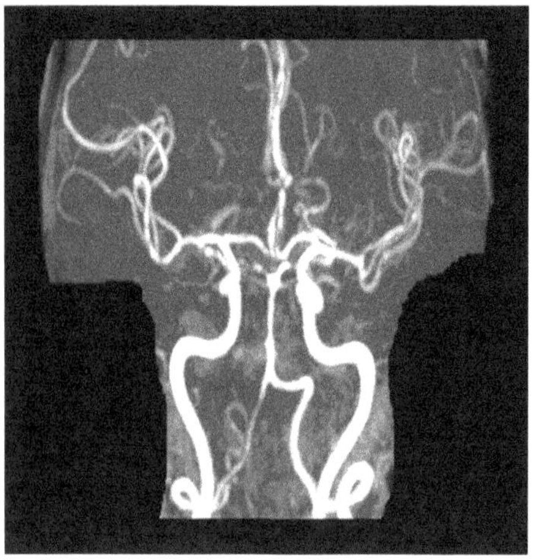

Figure 2: MRA showing multiple luminal narrowing beaded pattern in most vessels (anterior cerebral arteries, posterior inferior M2 division of the right middle cerebral artery, and posterior cerebral arteries).

conversion within the right parietal parasagittal lesion. MRA of the brain (Figure 2) without contrast further revealed multiple long and short segments of luminal narrowing with a beaded pattern in the anterior cerebral arteries, posterior inferior M2 division of the right middle cerebral artery, and posterior cerebral arteries indicating vasculitis as the etiology. CRP was more than 40 mg/dl. dsDNA and ANCA testing were both negative. A thromboembolic phenomenon was ruled-out as transthoracic echocardiography showed no evidence of valvular disease, vegetation, patent foramen ovale, or thrombosis. Also, carotid Doppler showed no significant carotid stenosis.

We withheld further chemotherapy, and a short course of dexamethasone IV was started and later switched to prednisone PO before discharge. She also received anticoagulation with apixaban. After outpatient follow-up, she resumed carfilzomib, cyclophosphamide, and dexamethasone regimen, which responded briefly as M spike returned to near baseline but later developed myelomatous meningitis. As a result, she received intrathecal methotrexate and cytarabine and commenced salvage therapy with DCEP (dexamethasone, cyclophosphamide, etoposide, and cisplatin). Three weeks after receiving the first cycle, she was admitted for severe pancytopenia, septic shock with *Klebsiella* bacteremia, acute respiratory distress syndrome (ARDS), and gastrointestinal bleeding secondary to thrombocytopenia and apixaban use. Unfortunately, she died from multiorgan failure.

3. Discussion

There have been no prior reports of stroke in a patient with relapsed multiple myeloma treated with carfilzomib, lenalidomide, and dexamethasone regimen [8, 9]. However, the lenalidomide and dexamethasone regimen approved for patients with newly diagnosed multiple myeloma has an increased risk for arterial thromboembolism, including stroke and myocardial infarction [16, 17]. Lenalidomide carries a black box warning for thromboembolic risks, and thromboprophylaxis with either low-molecular-weight heparin, warfarin, or low-dose aspirin is recommended for patients treated with a lenalidomide-based regimen [18–20]. Our patient, however, had a stroke with cerebral vasculitis being the underlying etiology.

Although the KRd regimen may have a promising safety profile from previous clinical trials, we expect that market surveillance will offer more data about rare or idiosyncratic adverse effects. We hope that such knowledge will identify patients who are at high risk and provide preventive measures to improve their quality of life.

Conflicts of Interest

The authors declare that they have no conflicts of interest.

References

[1] A. J. Cowan, C. Allen, A. Barac et al., "Global burden of multiple myeloma," *JAMA Oncology*, vol. 4, no. 9, p. 1221, 2018.

[2] C. Gerecke, S. Fuhrmann, S. Strifler, M. Schmidt-Hieber, H. Einsele, and S. Knop, "The diagnosis and treatment of multiple myeloma," *Deutsches Äerzteblatt International*, vol. 113, no. 27-28, pp. 470–476, 2016.

[3] S. Jewell, Z. Xiang, A. Kunthur, and P. Mehta, "Multiple myeloma: updates on diagnosis and management," *Federal Practitioner*, vol. 32, no. Suppl 7, pp. 49S–56S, 2015.

[4] S. V. Rajkumar, "Multiple myeloma: 2014 update on diagnosis, risk-stratification, and management," *American Journal of Hematology*, vol. 89, no. 10, pp. 998–1009, 2014.

[5] O. Landgren and K. Iskander, "Modern multiple myeloma therapy: deep, sustained treatment response and good clinical outcomes," *Journal of Internal Medicine*, vol. 281, no. 4, pp. 365–382, 2017.

[6] S. Lonial and K. C. Anderson, "Association of response endpoints with survival outcomes in multiple myeloma," *Leukemia*, vol. 28, no. 2, pp. 258–268, 2014.

[7] U. Vitolo, A. Chiappella, S. Franceschetti et al., "Lenalidomide plus R-CHOP21 in elderly patients with untreated diffuse large B-cell lymphoma: results of the REAL07 open-label, multicentre, phase 2 trial," *The Lancet Oncology*, vol. 15, no. 7, pp. 730–737, 2014.

[8] D. S. Siegel, M. A. Dimopoulos, H. Ludwig et al., "Improvement in overall survival with carfilzomib, lenalidomide, and dexamethasone in patients with relapsed or refractory multiple myeloma," *Journal of Clinical Oncology*, vol. 36, no. 8, pp. 728–734, 2018.

[9] A. K. Stewart, S. V. Rajkumar, M. A. Dimopoulos et al., "Carfilzomib, lenalidomide, and dexamethasone for relapsed multiple myeloma," *New England Journal of Medicine*, vol. 372, no. 2, pp. 142–152, 2015.

[10] W. Li, R. F. Cornell, D. Lenihan et al., "Cardiovascular complications of novel multiple myeloma treatments," *Circulation*, vol. 133, no. 9, pp. 908–912, 2016.

[11] V. Kotla, S. Goel, S. Nischal et al., "Mechanism of action of lenalidomide in hematological malignancies," *Journal of Hematology & Oncology*, vol. 2, no. 1, p. 36, 2009.

[12] M. A. Dimopoulos, A. Palumbo, M. Attal et al., "Optimizing the use of lenalidomide in relapsed or refractory multiple myeloma: consensus statement," *Leukemia*, vol. 25, no. 5, pp. 749–760, 2011.

[13] M. Breccia, L. Cannella, R. Latagliata et al., "Unexpected erythroid and cytogenetic responses after discontinuation of a short course of lenalidomide as a result of severe skin rash in a patient with 5q syndrome," *Journal of Clinical Oncology*, vol. 29, no. 14, pp. e402–e403, 2011.
[14] N. W. van de Donk, G. Görgün, R. W. Groen et al., "Lenalidomide for the treatment of relapsed and refractory multiple myeloma," *Cancer Management and Research*, vol. 4, pp. 253–268, 2012.
[15] H. P. Sviggum, M. D. P. Davis, S. V. Rajkumar, and A. Dispenzieri, "Dermatologic adverse effects of lenalidomide therapy for amyloidosis and multiple myeloma," *Archives of Dermatology*, vol. 142, no. 10, pp. 1298–1302, 2006.
[16] P. Shridhar, R. Khalil, D. Lasorda, and Y. Chun, "Lenalidomide induced stroke in multiple myeloma," *Journal of Integrative Cardiology*, vol. 2, no. 6, 2016.
[17] A. Hinduja, K. Limaye, R. Ravilla et al., "Spectrum of cerebrovascular disease in patients with multiple myeloma undergoing chemotherapy-results of a case control study," in *PLoS One*, J. Hendrikse, Ed., vol. 11, no. 11, Article ID e0166627, 2016.
[18] S. P. Menon, S. V. Rajkumar, M. Lacy, P. Falco, and A. Palumbo, "Thromboembolic events with lenalidomide-based therapy for multiple myeloma," *Cancer*, vol. 112, no. 7, pp. 1522–1528, 2008.
[19] E. Zamagni, A. Brioli, P. Tacchetti, B. Zannetti, L. Pantani, and M. Cavo, "Multiple myeloma, venous thromboembolism, and treatment-related risk of thrombosis," *Seminars in Thrombosis and Hemostasis*, vol. 37, no. 3, pp. 209–219, 2011.
[20] M. P. Cruz, "Lenalidomide (revlimid): a thalidomide analogue in combination with dexamethasone for the treatment of all patients with multiple myeloma," *P & T*, vol. 41, no. 5, pp. 308–313, 2016.

26

Heat Stroke: A Medical Emergency Appearing in New Regions

Sofie Søndergaard Mørch,[1] Johnny Dohn Holmgren Andersen,[2] and Morten Heiberg Bestle[3]

[1]*Department of Anaesthesiology and Intensive Care, Bispebjerg Hospital, Bispebjerg Bakke 23, 2400 København NV, Denmark*
[2]*Department of Anaesthesiology and Intensive Care, Hvidovre Hospital, Kettegård Alle 30, 2650 Hvidovre, Denmark*
[3]*Department of Anaesthesiology and Intensive Care, Nordsjællands Hospital, Dyrehavevej 29, 3400 Hillerød, Denmark*

Correspondence should be addressed to Sofie Søndergaard Mørch; sofiesmorch@gmail.com

Academic Editor: Kenneth S. Waxman

Heat stroke is an acute, life-threatening emergency characterized clinically by elevated body temperature and central nervous system dysfunction. Early recognition and treatment including aggressive cooling and management of life-threatening systemic complications are essential to reduce morbidity and mortality. This case report describes two Danish patients diagnosed with heat stroke syndrome during a heat wave in the summer of 2014. Both patients were morbidly obese and had several predisposing illnesses. However since heat stroke is a rare condition in areas with temperate climate, they were not diagnosed until several days after admittance; hence treatment with cooling was delayed. Both patients were admitted to the intensive care unit, where they were treated with an external cooling device and received treatment for complications. Both cases ended fatally. As global warming continues, more heat waves will occur in previously cooler regions. Therefore it is important to raise awareness of heat stroke since outcome depends on early recognition and rapid cooling.

1. Introduction

Classic heat stroke (HS) is an unusual diagnosis in countries with temperate climate. However, as global warming has resulted in a higher frequency of heat waves, an increase in weather-related heat deaths is seen [1–5].

Heat illnesses cover a spectrum of syndromes culminating with the acute, life-threatening emergency of HS that carries a high mortality [2, 3, 6–12]. HS is traditionally defined as a high core temperature accompanied by encephalopathy [6, 10–13]. An alternative definition that takes into consideration the pathophysiology is gaining recognition. This defines HS as hyperthermia associated with a systemic inflammatory response leading to multiorgan dysfunction in which encephalopathy predominates [11, 14].

Two forms of HS are recognized. Exertional HS primarily affects young and healthy athletic patients exercising vigorously in hot and humid climates until the body's normal thermoregulatory mechanisms are overwhelmed. Exertional HS is characterized by rapid onset and is frequently associated with a high core temperature [2, 3, 6, 7, 9, 10, 12, 13, 15].

Classic (passive or nonexertional) HS is caused by environmental exposure and occurs in young children, in elderly patients or in patients with underlying chronic illnesses, who are exposed to extreme environmental conditions. Classic HS can develop slowly over several days [2, 3, 7, 9, 10, 12, 13, 15].

HS occurs when the body ceases to dissipate heat adequately because of extreme environmental conditions or increased endogenous heat production [15]. When the body's thermoregulatory mechanisms are exceeded and fail, a variable degree of organ failure may occur [15]. Furthermore complex immunological and inflammatory processes that resemble SIRS (systemic inflammatory response syndrome) contribute to the illness [2, 3, 6, 10–14]. Rapid diagnosis and prompt cooling are pivotal, since the condition triggers a cascade of metabolic events that may progress to irreversible injury or death [2, 4, 6, 13]. In-hospital mortality for classical HS ranges from 10 to 65% [2].

This case report describes two Danish patients suffering from HS that was initially overlooked at hospital admission. Both patients report one week's malaise, elevated temperature, and symptoms suggesting cerebral dysfunction.

Written informed consent was obtained from relatives for publication of this case report.

2. Case Presentation

Patient 1 was a 64-year-old woman with a premedical history of unspecified mental disorder, musculoskeletal pain, and severe obesity (145 kg, BMI 57). She appeared neglected and was described as tending to isolate herself at home.

At the hospital admission she presented with Glasgow Coma Score (GCS) 5-6, hypotension, tachycardia, and divergent, fixed dilated pupils. Arterial blood gas analyses showed metabolic acidosis (pH 7.15, lactate 4.6 mmol/L, BE −11 mmol/L). Sepsis was suspected on the background of aspiration pneumonia and treatment was initiated with antibiotics and fluid replacement, soon after she was intubated and transferred to the intensive care unit (ICU).

Primary findings in the ICU were GCS 3, tachycardia (130 beats/minute), tachypnoea, hyperthermia (39.9°C), and decreased urine output. The initial wide panel of blood tests were normal except INR 1.3, potassium 2.9 mmol/L, glucose 13.3 mmol/L, troponin T 10300 ng/L, and a normal CK-MB. Nasogastric aspiration contained coffee-grounds and a urine test strip revealed presence of blood, protein, nitrite, and glucose. A neurological evaluation and a head CT-scan were performed; both were normal.

During the first days after admission a large urine output, hyperthermia, and setting sun eye phenomenon were observed. Oxygen demand increased and cooling with ice and fanning were initiated. MRI, lumbar puncture, and EEG were all normal. Microbiological tests showed no sign of infection.

The fifth day after ICU admission, HS syndrome was suspected and active cooling was intensified using a thermoregulatory device with cooling pads. The patient started to recover and the dose of cardiac inotropes was gradually reduced and then ceased. For the first time since admission some levels of contact were described. An infection with *Staphylococcus* bacteria halts improvement and her level of consciousness fell. A neurologic examination revealed an abnormal EEG and positive Babinski sign. On day 21 a PET-CT was conducted, showing globally reduced, cortical metabolic activity. It was therefore decided not to escalate treatment. The patient was extubated and died 34 days after hospital admission.

Patient 2 was a 74-year-old man suffering from heart failure, chronic atrial fibrillation, severe venous insufficiency, leg ulcers, type 2 diabetes, chronic obstructive lung disease, and severe obesity (160 kg, BMI 49). At hospital admission the patient was confused with delayed response time. Furthermore he presented with atrial fibrillation (140 beats/minute), hyperthermia (39.0°C), and elevated blood levels of creatinine. He was tachypnoeic with low oxygen saturation (91%). A urine test strip showed presence of blood, protein, and ketone bodies. Initial treatment included fluid therapy and antibiotics on the suspicion of sepsis. The patient was transferred to telemetry in the cardiology department where treatment with digoxin was initiated.

During the following days urine output increased, but his level of consciousness decreased and he developed myoclonia. Due to accumulation of carbon dioxide he was transferred to the ICU, where intubation and mechanical ventilation were initiated. At admission GCS score was 3, pupil reactions were sluggish, and muscle spasms in the upper body were observed. Blood tests were normal except an increasing INR.

During the first days in the ICU the patient improved with decreasing demand of oxygen and cardiac inotropes. Analysis of the cerebrospinal fluid and a head CT were both normal. Microbiological tests showed no sign of infection. Despite fanning and cold fluids the patient still had an elevated temperature and cooling was intensified using a thermoregulatory device with cooling pads. On day 5 the patient's temperature normalized and he gained consciousness. On day 7 the diagnosis of HS syndrome was suspected. The patient stabilized and was extubated, but he still received intermittent cooling. The patient developed hypercapnia and was reintubated and later a tracheostomy was performed. Due to anuria dialysis was performed until he regained his kidney function on day 23. The patient was again stabile and interacting with family and staff. Unfortunately the patient was infected with pneumonia. His overall condition thereafter gradually declines and he died 55 days after admission.

3. Discussion

Several factors predispose to the development of HS (Table 1). Both patients described above were morbidly obese, which is a risk factor for HS due to more insulation and a lower surface area-to-volume ratio resulting in less capacity for dissipating heat [8]. Furthermore Patient 1 had an unspecified mental disorder and tended to isolate herself in her home. Patient 2 suffered from cardiovascular disease, diabetes, and COLD.

Both patients presented with the two cardinal features of HS: hyperthermia and central nervous system dysfunction, although they were both faulty diagnosed at the hospital admittance.

The reason can be that HS is a systemic disorder that can mimic other medical conditions such as meningitis, encephalitis and septic shock, and myocardial infarction [2, 9]. These differential diagnoses were all examined and tested but excluded as test results came back normal. The patients were treated symptomatically since HS was not suspected until several days after admittance.

Contributing to the delayed diagnosis is the fact that classical HS is a very unusual cause of hyperthermia in temperate regions. But accompanying the rise in average global temperature is a rise in the frequency, intensity, and duration of heat waves and thereby weather-related deaths [3–5]. An increased awareness of HS is necessary not only in warmer regions, where the increased frequency and severity of heat waves probably will result in more cases, but also in

Table 1: Predisposing factors to classic heat stroke [1–3, 6, 8–15].

Age	Young children and individuals over 65 years
Diseases	Dermatologic conditions, infection, and endocrine disorders that increase endogenous heat production, cardiovascular disease, obesity, dehydration, pulmonary disease, neurologic disease, psychiatric illness, and previous history of heat-related illnesses[1]
Medicine	Beta-blockers, diuretics, calcium channel blockers, laxatives, anticholinergic drugs, salicylates, thyroid agonists, benzatropine, trifluoperazine, ephedra, certain diet pills, butyrophenones, alpha agonists, inhaled anaesthetics, monoamine oxidase inhibitors, and sympathomimetic medications
Drugs	Alcohol, cocaine, amphetamine, and derivatives, PCP and LSD
Social	Immobilization, isolation, being unable to care for oneself, low socioeconomic status, residing in upper floors in tall buildings, no air-condition at home, and being unable to secure a cooler environment for a few hours daily
Exposure	Prolonged sun exposure, recent move from a temperate to a hot climate, hot environments, and wearing excessive or protective clothing limiting heat dissipation

[1]Previous history of heat related illness is suspected to be a predisposing factor.

regions where this HS was previously an unusual diagnosis due to cooler climate and few heat waves.

HS is a medical emergency and it is essential that doctors recognize the signs and initiate treatment rapidly to reduce morbidity and increase survival. Decreasing the core temperature below 38.9°C within 30 min of presentation significantly improves survival [3, 12]. In this case cooling was not initiated until more than 24 hours after arrival at the hospital and this may have influenced outcome. On the contrary, the delayed cooling may instead have exacerbated the conditions of the patients: elevated temperature several days after debut of the syndrome is more likely due to fever than hyperthermia. Since fever represents an increase in the set-point, cooling was probably ineffective and may even have aggravated the condition.

4. Conclusion

These cases demonstrate the importance of keeping heat related diseases in mind when ambient temperatures rise above normal. HS is a very rare diagnosis in Northern Europe and this is probably the main reason for the delayed diagnoses which might have contributed to the fatality of the cases. As climate models predict an increased frequency and severity of heat waves the incidence of heat stroke is expected to rise.

It is our hope that this case report will increase the awareness of heat stroke in all temperate areas of the world, since more cases may appear as the temperature rises.

Conflicts of Interest

The authors declare that they have no conflicts of interest.

References

[1] A. Bouchama, M. Dehbi, G. Mohamed, F. Matthies, M. Shoukri, and B. Menne, "Prognostic factors in heat wave-related deaths: a meta-analysis," *Archives of Internal Medicine*, vol. 167, no. 20, pp. 2170–2176, 2007.

[2] L. R. Leon and A. Bouchama, "Heat stroke," *Comprehensive Physiology*, vol. 5, pp. 611–647, 2015.

[3] T. P. Yeo, "Heat stroke: a comprehensive review," *AACN clinical issues*, vol. 15, no. 2, pp. 280–293, 2004.

[4] A. Bouchama, M. Dehbi, and E. Chaves-Carballo, "Cooling and hemodynamic management in heatstroke: practical recommendations," *Critical Care*, vol. 11, no. 3, article R54, 2007.

[5] W. L. Kenney, D. H. Craighead, and L. M. Alexander, "Heat waves aging and human cardiovascular health," *Medicine and Science in Sports and Exercise*, vol. 46, no. 10, pp. 1891–1899, 2014.

[6] G. S. Lipman, K. P. Eifling, M. A. Ellis, F. G. Gaudio, E. M. Otten, and C. K. Grissom, "Wilderness medical society practice guidelines for the prevention and treatment of heat-related illness: 2014 update," *Wilderness and Environmental Medicine*, vol. 25, no. 4, pp. S55–S65, 2014.

[7] J. G. Mattis and A. M. Yates, "Heat stroke: helping patients keep their cool," *The Nurse Practitioner*, vol. 36, no. 5, pp. 48–52, 2011.

[8] T. A. Waters, "Heat illness: tips for recognition and treatment," *Cleveland Clinic Journal of Medicine*, vol. 68, no. 8, pp. 685–687, 2001.

[9] R. Sucholeiki, "Heatstroke," *Seminars in Neurology*, vol. 25, no. 3, pp. 307–314, 2005.

[10] W. F. Atha, "Heat-related illness," *Emergency Medicine Clinics of North America*, vol. 31, no. 4, pp. 1097–1108, 2013.

[11] A. Bouchama and J. P. Knochel, "Heat stroke," *The New England Journal of Medicine*, vol. 346, no. 25, pp. 1978–1988, 2002.

[12] H. Grogan and P. M. Hopkins, "Heat stroke: implications for critical care and anaesthesia," *British Journal of Anaesthesia*, vol. 88, no. 5, pp. 700–707, 2002.

[13] L. R. Leon and B. G. Helwig, "Heat stroke: role of the systemic inflammatory response," *Journal of Applied Physiology*, vol. 109, no. 6, pp. 1980–1988, 2010.

[14] Y. Epstein and W. O. Roberts, "The pathopysiology of heat stroke: an integrative view of the final common pathway," *Scandinavian Journal of Medicine and Science in Sports*, vol. 21, no. 6, pp. 742–748, 2011.

[15] D. Widodo, "Heat stroke," *Acta Medica Indonesiana*, vol. 37, pp. 39–42, 2005.

27

A Case of Cardiac Calcified Amorphous Tumor Presenting with Concomitant ST-Elevation Myocardial Infarction and Occipital Stroke and a Brief Review of the Literature

Kyaw Kyaw,[1] Htun Latt,[2] Sammy San Myint Aung,[1] and Chanwit Roongsritong[1]

[1]*Institute for Heart and Vascular Health, Renown Regional Medical Center, 1500 E. 2nd St. No. 302, Reno, NV 89502, USA*
[2]*Department of Internal Medicine, University of Nevada-Reno, School of Medicine, 1155 Mill St. No. W11, Reno, NV 89502, USA*

Correspondence should be addressed to Kyaw Kyaw; drkyawkyawmd@gmail.com

Academic Editor: Assad Movahed

Cardiac calcified amorphous tumor (CAT) is an extremely rare benign intracavitary tumor of the heart. It may mimic other cardiac tumors and can present with signs or symptoms of systemic embolization. There are limited data regarding CAT in the literature. We report a case of a 68-year-old woman with a cardiac CAT and mitral annular calcification (MAC), who presented with acute ST-elevation myocardial infarction (STEMI) and occipital stroke. After extensive review of the literature, we believe that this case is possibly the first description of a cardiac CAT presenting with STEMI. The CAT was surgically removed, and the diagnosis was confirmed by histology. The patient tolerated the surgery and reported no events at 6-month follow-up.

1. Introduction

Cardiac calcified amorphous tumor (CAT) is a rare benign intracavitary tumor of the heart. Like other cardiac tumors, CAT may present with dyspnea, syncope, and pulmonary or systemic embolization and obstruction [1–4]. Herein, we are reporting a case of CAT with mitral annular calcification, who presented with acute ST-elevation myocardial infarction (STEMI) and occipital stroke. To the best of our knowledge, our case perhaps is the first description of a cardiac CAT presenting with STEMI.

2. Case Presentation

A 68-year-old woman with a 40-pack-year smoking history but no known medical problem was brought in by ambulance for sudden onset of persistent, severe left-sided chest pain without radiation. The patient also reported a new onset of blurred vision. She denied history of hypertension, dyslipidemia, diabetes mellitus, coronary artery disease (CAD), or chronic kidney disease or family history of premature CAD. Initial vital signs were normal with oxygen saturation of 98% on 2-liter supplemental oxygen via nasal cannula. Physical examination was benign, without murmur or abnormal heart sounds. There were no focal neurological deficits or signs of peripheral embolization noted. Initial electrocardiogram (EKG) showed 1-2 mm ST elevation in inferior leads (II, III, and aVF) with reciprocal ST depression in leads I and aVL (Figure 1). Oral aspirin and sublingual nitroglycerin were given immediately. Intravenous heparin was also initiated. Emergent coronary angiography showed an occlusion in one of the acute marginal branches of the right coronary artery and slow flow in the posterior descending artery. There was no other significant CAD (Figure 2). Left ventricular wall motion and systolic function were normal. Subsequent transthoracic echocardiogram (TTE) showed a 1.2×1.2 cm mobile mass attached to the base of the posterior mitral valve leaflet on ventricular aspect (Figure 3). Of note, the mitral annulus also appeared rather echogenic. No thrombus was noted in left atrium or left ventricle during TTE or transesophageal echocardiogram (TEE). Troponin I was 1.7 ng/ml on arrival. It increased to 26 ng/ml 10 hours later. Her workups, including complete

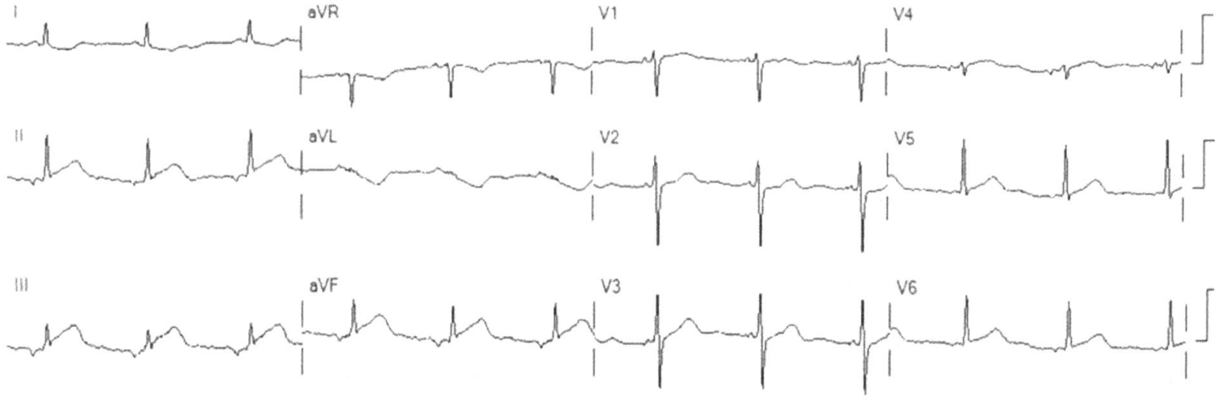

FIGURE 1: EKG showing ST elevation at II, III, and aVF with reciprocal ST depression at I and aVL.

blood count, prothrombin time/international normalized ratio, calcium, creatinine, liver function test, lipid panel, and hemoglobin A1c, were all normal. CT scan of the brain without contrast showed an infarct in the left occipital lobe (Figure 4). Cardiothoracic surgery was performed. A $1.2 \times 0.9 \times 0.2$ cm tan-pink-colored soft tissue mass was surgically removed without any complications. Histologic examination of the mass showed a nodule of amorphous debris and fibrinous material with histiocytes and multinucleated giant cells without organism, consistent with a cardiac CAT (Figure 5). Throughout the hospital stay, she was closely monitored in coronary care unit and subsequently on telemetry floor. No atrial arrhythmia was reported.

The patient recovered well without recurrent symptoms at her 6-month follow-up.

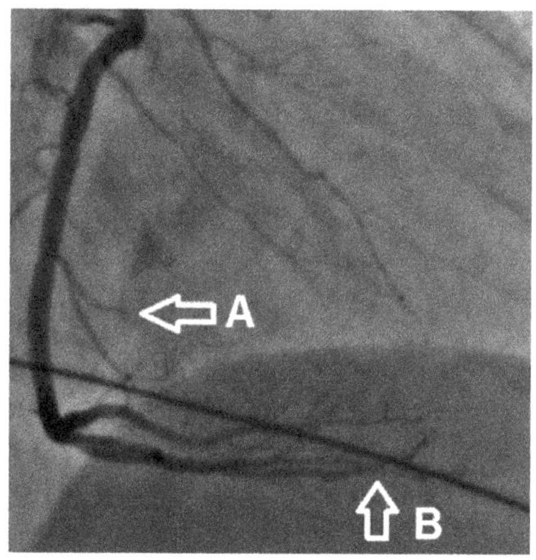

FIGURE 2: Coronary angiogram showing an occlusion of the small acute marginal branch (A) of the right coronary artery with slow flow in the posterior descending artery (B).

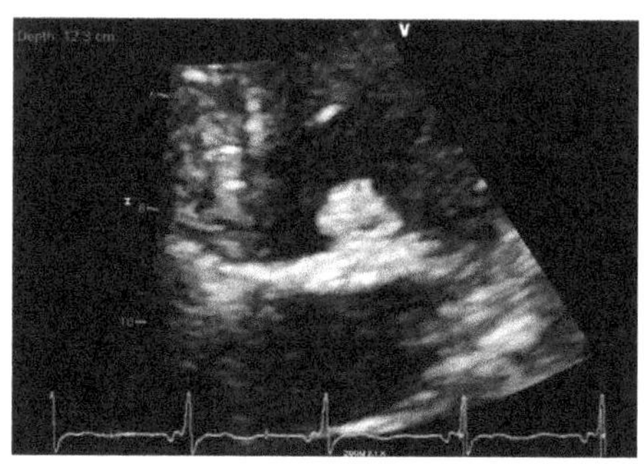

FIGURE 3: Transthoracic echocardiogram (TTE) showing a 1.2×1.2 cm mobile mass attached to the ventricular aspect of mitral valve and hyperechogenic mitral annulus.

3. Discussion

First introduced by Reynolds et al. in 1997, cardiac CAT is an extremely rare nonneoplastic primary tumor of the heart. It is characterized histologically by the features of calcified nodules and amorphous fibrinous materials [1]. CAT is usually discovered by cardiac imaging studies, but the definite diagnosis requires histological study of the tumor. ElBardissi et al. reported that the lifetime incidence of primary cardiac tumors (benign or malignant) was 0.02% based on 48 years of data collection, and only 8 of 323 cases (2.47%) of primary cardiac tumors were CAT [5]. There have so far been limited data on pathophysiology, treatment, and prognosis of CAT. The majority of CAT is seen in association with valvular heart disease (31%), end-stage renal disease (21%), mitral annular calcification (MAC) (14%), or diabetes mellitus (14%) [2]. Of interest, the MAC-related CAT tends to be highly mobile and more likely to embolize [6]. To date, there have been 13 reported cases of MAC-related CAT [6–11]. Most of them (9 cases) are associated with ESRD. MAC, a chronic fibrous degeneration of the mitral valve, is reportedly caused by abnormalities of calcium-phosphorus ($Ca\text{-}PO_4$) metabolism [7–9, 12]. MAC has been reported to increase the incidence and mortality of cardiovascular diseases but has not been linked to increased risk of myocardial infarction [13]. MAC is usually diagnosed based on hyperechoic mitral annulus on TTE. Our patient has normal renal function and serum calcium level. The echo densities of the tumor and mitral annulus in our patient are quite similar, suggesting the presence of MAC-like appearance on TTE. We felt that the MAC-like appearance on TTE in our patient and other reported cases

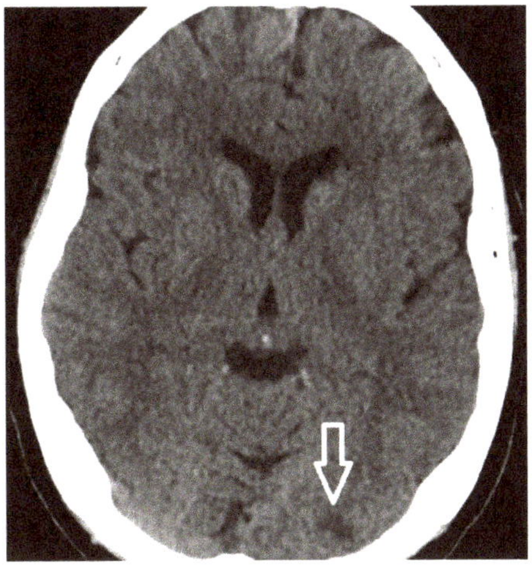

FIGURE 4: CT scan of the brain without contrast showing an infarct in the left occipital lobe.

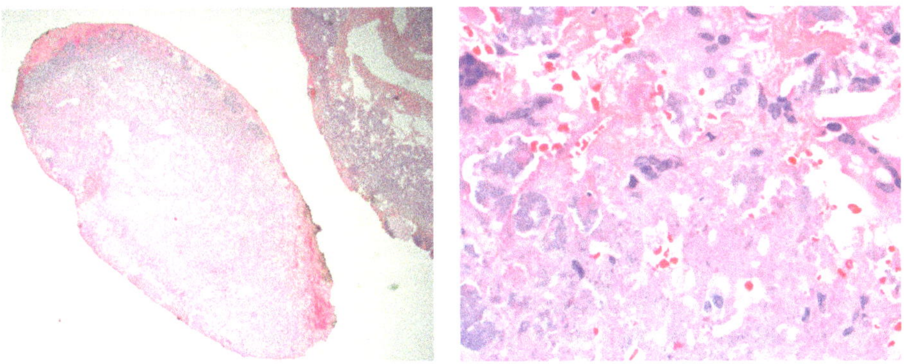

(a) (b)

FIGURE 5: Pathology specimens showing a nodule of amorphous debris and fibrinous material in low-power field (a) and histiocytes and multinucleated giant cells in high-power field (b).

without associated ESRD may have resulted from tumor infiltration into mitral valve annulus rather than from the conventional MAC process due to abnormal Ca-PO_4 metabolism. However, more studies are required to determine the exact underlying mechanism. Unfortunately, as in most patients who underwent surgical resection of the CAT, only the tumor was removed and biopsy of the mitral annulus was not performed in our patient. Surgical resection of the tumor is generally recommended to prevent embolization in most patients [6, 8–10, 14]. Our patient presented with concomitant blurred vision and STEMI, most likely due to the embolic phenomenon from the cardiac CAT.

The patient did not have any evidence of atrial arrhythmias on telemetry monitoring or intracardiac thrombus in TTE or TEE. Additionally, coronary angiogram showed isolated lesions at the third acute marginal branch and PDA of RCA and otherwise nonobstructive coronaries. Carotid ultrasound also showed normal bilateral vertebral and subclavian arteries, but there were mild stenoses (<50%) of bilateral internal carotid arteries (ICAs). Mild ICA stenoses could not explain the left occipital stroke as well. The occluded acute marginal branch of the right coronary artery was <1.5 mm in diameter angiographically. Therefore, no coronary intervention or aspiration was performed. The prognosis is generally good after complete removal of the mass lesion [15, 16]. The only recurrence was reported in a patient who received incomplete resection of the tumor [17]. Our patient tolerated the surgical procedure and has done well without any recurrent events at the six-month follow-up.

4. Conclusion

CAT of the heart is rare. Despite its benign nature, it can be highly mobile and consequently lead to systemic embolization, particularly in those with associated MAC. The prognosis is excellent with surgical resection in most patients. For those without ESRD or abnormal calcium metabolism, further studies may help determine whether cardiac CAT can involve the mitral annulus and result in an appearance similar to MAC on TTE.

Conflicts of Interest

The authors declare that there are no conflicts of interest regarding the publication of this paper.

References

[1] C. Reynolds, H. D. Tazelaar, and W. D. Edwards, "Calcified amorphous tumor of the heart (cardiac CAT)," *Human Pathology*, vol. 28, no. 5, pp. 601–606, 1997.

[2] Q. de Hemptinne, D. De Cannière, J. L. Vandenbossche, and P. Unger, "Cardiac calcified amorphous tumor: a systematic review of the literature," *IJC Heart & Vasculature*, vol. 7, pp. 1–5, 2015.

[3] N. Hussain, N. Rahman, and A. Rehman, "Calcified amorphous tumors (CATs) of the heart," *Cardiovascular Pathology*, vol. 23, no. 6, pp. 369–371, 2014.

[4] E. K. Choi, J. Y. Ro, and A. G. Ayala, "Calcified amorphous tumor of the heart: case report and review of the literature," *Methodist DeBakey Cardiovascular Journal*, vol. 10, no. 1, pp. 38–40, 2014.

[5] A. W. ElBardissi, J. A. Dearani, R. C. Daly et al., "Survival after resection of primary cardiac tumors," *Circulation*, vol. 118, no. 14, pp. S7–S15, 2008.

[6] Q. de Hemptinne, J .P. Bar, D. de Cannière, and P. Unger, "Swinging cardiac calcified amorphous tumour arising from a calcified mitral annulus in a patient with normal renal function," *BMJ Case Reports*, vol. 2015, p. bcr2014207401, 2015.

[7] T. Kawata, H. Konishi, A. Amano, and H. Daida, "Wavering calcified amorphous tumour of the heart in a haemodialysis patient," *Interactive Cardiovascular and Thoracic Surgery*, vol. 16, no. 2, pp. 219-220, 2012.

[8] S. Matsukuma, K. Eishi, K. Tanigawa et al., "Swinging calcified amorphous tumors with related mitral annular calcification," *Annals of thoracic surgery*, vol. 101, no. 4, pp. e103–e105, 2016.

[9] T. Takeuchi, K. Dohi, Y. Sato et al., "Calcified amorphous tumor of the heart in a hemodialysis patient," *Echocardiography*, vol. 33, no. 12, pp. 1926–1928, 2016.

[10] S. Katsuki, K. Ito, T. Tadokoro, T. Sasaguri, M. Hisahara, and M. Mohri, "Mitral annulus calcification-related calcified amorphous tumour trapped and extended by closing aortic valve," *European Heart Journal-Cardiovascular Imaging*, vol. 17, no. 5, p. 585, 2016.

[11] R. Nakamaru, H. Oe, K. Iwakura, T. Masai, and K. Fujii, "Calcified amorphous tumor of the heart with mitral annular calcification: a case report," *Journal of Medical Case Reports*, vol. 11, no. 1, p. 195, 2017.

[12] Y. Abramowitz, H. Jilaihawi, T. Chakravarty, M. J. Mack, and R. R. Makkar, "Mitral annulus calcification," *Journal of the American College of Cardiology*, vol. 66, no. 17, pp. 1934–1941, 2015.

[13] C. S. Fox, R. S. Vasan, H. Parise et al., "Mitral annular calcification predicts cardiovascular morbidity and mortality," *Circulation*, vol. 107, no. 11, pp. 1492–1496, 2003.

[14] M. AbbasiTeshnizi, A. Ghorbanzadeh, N. Zirak, B. Manafi, and A. Moeinipour, "Cardiac calcified amorphous tumor of the mitral valve presenting as transient ischemic attack," *Case Reports in Cardiology*, vol. 2017, Article ID 2376096, 3 pages, 2017.

[15] M. Kinoshita, H. Okayama, G. Kawamura et al., "A calcified amorphous tumor that developed on both sides of the atrioventricular valve annulus," *Journal of Echocardiography*, vol. 13, no. 4, pp. 148–150, 2015.

[16] F. Sabzi, H. Karim, B. Eizadi, R. Faraji, and N. Javid, "Calcified amorphous tumor of the heart with purple digit," *Journal of Cardiovascular and Thoracic Research*, vol. 6, no. 4, pp. 261–264, 2014.

[17] M. E. Fealey, W. D. Edwards, C. A. Reynolds, P. A. Pellikka, and J. A. Dearani, "Recurrent cardiac calcific amorphous tumor: the CAT had a kitten," *Cardiovascular Pathology*, vol. 16, no. 2, pp. 115–118, 2007.

28

Large Device-Related Thrombus Detected following Symptoms of Transient Ischemic Attack

Osayi Lawani[1] **and Edward Baptista**[2]

[1]*University of Houston College of Medicine/HCA Houston Healthcare, USA*
[2]*Vital Heart & Vein, USA*

Correspondence should be addressed to Osayi Lawani; osayimd@gmail.com

Academic Editor: Luigi Sciarra

As an independent risk factor for stroke, atrial fibrillation has been shown to be associated with a fivefold increase in the cause of embolic stroke in comparison to healthy individuals without atrial fibrillation. This risk may be compounded by other factors; however, the main probable cause of stroke leading from atrial fibrillation is thrombus formation in the left atrial appendage. In patients for whom anticoagulation is contraindicated, left atrial appendage occlusion has become a leading alternative option for therapeutic prevention of thromboembolism and stroke in patients with this condition. Unfortunately, these devices (particularly the WATCHMAN) have been associated with a 3-6% incidence of intracardiac thrombus development postimplantation. Some risk factors for the development of device-related thrombus are high platelet count, permanent atrial fibrillation, resistance to clopidogrel, and prior transient ischemic attack or stroke. Despite following an anticoagulant regimen, thrombus formation was reported in 5.6% of participants of a randomized clinical trial, and further analysis showed that some of these patients continued to develop either ischemic stroke or thromboembolism five years later as compared to patients without initial thrombus development. We present a case of an elderly male with prior history of stroke and transient ischemic attack who developed a large device-related thrombus five months following WATCHMAN FLX™ implantation. Currently, there are no specific recommendations on the management of this rare complication; however, we discuss possible consideration of initially prolonging anticoagulation therapy following implantation for high-risk individuals, as there is an increased possibility for thrombus formation in this population. Management options should continue to be studied for therapeutic benefit in streamlining postprocedural therapy and improve future outcomes in the use of left atrial appendage occlusion devices, as well as continual thrombus prevention.

1. Introduction

The incidence and prevalence of atrial fibrillation (AF) have increased greatly in the past 20 years as the population of elderly individuals continues to grow, with 75 years being the median age of patients with AF [1]. Currently, there are greater than two million Americans and eight million Europeans that are affected with this condition and is likely underestimated due to lack of notable symptoms [2]. Since the first confirmation of a relationship between an electrocardiogram with AF and a clinical irregularly irregular pulse was published by a group of European physicians in 1909, there has been a continual attempt to find various methods to eliminate or manage this disorder [3]. Management in non-rheumatic AF patients with a $CHA_2DS_2 - VASc\ score \geq 2$ consists of an antiarrhythmic agent along with common oral anticoagulants such as vitamin K antagonists, or direct oral anticoagulants via thrombin inhibition, or factor X_a inhibition as to prevent thrombosis [2, 4]. Additionally, in patients with a history of coronary artery disease and planned percutaneous coronary intervention, dual antiplatelet therapy with aspirin and a $P2Y_{12}$ receptor antagonist is included to prevent risk of thrombotic ischemic events and stent thrombosis [2].

In patients for whom anticoagulation is contraindicated, device implantation to close off the left atrial appendage

(LAA) is the next likely choice in intervention and has become a leading alternative option for therapeutic prevention of thromboembolism; several devices have been developed for this use (Table 1) [5]. Unfortunately, some of these devices have been associated with about a 3-6% incidence of intracardiac thrombus development postimplantation despite the use of anticoagulant therapy [6]. In this report, we present a case of an elderly male who was found to develop a large device-related thrombus in his left atrium five months following placement of a WATCHMAN device.

2. Case History

A 75-year-old male with a past medical history of paroxysmal atrial fibrillation, recent WATCHMAN FLX™ placement, coronary artery disease with three cardiac stents, hypertension, hyperlipidemia, bilateral carotid endarterectomies, recurrent transient ischemic attack (TIA), and two prior cerebrovascular accidents presented to our emergency department with complaints of left-sided numbness that began two hours prior to arrival.

Roughly eight months earlier, the patient experienced similar symptoms and was diagnosed with TIA. He had been taking apixaban 5 mg daily and clopidogrel 75 mg daily following previous cardiac stenting and asserted that he remained compliant with his prescriptions. A transthoracic echocardiogram (TTE) performed showed an ejection fraction of 55-60% and a mildly dilated left atrium. No defects or shunts were noted, and the foramen ovale was not patent. The patient was discharged home and advised to continue his prescriptions for apixaban and clopidogrel.

One month later, the patient returned to an emergency department with complaints of acute onset right-sided weakness and numbness. A magnetic resonance imaging (MRI) of the brain showed ischemic events in multiple territories, and a computed tomography (CT) angiogram of the neck vessels indicated a focal left (dominant) vertebral artery stenosis. Neurointerventional radiology was consulted, and a stenting of the left vertebral artery was performed. Telemetry showed atrial fibrillation with controlled ventricular response. The patient stated that he had remained compliant with taking apixaban and clopidogrel. A platelet $P2Y_{12}$ assay was performed to assess failure of therapy with clopidogrel and was negative. As there was no clear etiology to the diagnosed embolic stroke, a transesophageal echocardiogram (TEE) was ordered. The TEE was deferred to a later date due to patient preference. On discharge, apixaban was changed to rivaroxaban 20 mg daily, and the patient was instructed to continue taking clopidogrel and to follow-up out-patient with his primary cardiologist.

Exactly one month later, the patient was found to be in persistent AF during a follow-up appointment with his cardiologist. The patient also admittedly had several mechanical falls in the past few months. It was decided by his outpatient cardiologist that the patient would undergo implantation of a WATCHMAN FLX™ device for left atrial appendage closure under TEE guidance. The appendage, which was 22 mm in diameter, showed no clot within its interior prior to device implantation. A 27 mm device was ultimately placed more distally following a partial recapture after an initial attempt placed the device somewhat proximal to the opening. A tug test was satisfactory, and no leaks were noted. The patient was instructed to begin taking aspirin 81 mg daily, to continue taking clopidogrel and rivaroxaban, and to return in six weeks for a repeat TEE.

About two months later, the patient had a repeat TEE which showed a normal sized left atrium and a well-positioned WATCHMAN FLX™ without significant peri-device leak (<4 mm). No spontaneous echo contrast, new shunt, or evidence of thrombus was observed. As per protocol, the patient was instructed by his cardiologist to continue taking clopidogrel and aspirin daily, to discontinue use of rivaroxaban, and to follow-up within six months.

Over three months later, the patient presented to the emergency department at our hospital with complaints of left-sided numbness. It was the patient's first encounter at this facility as he was visiting family from out-of-town. Laboratory results at the time of admission were as follows: creatinine 1.2 mg/dL, calcium 8.6 mg/dL, rapid troponin 0.01 ng/ml, low-density lipoprotein 76.45 mg/dL, high-density lipoprotein 26 mg/dL, hemoglobin 14.7 g/dL, and a platelet count of 124×10^3/uL. Chest X-ray, head CT, brain MRI, and CT angiogram of the head and neck were unremarkable. The patient stated that he had been compliant with taking his prescribed clopidogrel and aspirin, as well as amlodipine 5 mg daily and carvedilol 6.25 mg twice a day. Causes of the patients' symptoms that may have mimicked a TIA (e.g., anxiety, seizure, migraine, and syncope) were unfounded following laboratory results and a bedside evaluation by neurology. As the etiology of the diagnosed TIA was unclear, cardiology was consulted, and a TEE was scheduled to reevaluate the positioning of his previously implanted WATCHMAN FLX™ device for leakage and to rule out any thrombus formation. The TEE showed an ejection fraction of 55-59%, a mildly dilated left atrium, and a well-positioned WATCHMAN FLX™ without peri-device leakage. Surprisingly, it was revealed that there was a large thrombus measuring 2.5×1.5 cm at the mouth of the LAA that was adherent to and covered the entire top of the WATCHMAN FLX™ device (Figures 1 and 2). No other structural cardiac defects were noted. The patient was promptly restarted on rivaroxaban and on discharge was instructed to follow-up out-patient with his cardiologist for continued management.

A little over two months later, the patient returned to his cardiologist for an outpatient follow-up. He denied any further complaints of stroke-like symptoms and continued to take rivaroxaban as prescribed. Another TEE was performed and showed a moderate to severely dilated left atrium. The WATCHMAN FLX™ device was noted in the LAA, as was a small mobile thrombus. The right atrium was also moderately dilated without evidence of thrombus. In comparison to the previous TEE performed over two months prior, the attached thrombus to the device was significantly smaller, but not completely dissolved (Figure 3). The patient was advised to continue rivaroxaban 20 mg daily and to follow-up with his cardiologist for continued surveillance.

Table 1: Devices for use in percutaneous left atrial appendage occlusion [5].

Device	Manufacturer	Design	Sizes (mm)	Sheath (F)	Approval status
Endocardial LAAO devices					
WATCHMAN	Boston Scientific	Single (lobe)	21, 24, 27, 30, 33	14	CE Mark (2005) FDA (2015)
WATCHMAN FLX			20, 24, 27, 31, 35	14	CE Mark (2019) FDA (2020)
Amplatzer Cardiac Plug	Abbot Vascular, formerly St. Jude Medical	Double (lobe and disc)	16, 18, 20, 22, 24, 26, 28, 30	9-13	CE Mark (2008)
Amplatzer Amulet			16, 18, 20, 22, 25, 28, 31, 34	12-14	CE Mark (2013)
WaveCrest	Biosense Webster, Inc. (Johnson and Johnson company)	Single (lobe)	22, 27, 32	12	CE Mark (2013)
Occlutech	Occlutech International AB	Single (lobe)	15, 18, 21, 24, 27, 30, 33, 36, 39	12, 14	CE Mark (2016)
LAmbre	Lifetech Scientific Co., Ltd.	Double (umbrella and cover)	16, 18, 20, 22, 24, 26, 28, 30, 32, 34, 36	8-10	CE Mark (2016); CFDA (2017)
Sideris transcatheter patch	Custom Medical Devices	Frameless, bioabsorbable, balloon-deliverable device	15-25	13	Undergoing clinical evaluation
Ultraseal	Cardia, Inc.	Double (bulb and sail)	16, 18, 20, 22, 24, 26, 28, 30, 32	10-12	CE Mark (2016)
SeaLA	Hangzhou Valued Medtech Co., Ltd.	Double (dual disc)	16, 18, 20, 22, 24, 26, 28, 30, 32, 34, 36	9-12	Undergoing clinical evaluation
LeFort	Lepu Medical Technology (Beijing) Co., Ltd.	Single (lobe)	21-33	—	Undergoing clinical evaluation
Pfm device	Pfm Medical	Single (disc), dual anchor	—	10-12	Undergoing clinical evaluation
Epicardial LAAO devices					
Lariat	SentreHeart, Inc.	Endoepidcardial	40 (W), (45 [W] lariat +) x 20 (H) x 70 (L)	12	CE Mark (2015); FDA 510(k) (2006), surgical use only
Sierra	Aegis Medical Innovations Inc.	Epicardial	Single size	20	Undergoing clinical evaluation

LAAO: left atrial appendage occlusion; CE Mark: Comformité Européenne Mark; CFDA: China Food and Drug Administration; FDA: United States Food and Drug Administration; W: width; H: height; L: length.

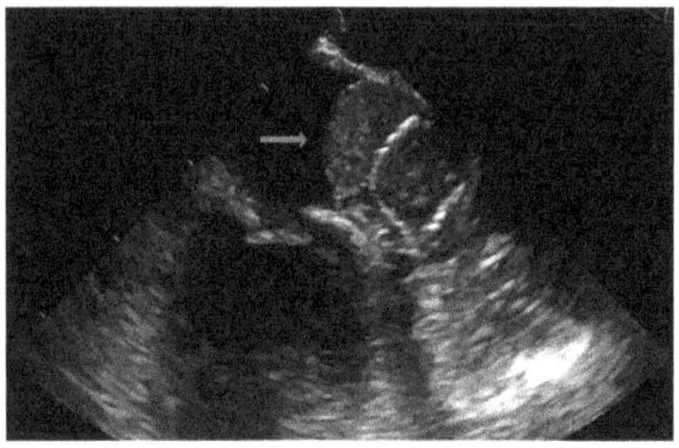

FIGURE 1: Transesophageal echocardiogram indicating a large thrombus located at the opening of the left atrial appendage covering an implanted WATCHMAN FLX™ device.

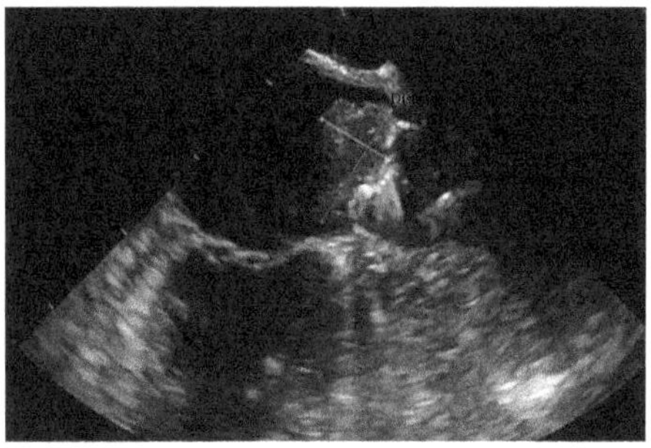

FIGURE 2: Transesophageal echocardiogram measuring a large thrombus within the left atrium atop an implanted WATCHMAN FLX™ device.

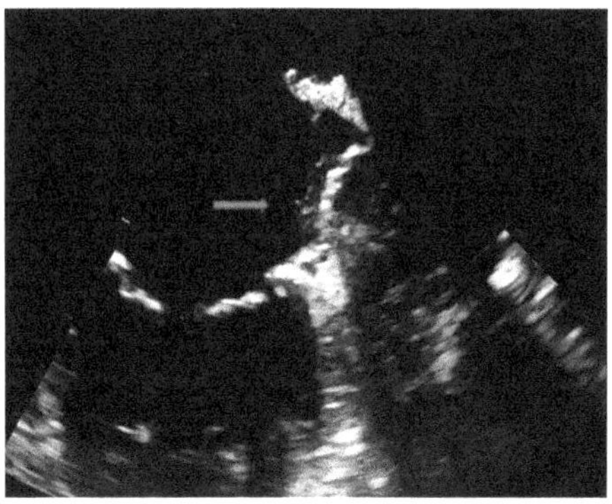

FIGURE 3: Repeat transesophageal echocardiogram showing a decrease in clot formation on a WATCHMAN FLX™ device within the left atrial appendage.

3. Discussion

As the left atrium dilates from continued fibrillation, there is more stasis and thrombus formation within the LAA [7]. Since the 1990s, interest in treating the LAA in AF patients increased with the advancement of the maze procedure, common use of TEE, and the development of percutaneous occlusion devices [8]. Left atrial appendage occlusion (LAAO) has been the primary method of stroke prevention in AF patients who have a contraindication to anticoagulation therapy, which includes increased risk for fall, lack of patient compliance, discontinuation of anticoagulants due to gastrointestinal bleed or recent stroke, or difficulty in maintaining a therapeutic window (as seen with warfarin use) [7, 8]. Based on both the PROTECT-AF and PREVAIL studies, the WATCHMAN has continually been a popular choice in AF treatment, as it was shown that using this device was not inferior to being on oral anticoagulation to prevent thromboembolism in AF [8].

Changes in the second version of the WATCHMAN FLX in comparison to its predecessor were evaluated during the PINNACLE FLX study and indicated that there was indeed a decreased incidence of complications and increased evidence of effective LAA closure at one year [9]. Device-related thrombosis (DRT) was only found in 3.7% of patients after 12 months of follow-up; however, it was attributed to both the change in the structure of the device and possibly the change in the 6-week postimplantation anticoagulation course regimen from warfarin and aspirin used in the PROTECT-AF and PREVAIL trials, to use of direct oral anticoagulants and aspirin [9]. It was also noted that the new antithrombotic regimen showed an absence of DRT in patients who were compliant with taking these medications [9]. This was not the case for the individual in this report, although his DRT could have had a multifactorial cause.

It is important to mention that although the patient in this report was discovered to have a DRT following a TIA, thrombus is not always associated with an embolic event and is usually an incidental finding. Risk factors for the development of DRT are high platelet count, resistance to clopidogrel, an elevated $CHADS_2$ and CHA_2DS_2-VASc score, decreased left ventricular ejection fraction, permanent AF, prior TIA or stroke, or device-specific issues (large mean device size or deep implantation) [10]. With regards to this case, the patient met at least three risk factors for thromboembolism formation. The pathophysiology of DRT can be directly related to elderly individuals with prior history of stroke, elevated CHA_2DS_s-VASc score, and vascular disease, all of which are indicated in an increased prothrombotic state [11]. DRT may also be induced by incomplete or deep implantation of the device by exposing areas of trabeculations [11]. Large devices also increase the risk for DRT due to having an increased fabric surface area [11]. The patient in this case had his device implanted deeply on a second attempt and also had a device placed that was 5 mm larger than the diameter of his LAA.

The most common cause of DRT has been noted to occur following the discontinuation of oral anticoagulant therapy [6]. At this time, there is no indication of which oral anticoagulant is preferred as one retrospective study suggested that there was no significant difference in developing DRT with the initial use of either vitamin K antagonists or direct oral anticoagulants [11]. What is known is that a recent analysis showed that after five years, about 25% of patients who were diagnosed with DRT from the PROTECT-AF and PREVAIL studies later developed either ischemic stroke or thromboembolism compared to patients without DRT, and that there was also a temporal association [11]. Although the incidence of DRT is about 3-7%, it is associated with a threefold increase in stroke risk [11].

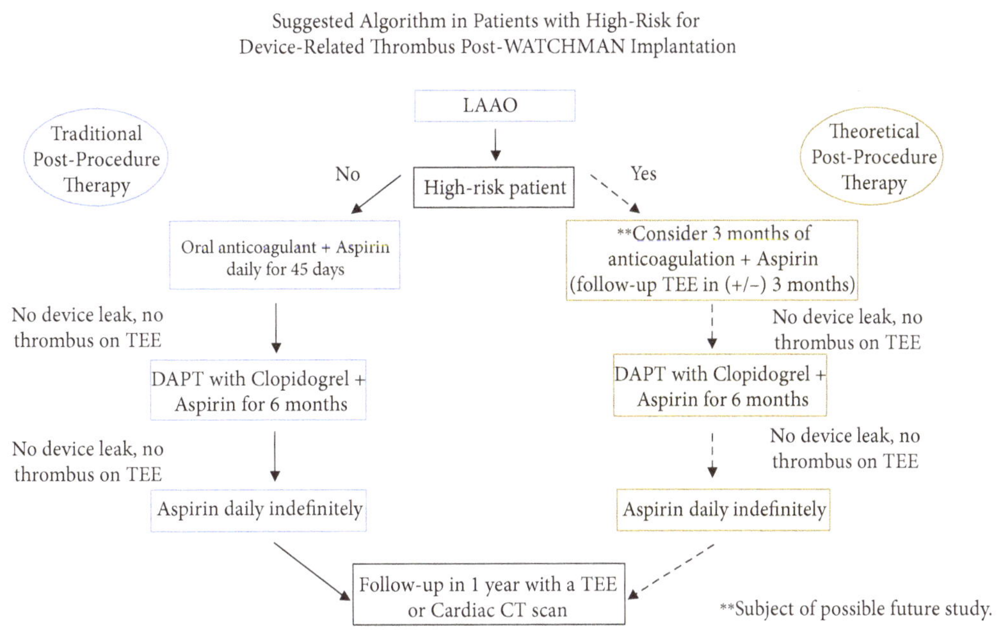

Figure 4: Suggested algorithm for assessment and treatment of a patient post-WATCHMAN placement who may be high risk for DRT. LAAO: left atrial appendage occlusion; TEE: transesophageal echocardiogram; DAPT: dual antiplatelet therapy; DRT: device-related thrombus; CT: computed tomography [11].

Furthermore, as there is usually resolution of DRT with the use of direct oral anticoagulation, there have been several accounts of recurrent DRT after anticoagulation was discontinued [12]. Consequently, more thoughtful consideration should be placed for patients that qualify for an LAAO device and have a significant history of stroke or thromboembolism.

For high-risk patients prior to LAAO device placement, it is proposed that anticoagulation continue for >45 days following implantation, then a repeat TEE is performed at a later date, and the patient can start dual antiplatelet therapy followed by aspirin indefinitely if there is no evidence of peri-device leaks or DRT [13]. Future studies should focus on an optional length of time a high-risk patient should stay on anticoagulation postimplantation as this is presently undetermined (Figure 4) [11].

Duration of use and choice of anticoagulant and antiplatelet regimen should be tailored for high-risk patients. In addition, it may be worth investigating whether $P2Y_{12}$ inhibitors other than clopidogrel should be used for patients who are prone to thromboembolism as they have better platelet aggregation inhibition during the device sealing process [13]. Previously, a DRT score based on predictors was suggested to assist in identifying individuals that would be at a high risk for thrombus development postdevice implantation. This would be helpful as it would potentially lead to finding whether factors related to anticoagulation, the patient, or the actual procedure contributed to the formation of DRT [12]. At this time, treatment strategies for high-risk individuals who may develop DRT have not been clinically proven and should be treated on a case-by-case basis.

4. Conclusion

Although the incidence of DRT following WATCHMAN implantation is relatively low, it does have a significant impact on how high-risk patients are viewed and considered for treatment. As the results of the ASAP-TOO trial will indicate whether anticoagulation is needed overall after device implantation, the incidence of DRT should continue to be further investigated, particularly for high-risk individuals. Prolonging anticoagulation or change in antiplatelet regimen should also continue to be studied for therapeutic benefit. One study suggested possible coating of the device in an antithrombotic agent to help in decreasing the risk of DRT development [12]. Integration of these changes into clinical practice will likely assist in streamlining postprocedural therapy as to keep up with achieving continual promising outcomes with the use of LAAO devices, as well as continual thrombus prevention.

Conflicts of Interest

The authors declare that they have no conflicts of interest.

Authors' Contributions

Osayi Lawani participated in conceptualization, data curation, investigation, visualization, and creation, review, and editing of the original draft. Edward Baptista provided supervision, methodology, validation, resources, and editing of original draft.

Acknowledgments

The authors would especially like to thank Dr. Justin Saunders, Patricia Dottery, Saadia Farehan, and Amanda Posada for their support.

References

[1] S. S. Chugh, J. L. Blackshear, W.-K. Shen, S. C. Hammill, and B. J. Gersh, "Epidemiology and natural history of atrial fibrillation: clinical implications," *Journal of the American College of Cardiology*, vol. 37, no. 2, pp. 371–378, 2001.

[2] D. Capodanno, H. Huber, R. Mehranet al. et al., "Management of Antithrombotic Therapy in Atrial Fibrillation Patients Undergoing PCI:," *Journal of the American College of Cardiology*, vol. 74, no. 1, pp. 83–99, 2019.

[3] T. Fazekas, "The concise history of atrial fibrillation," *Orvostörténeti Közlemények*, vol. 53, no. 3-4, pp. 37–68, 2007.

[4] O. de Backer, S. Arnous, N. Ihlemann et al., "Percutaneous left atrial appendage occlusion for stroke prevention in atrial fibrillation: an update," *Open Heart*, vol. 1, no. 1, article e000020, 2014.

[5] L. Asmarats and J. Rodes-Cabau, "The spectrum of devices for percutaneous left atrial appendage occlusion," *Cardiac Interventions Today*, vol. 12, no. 3, pp. 34–39, 2018.

[6] B. Hannawi, F. Beg, M. Valderrabano, and K. Kurrelmeyer, "Device-related thrombus: a reason for concern?," *Methodist Debakey Care*, vol. 15, no. 1, pp. 77–80, 2021.

[7] J. Romero, I. E. Perez, A. Krumerman, M. J. Garcia, and R. J. Lucariello, "Left atrial appendage closure devices," *Clinical Medicine Insights: Cardiology*, vol. 8, pp. CMC.S14043–CMC.S14052, 2014.

[8] S. Chatterjee, J. C. Alexander, P. J. Pearson, and T. Feldman, "Left atrial appendage occlusion: lessons learned from surgical and transcatheter experiences," *The Annals of Thoracic Surgery*, vol. 92, no. 6, pp. 2283–2292, 2011.

[9] S. Kar, S. K. Doshi, A. Sadhu et al., "Primary outcome evaluation of a next-generation left atrial appendage closure device," *Circulation*, vol. 143, no. 18, pp. 1754–1762, 2021.

[10] S. R. Dukkipati, S. Kar, D. R. Holmes et al., "Device-related thrombus after left atrial appendage closure," *Circulation*, vol. 138, no. 9, pp. 874–885, 2018.

[11] M. Turagam, V. Y. Reddy, and S. Dukkipati, "Device-related thrombus: understanding and managing the "Achilles heel" of LAA closure," in *American College of Cardiology*, 2018, June 2021, https://www.acc.org/latest-in-cardiology/articles/2018/09/14/09/54/device-related-thrombus.

[12] M. Alkhouli and D. R. Holmes, "Remaining challenges with transcatheter left atrial appendage closure," *Mayo Clinic Proceedings*, vol. 95, no. 10, pp. 2244–2248, 2020.

[13] P. Garot, B. Cormier, and J. Horvilleur, "Device-related thrombus after left atrial appendage closure," *International Cardiology Review*, vol. 14, no. 1, pp. 42–44, 2019.

29

Gamma-Glutamyl Transferase Levels in Patients with Acute Ischemic Stroke

Nurbanu Gurbuzer, Eren Gozke, and Zeliha Ayhan Basturk

Department of Neurology, FSM Teaching and Research Hospital, E-5 Uzeri, Bostanci, 34744 Istanbul, Turkey

Correspondence should be addressed to Eren Gozke; egozke@hotmail.com

Academic Editor: Janusz K. Rybakowski

Objective. The aim of this study was to investigate the relationship between gamma-glutamyl transferase (GGT) levels, cerebrovascular risk factors, and distribution of cerebral infarct areas in patients with acute ischemic stroke (AIS). *Patients and Methods.* Sixty patients with AIS and 44 controls who had not cerebrovascular disease were included in the study. The patients were divided into four groups according to the location of the infarct area and evaluated as for GGT levels and the presence of diabetes mellitus (DM), hypertension (HT), and hyperlipidemia (HL). *Results.* The frequency of DM, HT, and HL and gender distributions were similar. The mean GGT levels were significantly higher in patients with AIS and those with relatively larger areas of infarction ($P < 0.05$). Increased mean GGT levels were found in the subgroup with hypertension, higher LDL-cholesterol, and triglyceride levels among cases with AIS ($P < 0.05$). *Conclusion.* Higher GGT levels in AIS patients reinforce the relationship of GGT with inflammation and oxidative stress. The observation of higher GGT levels in patients with relatively larger areas of infarction is indicative of a positive correlation between increases in infarct areas and elevated GGT levels.

1. Introduction

Gamma-glutamyl transferase (GGT) mediates intracellular intake of extracellular glutathione which is an important component of antioxidant mechanisms. Glutathione is produced during normal metabolic processes and plays an important role in the protection of cells against oxidative stress. GGT has been used for years as an index of hepatic dysfunction and marker of alcohol use [1, 2]. In population-based studies, after exclusion of alcohol consumption, a positive correlation has been demonstrated between higher GGT levels and advanced age, male gender, increases in body mass index (BMI), smoking, sedentary life style, hypertension, tachycardia, hyperglycemia, increased LDL-cholesterol, and decreased HDL-cholesterol levels, hypertriglyceridemia, menopause, and oral contraceptive use [3, 4].

In this study, our aim was to investigate the relationship between serum GGT levels and several risk factors for cerebrovascular disease (CVD) and also distribution of cerebral infarct areas in patients with acute ischemic stroke (AIS).

2. Material and Method

Sixty patients hospitalized with the diagnosis of AIS and 44 CVD-naïve individuals who consulted to neurology polyclinic for other reasons were investigated. Patients with a history of chronic liver or renal disease, endocrine, and autoimmune diseases other than diabetes, alcoholics, smokers, those who had undergone surgical interventions related to coronary, carotid, or extremity arteries, or users of drugs which might alter GGT test results (lipid-lowering drugs, antibiotics) were excluded from the study. However diabetic and/or hypertensive patients continued to use the drugs for regulation of their glycemic state and blood pressure levels. The patients with newly onset angina, myocardial infarction, and advanced heart failure were not enrolled in the study. Levels of liver enzymes, bilirubin, and hepatic markers of all cases were within normal limits. Blood samples of AIS patients were obtained within twenty-four hours after stroke.

According to Bamford classification, stroke patients were divided into 4 groups based on the infarct area as total

Table 1: Demographic data of the cases with AIS and the control group.

	AIS $n = 60$	Control $n = 44$	P
Age (mean ± SD)	71.7 ± 9.9	69.5 ± 8.7	0.065
Age range	51–90	50–82	
	AIS n (%)	Control n (%)	P
Gender			
Male	32 (53%)	19 (43%)	0.273
Female	28 (47%)	25 (57%)	

Student's t-test.
AIS: acute ischemic stroke.

Table 2: Mean GGT levels in cases with AIS according to infarction area.

Infarction area	n (%)	GGT mean ± SD (IU/L)	P
LACI	15 (25.0%)	16.0 ± 6.1	**0.044***
PACI	21 (35.0%)	26.7 ± 15.3	
POCI	16 (26.7%)	24.4 ± 11.1	
TACI	8 (13.3%)	25.8 ± 3.1	

Kruskal-Wallis test.
LACI: lacunar infarctions, PACI: partial anterior circulation infarctions, POCI: posterior circulation infarctions, and TACI: total anterior circulation infarctions.
*Statistically significant (mean GGT level in the LACI group was significantly lower than other groups).

Table 3: Mean GGT levels in cases with AIS according to gender and risk factors.

	n	GGT mean ± SD (IU/L)	P
Gender			
Female	28	23.18 ± 13.98	0.918
Male	32	23.50 ± 9.910	
LDL cholesterol			
<129	24	17.25 ± 8.330	**0.00***
>129	36	27.42 ± 12.21	
Triglyceride			
>150	27	27.00 ± 8.350	**0.03***
<150	33	20.36 ± 13.50	
HDL cholesterol			
>40	15	27.13 ± 17.87	0.155
<40	45	22.09 ± 8.970	
Total cholesterol			
>200	22	23.86 ± 7.580	0.801
<200	38	23.05 ± 13.83	
Diabetes mellitus			
(−)	37	21.49 ± 8.620	0.124
(+)	23	26.35 ± 15.50	
Hypertension			
(−)	7	14.14 ± 2.670	**0.028***
(+)	53	24.57 ± 12.08	

Chi-square test.
*Statistically significant.

anterior circulation infarcts (TACI), partial anterior circulation infarcts (PACI), lacunar infarcts (LACI), and posterior circulation infarcts (POCI). In the patient and the control groups, study participants were evaluated as for the presence of diabetes mellitus (DM), hypertension (HT), hyperlipidemia (HL), and alterations in serum GGT levels. GGT was analyzed using a spectrophotometric method, and values ranging between 7 and 60 U/L were considered to be within physiologic limits.

In the statistical analysis Student's t-test, independent samples t-test, Mann Whitney U test, chi-square test, and Kruskal-Wallis test were performed. The significance level was evaluated at $P < 0.05$.

3. Results

Demographic data are seen in Table 1. A significant difference was not found between groups regarding mean ages and gender distribution. The frequencies of hypertension, diabetes mellitus, and hyperlipidemia in the cases with AIS and controls were comparable (88.3 versus 88.6%, 38.3 versus 38.6%, and 36.6 versus 40.9%, resp.). Mean GGT level in the AIS group was found to be significantly higher relative to the control group (23.3 ± 11.8 versus 15.0 ± 5.7 IU/L; $P < 0.000$). The cut-off value for GGT was calculated as 26.4 IU/L. Mean GGT level in the AIS group did not differ between female and male cases (23.1 ± 13.9 versus 23.5 ± 9.9 IU/L, resp.; $P > 0.05$). The lowest and the highest GGT levels were detected in the LACI and PACI groups, respectively. Mean GGT levels were significantly higher in TACI, PACI, and POCI groups than in LACI group (Table 2). Increased GGT level was found in the subgroup with hypertension, higher LDL-cholesterol, and triglyceride levels among cases with AIS (Table 3).

4. Discussion

Although gamma-glutamyl transferase is mostly found within cytosoles, it is also present on cellular membrane in considerable amounts and plays a role in intracellular ingress of amino acids and peptides in the form of γ-glutamyl peptides. Glutathione is its most important substrate. This tripeptide is a thiol derivative which is the most important nonprotein intracellular component and functions as a primary determinant of cellular redox mechanisms. In conditions giving rise to cellular stress, intracellular glutathione levels decrease. Decreased intracellular glutathione levels induce formation of GGT enzyme so as to maintain preexisting levels. Increased oxidative stress enhances requirement for glutathione. In the presence of inadequate amounts of glutathione, oxidative stress exerts more harmful effects [5–7]. The mechanism of the relationship between cardiovascular and cerebrovascular risk factors and GGT level is not fully known. According to a currently entertained theory, oxidative stress and related decrease in glutathione levels induce activity of GGT. Independent of alcohol consumption and presence of a liver disease, the predictive role of GGT activity in the development of new cases of diabetes, hypertension, and ischemic stroke has been established [8–12].

The Vorarlberg Health Monitoring and Promotion Program (VHM&PP) study conducted by Ruttmann et al. in Austria is the largest scale prospective study performed up to date [13]. This epidemiologic study has investigated the association between GGT and cardiovascular mortality. In this survey study an independent but significant association between GGT levels and cardiovascular mortality in both female and male cohorts was found. In the male patient cohort, a significant correlation between GGT and cardiovascular disease and ischemic and hemorrhagic stroke was present. In the same study, the correlation between GGT and cardiovascular disease was observed, but a statistically significant correlation between GGT levels and stroke (both hemorrhagic and ischemic types) could not be detected. Besides, prognostic significance of GGT was more prominently observed in patients younger than 60 years of age. Also in our study GGT levels were statistically significantly higher in the ischemic stroke group relative to the control group. However distribution of increased GGT values in the female and male patient groups did not differ significantly.

A multicenter prospective epidemiologic study (CARDIA, The Coronary Artery Risk Development in Young Adults) investigated 5115 individuals aged between 17 and 35 years. CARDIA study revealed correlations among normal GGT levels, diabetes, and hypertension [14]. The investigators also reported potential role of oxidative stress as a risk factor for the development of diabetes and hypertension and concluded that GGT is a sensitive early stage predictor of oxidative stress. In our study, a statistically significant difference was not observed between patients with or without diabetes; however, significant increases in GGT levels were noted in hypertensive patients. Besides significantly higher GGT levels were detected in patients with increased LDL-cholesterol and triglyceride levels.

D'Ambrosio et al. reported that increased gamma-glutamyl transferase levels predict functional impairment in elderly adults after ischemic stroke [15]. Korantzopoulos et al. also found positive correlation between serum gamma-glutamyl transferase and acute ischemic nonembolic stroke in the elderly subjects [16]. The role played by oxidative stress, subclinical inflammation in the pathophysiology of cardiovascular diseases, and development of stroke is already acknowledged. Mechanisms related to oxidative stress and subclinical inflammation can account for the role of GGT in the development of cerebrovascular disease [5, 17–20]. Increased GGT levels can play a pathogenetic role in the evolution and instability of atherosclerotic plaques in different vascular regions [21].

In our study, significantly higher GGT levels were detected in the AIS group relative to the control group. Besides, statistically significantly higher levels of GGT in cases with hypertension, increased LDL-cholesterol, and triglyceride levels suggest the role of oxidative stress. GGT might increase secondary to arterial wall inflammation and resultant arterial wall thickening, and higher GGT levels might protect arterial wall against oxidative stress as well.

In conclusion, higher GGT levels in AIS patients relative to the control group reinforce the relationship of GGT with inflammation and oxidative stress. Detection of relatively higher levels of GGT in AIS patients with hypertension, increased LDL-cholesterol, and triglyceride levels indicates the presence of a positive correlation between GGT levels, oxidative stress, and inflammation. When compared with the LACI group of patients with relatively smaller lacunar infarcts, observation of higher GGT levels in TACI, PACI, and POCI groups with relatively larger areas is indicative of a positive correlation between increases in infarct areas and elevated GGT levels. Future studies can better reveal the possible role of GGT in the prediction of oxidative stress and mild degrees of chronic inflammation.

Conflict of Interests

The authors declare that there is no conflict of interests regarding the publication of this paper.

References

[1] J. B. Whitfield, "Gamma glutamyl transferase," *Critical Reviews in Clinical Laboratory Sciences*, vol. 38, no. 4, pp. 263–355, 2001.

[2] B. W. Karlson, O. Wiklund, P. Hallgren, M. Sjölin, J. Lindqvist, and J. Herlitz, "Ten-year mortality amongst patients with a very small or unconfirmed acute myocardial infarction in relation to clinical history, metabolic screening and signs of myocardial ischaemia," *Journal of Internal Medicine*, vol. 247, no. 4, pp. 449–456, 2000.

[3] D. J. Kim, J. J. Noh, N. H. Cho et al., "Serum γ-glutamyltransferase within its normal concentration range is related to the presence of diabetes and cardiovascular risk factors," *Diabetic Medicine*, vol. 22, no. 9, pp. 1134–1140, 2005.

[4] Y. Shimizu, H. Imano, T. Ohira et al., "γ-glutamyltranspeptidase and incident stroke among japanese men and women: the circulatory risk in communities study (CIRCS)," *Stroke*, vol. 41, no. 2, pp. 385–388, 2010.

[5] D. Lee, R. Blomhoff, and D. R. Jacobs Jr., "Is serum gamma glutamyltransferase a marker of oxidative stress?" *Free Radical Research*, vol. 38, no. 6, pp. 535–539, 2004.

[6] A. Paolicchi, G. Minotti, P. Tonarelli et al., "γ-Glutamyl transpeptidase-dependent iron reduction and LDL oxidation: a potential mechanism in atherosclerosis," *Journal of Investigative Medicine*, vol. 47, no. 3, pp. 151–160, 1999.

[7] J. Yamada, H. Tomiyama, M. Yambe et al., "Elevated serum levels of alanine aminotransferase and gamma glutamyltransferase are markers of inflammation and oxidative stress independent of the metabolic syndrome," *Atherosclerosis*, vol. 189, no. 1, pp. 198–205, 2006.

[8] E. Ikai, R. Honda, and Y. Yamada, "Serum gamma-glutamyl transpeptidase level and blood pressure in nondrinkers: A possible pathogenetic role of fatty liver in obesity-related hypertension," *Journal of Human Hypertension*, vol. 8, no. 2, pp. 95–100, 1994.

[9] Y. Yamada, E. Ikai, I. Tsuritani, M. Ishizaki, R. Honda, and M. Ishida, "The relationship between serum γ-glutamyl transpeptidase levels and hypertension: common in drinkers and nondrinkers," *Hypertension Research*, vol. 18, no. 4, pp. 295–301, 1995.

[10] P. Jousilathi, E. Vartiainen, H. Alho, K. Poikolainen, and P. Sillanaukee, "Opposite association of carbohydrate deficient transferrin and gama-glutamyltransferase with prevalent coronary heart disease," *Archives of Internal Medicine*, vol. 162, no. 7, pp. 295–301, 2002.

[11] I. J. Perry, S. G. Wannamethee, and A. G. Shaper, "Prospective study of serum γ-glutamyltransferase and risk of NIDDM," *Diabetes Care*, vol. 21, no. 5, pp. 732–737, 1998.

[12] N. Nakanishi, K. Nishina, W. Li, M. Sato, K. Suzuki, and K. Tatara, "Serum γ-glutamyltransferase and development of impaired fasting glucose or type 2 diabetes in middle-aged Japanese men," *Journal of Internal Medicine*, vol. 254, no. 3, pp. 287–295, 2003.

[13] E. Ruttmann, L. J. Brant, H. Concin, G. Diem, K. Rapp, and H. Ulmer, "γ-glutamyltransferase as a risk factor for cardiovascular disease mortality: An epidemiological investigation in a cohort of 163 944 Austrian adults," *Circulation*, vol. 112, no. 14, pp. 2130–2137, 2005.

[14] D. H. Lee, D. R. Jacobs, M. Gross et al., "γ-Glutamyltransferase is a predictor of incident diabetes and hypertension: the coronary artery risk development in young adults (CARDIA) study," *Clinical Chemistry*, vol. 49, no. 8, pp. 1358–1366, 2003.

[15] D. D'Ambrosio, G. Gargiulo, D. Della-Morte et al., "Gamma-glutamyltransferase predicts functional impairment in elderly adults after ischemic stroke," *Journal of the American Geriatrics Society*, vol. 61, no. 6, pp. 1040–1041, 2013.

[16] P. Korantzopoulos, P. Tzimas, K. Kalantzi et al., "Association between serum gamma-glutamyltransferase and acute ischemic non-embolic stroke in elderly subjects," *Archives of Medical Research*, vol. 40, no. 7, pp. 582–589, 2009.

[17] D. H. Lee, M. H. Ha, J. H. Kim et al., "Gamma-glutamyltransferase and diabetes—a 4 year follow-up study," *Diabetologia*, vol. 46, no. 3, pp. 359–364, 2003.

[18] M. Emdin, A. Pompella, and A. Paolicchi, "Gamma-glutamyltransferase, atherosclerosis, and cardiovascular disease: triggering oxidative stress within the plaque," *Circulation*, vol. 112, no. 14, pp. 2078–2080, 2005.

[19] H. Brenner, D. Rothenbacher, V. Arndt, S. Schuberth, E. Fraisse, and T. M. Fliedner, "Distribution, determinants, and prognostic value of γ-glutamyltransferase for all-cause mortality in a cohort of construction workers from Southern Germany," *Preventive Medicine*, vol. 26, no. 3, pp. 305–310, 1997.

[20] A. Pompella, M. Emdin, C. Passino, and A. Paolicchi, "The significance of serum gamma-glutamyltransferase in cardiovascular diseases," *Clinical Chemistry and Laboratory Medicine*, vol. 42, no. 10, pp. 1085–1091, 2004.

[21] M. Emdin, C. Passino, L. Donato, A. Paolicchi, and A. Pompella, "Serum γ-glutamyltransferase as a risk factor of ischemic stroke might be independent of alcohol consumption," *Stroke*, vol. 33, no. 4, pp. 1163–1164, 2002.

30

Medicolegal Considerations withIntravenous Tissue Plasminogen Activator in Strok: A Systematic Review

Archit Bhatt, Adnan Safdar, Dhara Chaudhari, Diane Clark, Amber Pollak, Arshad Majid, and Mounzer Kassab

Providence Brain and Spine Institute, Portland, OR 97225, USA

Correspondence should be addressed to Archit Bhatt; architbhatt@gmail.com

Academic Editor: Thilo Hölscher

Background. Intravenous tPA (tissue plasminogen activator) therapy remains underutilized in patients with Acute Ischemic Stroke (AIS). Anecdotal data indicates that physicians are increasingly liable for administering and for failure to administer tPA. *Methods.* An extensive search of Medline, Embase, Westlaw, LexisNexis Legal, and Google Scholar databases was performed. Case studies that involved malpractice litigation in ischemic stroke and thrombolytic therapy were analyzed systematically. *Results.* We identified 789 ischemic stroke litigation cases, of which 46 cases were related to intravenous tPA and stroke litigation. Case descriptions of 40 cases were available. Data for verdicts were available for 38 patients. The most frequent plaintiff claim was related to failure to administer intravenous tPA (38, 95%). Only 2 (5.0%) claim involved complications of treatment with tPA. Hospitals were defendants in majority of the 36 cases. Physicians were involved in 33 cases. While ED physicians were involved in 25 (60.52%) cases, neurologists were involved in 8 (20.0%) cases. There were 26 (65%) defendant-favored and 12 (30%) plaintiff-favored verdicts. *Conclusion.* Physicians and hospitals are at an increased risk of litigation in patients with AIS when in IV-tPA is being considered for treatment. While majority of the cases litigated were cases where tPA was not administered, only about 1 in 20 cases was litigated when complications occurred.

1. Introduction

Acute Ischemic Strokes (AIS) is the number one cause of morbidity and third leading cause of mortality in the developed world behind heart disease and cancer. Approximately 795,000 cases of strokes occur annually in the United States, of which 610,000 are first ever strokes. Prior to 1995, there was no FDA-approved thrombolytic treatment available for AIS. Between 1991 and 1995, a NINDS sponsored randomized trial [1] was conducted to assess the safety and efficacy of recombinant tissue plasminogen activator (tPA) in patients with AIS, within 3 hours of stroke onset. The results showed that tPA-treated stroke patients were 32 percent more likely to show minimum or no disability at 3 months (odds ratio 1.7, CI 1.2–2.6, NNT 8, NNH 16, and ARR 12%), compared to patients who did not get tPA. Symptomatic intracerebral hemorrhage within 36 hours after the onset of stroke occurred not only in 6.4 percent of patients given tPA but also 0.6 percent of patients given placebo ($P < 0.001$). Mortality at three months was 17 percent in the tPA group and 21 percent in the placebo group ($P = 0.30$). Over subsequent years, two trials [2, 3] evaluated tPA within 0–6 hours, showing that tPA isnot efficacious in the expanded time window. However, tPA has recently been shown to be effective in a selected group of stroke patients between 0 and 4.5 hours [4].

A joint report by AHA stroke council and AAN quality standards committee states that tPA should be considered in patients with ischemic stroke within 3 hours [5]. In 2002, the American Academy of Emergency Medicine [6] position statement raised concerns about the risk and benefit ratio of tPA in stroke and debate over whether tPA should be considered standard of care. The statement argued that the National Institute of Neurological Disorders and Stroke (NINDS) study suggested that 8 out of 18 (44%) stroke patients who receive tPA according to a strict protocol recover by three months after the event without significant disability.

Whereas, 6 out of 18 (33%) stroke patients (one-third) recover substantially, regardless of treatment, they also indicated that 1 out of 18 patients have a symptomatic bleeding complication.

Malpractice is defined as "the failure to meet a standard of care or standard of conduct that is recognized by a profession reaches the level of malpractice when a client or patient is injured or damaged because of error." The burden of the proof or preponderance of evidence is on the plaintiff, in any medical malpractice litigation. In other words, if a jury believes there is at least 51 percent likelihood that a defendant was negligent or liable, the plaintiff has met its burden of proof and will prevail. This is particularly helpful when juries cannot decide between the testimonies of two expert witnesses presenting opposite opinions or views.

In the United States, AIS is the number one cause of disability and morbidity thus attracting medical litigation. A study reviewing malpractice cases in New York State showed that severity of the patient's disability, not the occurrence of an adverse event due to medical negligence, was predictive of payment to the plaintiff [7]. Frivolous medical malpractice lawsuits are common; consequently, exorbitant amount of human and financial resources is utilized, even if the case eventually is ruled in favor of the defendant [8].

According to the 2009 PIAA Risk Management Review: Neurology Edition (available at http://www.piaa.us) [9], for the year 2008, neurology and neurosurgery had the highest average indemnity of the 28 specialties included in the PIAA review. In the case of tPA and stroke, medical litigation works as a double-edged sword. Frequently reasons cited for litigation in the court of law include lost opportunity to give tPA or adverse events related to tPA. Recent reviews [10, 11] have emphasized that physicians are at risk for malpractice suits both when administering and not administering tPA to AIS patients. Disinclination to use tPA by physicians for legal or clinical reasons may potentially lead to medical malpractice litigation.

To date, no systematic reviews have been performed, which evaluate malpractice and thrombolytic therapy in ischemic stroke patients. The objective of this review is to do a systematic evaluation of malpractice cases published in major medical and legal databases.

2. Methods

2.1. Protocol. A robust systematic review protocol (Figure 1) was prepared. We searched Medline, Embase, Google Scholar, LexisNexis Legal, and Westlaw databases in order to identify cases, which involved malpractice litigation and tPA in ischemic stroke. LexisNexis Legal is a comprehensive database, which covers state as well as federal law cases in the USA Westlaw is a legal attorney database providing information on cases noted by practicing attorneys. In an attempt of completeness, we searched all state case, Health law case, Tort law case, Professional Malpractice case, and all federal case databases that fall within the Westlaw database.

2.2. Search Terms. We used 3 different search terms to be specific to our search, namely, "tPA, stroke, and malpractice," "clot busting, stroke, and malpractice," and "stroke and malpractice."

Table 1: Malpractice claims.

Claim	Cases (n, %)	Verdict in favor of (n, %)
Failure to treat with tPA	28, 70%	Of 28 Defendant: 19, 67.9% Plaintiff: 7, 25% NA: 2, 7.1%
Complication as a result of giving tPA	2, 5%	Of 2 Defendant: 1, 50% Plaintiff: 1, 50%
Failure to diagnose	10, 25%	Of 10 Defendant: 6, 60% Plaintiff: 4, 40%
Total claims	40	Defendant: 26, 65% Plaintiff: 12, 30% NA: 2, 5%

2.3. Search Results in Each Database. Using the terms "tPA, stroke, and malpractice" yielded 5 results in Medline, 40 in LexisNexis Legal, and 1383, 987, 984, 1063, and 576 results in All State law, Health law, Tort Law case, Professional Malpractice case, and all federal case databases, respectively (all of which are part of Westlaw database). The term "clot busting, stroke, and malpractice" did not show up any results in Medline but gave 13 results in LexisNexis Legal, and 2258, 1703, 1691, 1814, and 783 in All State law, Health Law, Tort law, Professional malpractice case, and all federal case databases of Westlaw. The term "stroke and malpractice" gave us 77 results in Medline, 999 in LexisNexis Legal, and 1370, 980, 976, 1053, and 558 search results in All State Law, Health Law, Tort Law, Professional Malpractice case, and all federal case databases. The Google scholar and Embase database results were subsumed in the Medline search results.

Finally, we identified 789 stroke cases with malpractice suits. AB and DC reviewed case summaries of all cases with the objective to retrieve malpractice lawsuits involving use or nonuse of intravenous tPA in AIS. Finally, 46 cases were identified, and full review was carried out by three reviewers (AB, DC, and AS).

3. Results

We identified 789 ischemic stroke cases involved in litigation. We were able to identify 46 cases related to tPA use in stroke patients between the years 1999 and 2010, of which data was available for 40 cases related to tPA in stroke. However, verdicts were only available for 38 cases. We categorized medico-legal characteristics depending on the malpractice claims and related verdicts (Table 1), hospital/physician characteristics (Table 2), factors favoring defendants (Table 3), and factors favoring plaintiffs (Table 4).

3.1. Malpractice Claims. The most frequent malpractice claims by the plaintiff were failure to treat with tPA (28, 70%) and failure to diagnose stroke, claiming a lost opportunity to

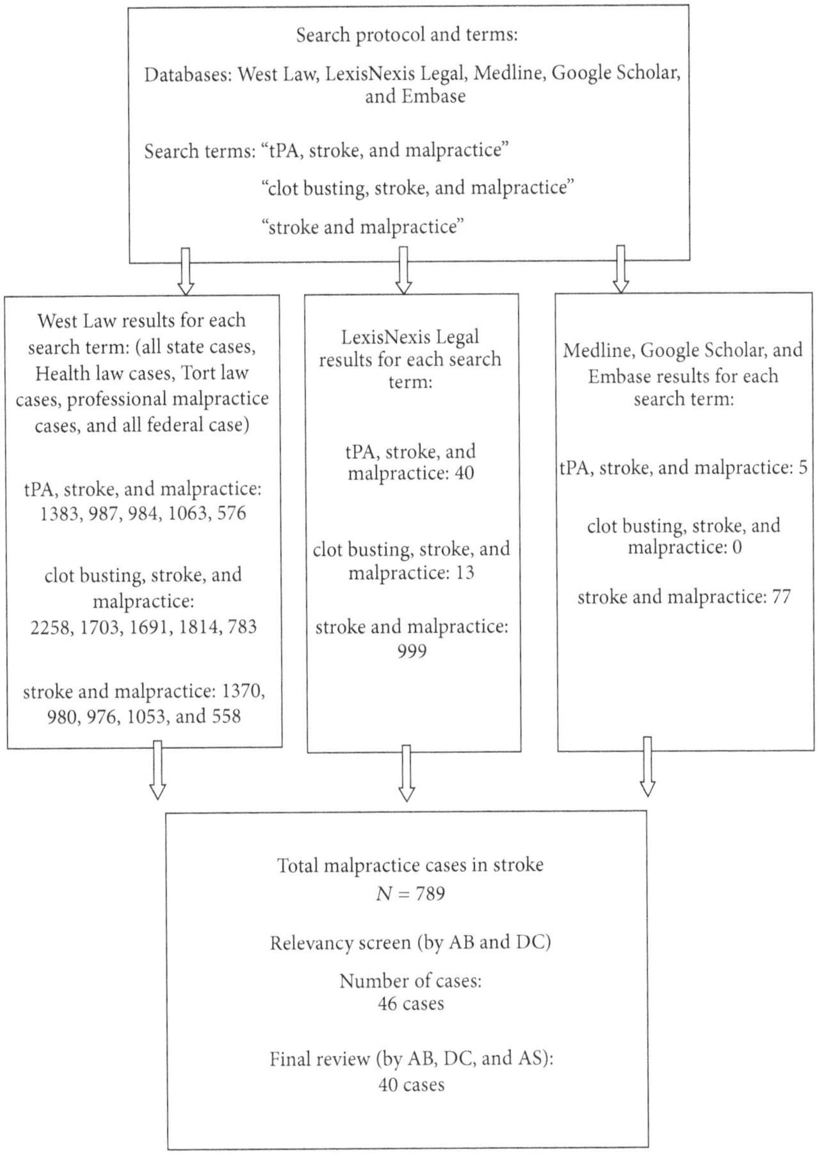

Figure 1

give tPA (10, 25%). Only 2 (5.0%) patients had claims involved complications of treatment with tPA. Of all cases, where verdicts were available, in 90% cases (n = 36) hospital was the defendant. There were 12 (30%) cases where only hospitals were defendants. Out of the 36 (90%) cases involving the hospitals, 28 (75%) were community hospitals, and 9(25%) were university or university affiliated. ED physicians were involved in 25 (60.52%) cases and neurologists participated in 8 (20.0%) cases. In a minority of cases 7 (17.5%), other physicians such as internists, neurosurgeons, and ICU physicians were involved. However, multiple physicians were involved in 11 (27.5% of cases). There were 5 (12.5%) cases where stroke occurred during the hospital stay.

3.2. Factors Favoring the Defendant. Factors favoring the defendant incuded proper documentation of contraindications and discussion regarding risks and benefits (50%), expert witness testimony (25%), duration of symptoms beyond 3 hr at the time of presentation (15.6%), informed consent (6.3%), no specific time of onset of symptoms (6.3%), tPA protocol in hospital (9.4%), and tPA not available in hospital (3.1%).

3.3. Factors Favoring the Plaintiff. Among all malpractice claims, factors favoring the plaintiff were failure to treat with tPA (67.5%), failure to diagnose (20%), failure to transfer to an institution where thrombolysis can be given (20%), no informed consent or proper documentation regarding contraindication (7.5%), delay in evaluating the patient by a doctor (12.5%) obtaining tests (10%), failure to perform proper medical exam (5%), failure to recommend tPA as a treatment (10%), and complications as a result of tPA treatment (5%).

TABLE 2: Physician/facility involved.

Faculty/facility involved	Cases (*n*, %)	Verdict in favor of (*n*, %)
ED physician involved	25, 62.5%	Defendant: 21, 84% Plaintiff: 4, 16%
Neurologist involved	8, 20%	Defendant: 6, 75% Plaintiff: 2, 25%
Other (PCP, hospitalist, ICU, and neurosurgeon)	7, 17.5%	Defendant: 5, 71.4% Plaintiff: 1, 14.3% NA: 1, 14.3%
Multiple physicians involved	11, 27.5%	Defendant: 10, 90.9% Plaintiff: 1, 9.1%
Only hospital involved	12, 30%	Defendant: 4, 33.3% Plaintiff: 7, 58.3% NA: 1, 8.3%
Hospital involved	36, 90%	Defendant: 22, 61.1% Plaintiff: 13, 36.1% NA: 1, 2.8%
Type of hospital involved	Of total 36, Community hospital: 27, 75% University Hospital: 9, 25%	Community hospital: defendant: 17, 62.9% plaintiff: 10, 37.03% University hospital: defendant: 5, 55.6% plaintiff: 3, 33.3% NA: 1, 11.1%
In hospital strokes	5 of total 40, 12.5%	Defendant: 2, 40% Plaintiff: 2, 40% NA: 1, 20%

TABLE 3: Frequency of factors favoring defendant.

Factors favoring defendants	Number of cases (total: 320), percentage (%) of cases	Verdict
Documented contraindication/discussion with the family	16, 50%	Defendant: 12, 75% Plaintiff: 4, 25%
Expert witness	8, 25%	Defendant: 8, 100% Plaintiff: 0
Beyond 3 hrs when diagnosed	5, 15.6%	Defendant: 2, 40% Plaintiff: 2, 40% NA: 1, 20%
"TPA protocol in hospital"	3, 9.4%	Defendant: 1, 33.3% Plaintiff: 2, 66.7%
Informed consent	2, 6.3%	Defendant: 2, 100% Plaintiff: 0
Discussion with patient and family	2, 6.3%	Defendant: 2, 100% Plaintiff: 0
No specific time of onset of symptoms	2, 6.3%	Defendant: 2, 100% Plaintiff: 0
tPA not available in hospital	1, 3.1%	Defendant: 1, 100% Plaintiff: 0
Timely transfer to other hospital	3, 9.3%	Defendant: 3, 100% Plaintiff: 0

4. Discussion

Our review indicates that hospitals, ED physicians, neurologists, and sometimes other physicians at the forefront of stroke management are always at risk for medical litigation. It appears from the case descriptions that not treating with tPA (38, 95% cases) is the main causative factor for litigations as 38 out of 40 cases reviewed did not receive tPA (i.e., the standard of care). Reasons of litigation were mostly preventable. Major plaintiff arguments in these cases were failure to diagnose ischemic stroke, inadequate documentation why tPA was not given, failure to transfer to a facility where tPA can be given, and delay in physician or CT evaluation. Our analysis showed that only two cases were related to complications of tPA, out of which 1 was ruled in favor of plaintiff and 1 in favor of defendant. Early data [12] have suggested that only 50% of neurologists were actually giving tPA. Early data also show that tPA is used by less than 2% of the community hospitals [13]; this number has probably increased as a result of comprehensive efforts by JCAHO [10]. Despite ongoing efforts, only 5–10% patients with stroke receive tPA [14]. As a result of perceived complications (e.g., intracranial hemorrhage), surveys have also shown that lack of benefits [15] and medico legal concerns were reported as barrier [11] to give tPA. A review suggested that physician reimbursement for the evaluation and treatment of acute stroke, when compared with other diagnoses commonly treated by neurologists, is relatively low in both the USA and Canada. Health policy decision makers in the USA and Canada should be made aware of the importance of providing a more balanced plan to provide medical care to stroke patients [16]. In addition, the familiarity and comfort among nonneurology physicians (NNPs) with the administration of tPA is still relatively low in rural settings [17]. Our review showed that even hospitalists, neurosurgeons, or PCPs can

TABLE 4: Frequency of factors favoring Plaintiff.

Factors favoring plaintiff	Number of cases (total: 40), percentage (%) of cases	Verdict
Failure to treat with tPA	27, 67.5%	Defendant: 18, 66.7% Plaintiff: 7, 25.9% NA: 2, 7.4%
Failure to diagnose	8, 20%	Defendant: 6, 75% Plaintiff: 2, 25%
Failure to transfer	8, 20%	Defendant: 5, 62.5% Plaintiff: 3, 42.9%
Delay in attending patient by ED physician or neurologist	5, 12.5%	Defendant: 3, 60% Plaintiff: 2, 40%
Failure to recommend tPA as a treatment option	4, 10%	Defendant: 4, 100% Plaintiff: 0
Delay in getting test (CT-scan)	4, 10%	Defendant: 3, 75% Plaintiff: 1, 25%
NO informed consent	3, 7.5%	Defendant: 2, 66.7% Plaintiff: 1, 33.3%
Complications of treatment with tPA	2, 5%	Defendant: 1, 50% Plaintiff: 1, 50%
Failure to perform proper complete exam	2, 5%	Defendant: 0 Plaintiff: 2, 100%

be defendants, if they are the only physicians taking care of the patient. Out of 6 cases where nonneurology non-ED physicians were involved, 5 were defendant favored compared to 1 plaintiff favored verdict. On a positive note, more recently, telemedicine efforts has been safely instituted in evaluation of AIS and has increased tPA rates in outlying hospitals in an effective and safe manner [18]. In our review, all 3 cases consisting of timely transfer to outside facilities were ruled in favor of the defendants. The most common reason for transfer was absence of neurology expertise and/or tPA protocol in the hospital. Conversely, 8 cases involved a delay in transfer with 3 cases (42%) being ruled in favor of the plaintiff. These methods potentially reduce legal liability especially in transfer cases. Among all cases reviewed, it was noticed that two thirds of the defendants received a favorable verdict. Informed consent, proper documentation of discussion with family, tPA protocol in place, time of transfer, time of onset of symptoms, and timely transfer were important factors in verdicts favoring the defendants. Risks and benefits associated with tPA as well as limited treatment window timeframe should be explained thoroughly, and patients' decision should be properly documented including transfer time. In 90% of cases, a hospital was the defendant. Hospitals, even those of a smaller size, should take initiatives and invest in human resources to facilitate thrombolytic therapy for AIS in the hospital. We found that ED physicians were more likely to be defendants than neurology physicians. However, rate of defendant-favored verdicts was similar on both sides (ED—84% and neurologist—75%). In 1 out of 4 cases, more than one physician is involved.

Expert witness testimony on the plaintiff side frequently argued that according to NINDS trial, there is a >51 percent chance that the patient will improve if the patient received tPA. However, expert testimony from the defendant side frequently argued that there is only a 32 percent greater chance that the patient would improve. Taking the legal definition of malpractice, the plaintiff needs to prove that the "patient is more likely to improve than not," and in other words the emphasis is on the chance of improvement and not the actual percentage. In short, in cases where thrombolysis was not given, argument for lack of efficacy of tPA by any defendant was not a very solid argument by defense expert witnesses, and usually these cases were ruled in favor of plaintiffs.

That brings us to the next point, is tPA in fact standard of care? Malpractice claims against physicians are difficult to measure, and physicians might be able to avoid liability by understanding the standard of care regarding tPA. A review has suggested that once an "experimental and risky to give drug" can eventually become a "standard of care" [11]. Emerging local stroke centers in the community have changed the concept of standard of care from nationwide to community and put expectations of elevated criteria on medical personnel and other hospitals in the community [10]. Overall, physicians are judged by standard of practice in their *community* or *similar communities*. However, that concept is changing, and standard of care may be judged by care that could be provided by a physician under *similar circumstances*.

5. Conclusion

Our review also indicates that hospitals and ED physicians are involved in a majority of these litigation cases. The review shows that having hospital-ED-based protocols for tPA administration, transfer protocols to appropriate care facility, clear discussion and documentation of treatment options by physicians, and early involvement of a neurologist may provide optimal milieu for selecting intravenous thrombolysis candidates for patients with AIS. While the majority of the cases litigated were cases where tPA was not administered, only minority of cases were litigated when complications occurred.

References

[1] J. R. Marler, "Tissue plasminogen activator for acute ischemic stroke," *The New England Journal of Medicine*, vol. 333, no. 24, pp. 1581–1587, 1995.

[2] C. Fieschi, W. Hacke, M. Kaste, D. Toni, and E. Lesaffre, "Thrombolytic therapy for acute ischaemic stroke. ECASS Study Group," *Lancet*, vol. 350, no. 9089, pp. 1476–1477, 1997.

[3] W. M. Clark, S. Wissman, G. W. Albers, J. H. Jhamandas, K. P. Madden, and S. Hamilton, "Recombinant tissue-type plasminogen activator (Alteplase) for ischemic stroke 3 to 5 hours after symptom onset the ATLANTIS study: a randomized controlled trial," *Journal of the American Medical Association*, vol. 282, no. 21, pp. 2019–2026, 1999.

[4] W. Hacke, M. Kaste, E. Bluhmki et al., "Thrombolysis with alteplase 3 to 4.5 hours after acute ischemic stroke," *The New England Journal of Medicine*, vol. 359, no. 13, pp. 1317–1329, 2008.

[5] H. P. Adams Jr., T. G. Brott, A. J. Furlan et al., "Guidelines for thrombolytic therapy for acute stroke: a supplement to the guidelines for the management of patients with acute ischemic stroke. A statement for healthcare professionals from a special writing group of the Stroke Council, American Heart Association," *Circulation*, vol. 94, no. 5, pp. 1167–1174, 1996.

[6] "Position statement of the american academy of emergency medicine on the use of intravenous thrombolytic therapy in the treatment of stroke," http://www.aaem.org/em-resources/position-statements/2002/thrombolytic-therapy.

[7] T. A. Brennan, C. M. Sox, and H. R. Burstin, "Relation between negligent adverse events and the outcomes of medical-malpractice litigation," *The New England Journal of Medicine*, vol. 335, no. 26, pp. 1963–1967, 1996.

[8] D. M. Studdert, M. M. Mello, A. A. Gawande et al., "Claims, errors, and compensation payments in medical malpractice litigation," *The New England Journal of Medicine*, vol. 354, no. 19, pp. 2024–2033, 2006.

[9] *Piaa Risk Management Review*, Neurology edition, 2009.

[10] M. I. Weintraub, "Thrombolysis (tissue plasminogen activator) in stroke: a medicolegal quagmire," *Stroke*, vol. 37, no. 7, pp. 1917–1922, 2006.

[11] B. A. Liang and J. A. Zivin, "Empirical characteristics of litigation involving tissue plasminogen activator and ischemic stroke," *Annals of Emergency Medicine*, vol. 52, no. 2, pp. 160–164, 2008.

[12] I. L. Katzan, C. A. Sila, and A. J. Furlan, "Community use of intravenous tissue plasminogen activator for acute stroke: results of the brain matters stroke management survey," *Stroke*, vol. 32, no. 4, pp. 861–864, 2001.

[13] I. L. Katzan, A. J. Furlan, L. E. Lloyd et al., "Use of tissue-type plasminogen activator for acute ischemic stroke: the Cleveland area experience," *Journal of the American Medical Association*, vol. 283, no. 9, pp. 1151–1158, 2000.

[14] M. J. Reeves, S. Arora, J. P. Broderick et al., "Acute stroke care in the us: results from 4 pilot prototypes of the paul coverdell national acute stroke registry," *Stroke*, vol. 36, pp. 1232–1240, 2005.

[15] D. L. Brown, W. G. Barsan, L. D. Lisabeth, M. E. Gallery, and L. B. Morgenstern, "Survey of emergency physicians about recombinant tissue plasminogen activator for acute ischemic stroke," *Annals of Emergency Medicine*, vol. 46, no. 1, pp. 56–60, 2005.

[16] D. Kleindorfer, M. D. Hill, D. Woo et al., "A description of Canadian and United States physician reimbursement for thrombolytic therapy administration in acute ischemic stroke," *Stroke*, vol. 36, no. 3, pp. 682–687, 2005.

[17] L. L. Edwards, "Using tPA for acute stroke in a rural setting," *Neurology*, vol. 68, no. 4, pp. 292–294, 2007.

[18] M. A. Pervez, G. Silva, S. Masrur et al., "Remote supervision of IV-tPA for acute ischemic stroke by telemedicine or telephone before transfer to a regional stroke center is feasible and safe," *Stroke*, vol. 41, no. 1, pp. e18–e24, 2010.

31

Short-Term Outcome in Stroke Patients with or without Atrial Fibrillation: A Retrospective Case-Control Study

Antonino Sant'Angelo,[1] Sergio Bagnato,[1] Cristina Boccagni,[1] Vincenzo Guardabasso,[2] and Giuseppe Galardi[1]

[1] *Rehabilitation Department, Fondazione Istituto "San Raffaele-G. Giglio", 90015 Cefalù (PA), Italy*
[2] *Azienda Policlinico-Vittorio Emanuele, University of Catania, 95123 Catania, Italy*

Correspondence should be addressed to Antonino Sant'Angelo, antonino.santangelo@hsrgiglio.it

Academic Editors: K.-H. Lin and K. Nas

Background. Patients with cardioembolic stroke due to atrial fibrillation (CE/AF stroke) seem to have a poorer functional recovery than those with non cardioembolic stroke. This may be ascribed to the heterogeneity between the samples of patients with and without CE/AF stroke. *Aim.* To compare the short-term outcome of patients with CE/AF stroke and with non-CE/AF stroke of same gender and similar age and level of disability and comorbidity. *Methods.* The functional independence measure (FIM) of 40 consecutive patients with CE/AF stroke was retrospectively evaluated at admission and discharge in our rehabilitation department. Each "case" was matched with a patient ("control") of the same sex and similar age and FIM score at admission, affected by non-CE/AF stroke admitted to our department in the same period. *Results.* FIM score at admission and discharge was respectively 51.9 ± 20.3 and 75.7 ± 21.2 in patients with CE/AF stroke and 54.9 ± 19 and 73.9 ± 22.7 in patients with non-CE/AF stroke; no significant difference was found between the groups. Multivariate analysis showed an effect of the rehabilitation treatment and age on FIM score, whereas no effect was attributable to AF. *Conclusions.* The short-term outcome is similar in patients with and without CE/AF stroke.

1. Introduction

Cardioembolic (CE) strokes account for 25 to 30% of ischemic strokes among white populations [1], most of which are associated with atrial fibrillation (AF). In fact AF is the most common persistent cardiac arrhythmia [2], and its prevalence has been estimated at 1% in the general population [3, 4], ranging from about 1% in people aged between 55 and 59 years to 9–13% in people older than 80 years [4–6].

Previous studies have reported that CE stroke associated with AF (CE/AF stroke) has a poorer prognosis in terms of survival because of the higher risk of early stroke recurrence, the larger volume of the infarct, the existing cardiac disease causing the arrhythmia, and the older age of patients compared to those with other ischemic strokes [7–9]. It has been also reported that patients with CE/AF stroke display a worse functional recovery than those with non-CE/AF stroke [7]. However, such a finding was drawn from the comparison of heterogeneous samples of patients. Hence, it has not been conclusively established the functional outcome of patients with CE/AF stroke. The aim of our study was to compare the short-term outcome of patients with or without CE/AF stroke after removing some confounding factors, such as different sex, age, and level of disability. Therefore, we used the Functional Independence Measure (FIM) instrument [10] in a retrospective case-control study to compare the short-term outcome of patients with a CE/AF stroke matched with non-CE/AF stroke patients of same sex and similar age and level of disability.

2. Materials and Methods

This retrospective case-control study was conducted on clinical records of patients admitted to our Rehabilitation department from January 2005 to June 2009 to carry out a standard neurorehabilitative treatment after an ischemic stroke.

We selected the clinical records of 40 patients ("cases"; 23 males, mean age 65.4 ± 9.1 years) with CE/AF stroke as supported by a 12-lead electrocardiogram (ECG) or Holter-ECG recorded during the acute phase. CE/AF stroke was diagnosed according to focal neurological symptoms and signs, with neuroradiological brain evidence of infarction associated with AF as the cardiac source of embolism, without evidence of large-artery disease by noninvasive vascular testing. The clinical record of each "case" was matched with that of a patient ("control") affected by non-CE/AF ischemic stroke (40 "controls"; 23 males, mean age 65.5 ± 8.9 years) with the same sex and similar age, level of disability and duration of disease.

Mean disease duration (DD) was expressed as the time interval (days) from stroke onset to admission to our department. Both groups had a similar length of hospitalization (LOH) and carried out the same standard rehabilitative treatment, consisting of 2 hours per day of kinesitherapy and occupational therapy, added to regular bed mobilization, chair transfers, and, when required, speech therapy and cognitive rehabilitation. During their stay in rehabilitation department the patients' physical burden of illness was measured by the severity index (SI) and comorbidity index (CI) of the Cumulative Illness Rating score (CIRS) [11]. The CIRS is a valid indicator of health status and a comprehensive comorbidity index among frail people [12]. CIRS uses a 5-point ordinal scales (score 1–5) to estimate the severity of pathology in each of 14 systems domains. Based on the ratings, two scores are derived: the SI (it is the mean of the scores of the first 13 categories, excluding psychiatric; it reflects the overall burden of illness, and it ranges 1–5) and the CI (it is calculated as the number of categories with a score of 3 or greater, excluding psychiatric; it reflects diversity of illnesses and it ranges 0–13).

2.1. Outcome Measure. The functional outcome was evaluated in each patient at admission and at discharge by means of the FIM instrument. It is a scale measuring a person's level of disability in terms of burden of care [13]. It was developed specifically to measure functional outcomes of rehabilitation [14]. FIM is a trademark of the Uniform Data System for Medical Rehabilitation, a division of UB Foundation Activities, Inc.

The FIM at admission and at discharge was administered by the patient's care team, consisting of a neurologist, a nurse, a physiotherapist and a psychologist/speech therapist, all experts and trained in its use. As this is a retrospective study, nobody knew the purpose of the present study at the time of the assessments.

2.2. Statistical Analysis. Descriptive statistics were computed and compared to confirm homogeneity of case and control groups before treatment. Analysis of variance (ANOVA) was used to compare results within patients before/after treatment, considering presence/absence of AF. A two-by-two ANOVA design, between-within subjects, was used. Statistical significance was set at the $P = 0.05$ level. Multiple linear regression was then used to compute the effect of each explanatory factor simultaneously adjusted for the effects of other factors. With this technique, so called confounding factors can be controlled separately. A linear model was construed, where the observed (dependent) variable was FIM. Explanatory factors (regressors) considered were: a numerical variable, *age* at time of hospital admission (expressed in years and tenths of year), and three "dummy" variables: *time* (before/after treatment), *case* (AF/no history of AF), and *sex* (male/female). Multiple linear regression was performed using Epi-info v. 3.5.1 (CDC, Atlanta, USA), suitable for dummy variables and that performs complete ANOVA calculations for significance of individual regressors and interaction terms. Results were expressed as units of FIM explained by each regressor (with 95% confidence intervals, CI). Statistical significance was set at the $P = 0.05$ level.

2.3. Ethics. The protocol was approved by the local Ethics Committee and has been performed in accordance with the ethical standards of Declaration of Helsinki. Data used for the study were those usually recorded in the medical file of patients only.

3. Results

Demographic and clinical characteristics of patients are reported in Table 1. Patients with and without CE/AF stroke were homogeneous regarding mean age, gender, mean disease duration, and mean LOH. Moreover CIRS (SI) and CIRS (CI) did not differ significantly between patients with and without CE/AF stroke. The difference in the level of disability at admission in the Rehabilitation Department and at discharge, as expressed by the FIM score, was not significant between groups (Table 1). ANOVA revealed a significant main effect of the within-subject factor (before/after treatment) (F 155.57; $P < 0.0001$). There were no significant effects either for the between-subjects factor (presence or absence of AF, $P = 0.89$) or for the interaction ($P = 0.16$) (Figure 1).

Multiple linear regression showed that *time* (before/after treatment), as expected, and *age* were significant factors ($P < 0.001$ and $P = 0.014$ resp.) in explaining FIM values, whereas *sex* was almost statistically significant ($P = 0.086$) and *case* was not a significant explanatory variable ($P = 0.84$). Results (Table 2) indicate the net effects of each variable on FIM values, simultaneously adjusted for all other factors:

(i) *time* caused an average increase of FIM after treatment of 21.35 (CI 15.05 to 27.65);

(ii) *age* explained an average loss of FIM of 4.5 per decade of age (−0.45 per year, CI −0.81 to −0.09), both before and after treatment;

(iii) *sex* explained a level of FIM lower by 5.67 as average in females versus males, with CI −12 to slightly above zero, indicating that this factor did not reach the $P < 0.05$ level of statistical significance ($P = 0.086$);

(iv) *case*, CE/AF stroke patients or matched controls, did not explain any significant difference in FIM average.

TABLE 1: Demographic and clinical characteristics of patients with (no. 40) and without (no. 40) CE/AF stroke undergoing a standard rehabilitation treatment.

Patients	Gender	Age	Affected hemisphere	DD (days)	LOH (days)	CIRS (SI)	CIRS (CI)	FIM (admission)	FIM (discharge)
CE/AF	23 males	65.4 ± 9.1	Right: 21 patients	32.3 ± 24.4	41.6 ± 13.4	1.1 ± 0.2	5.4 ± 1.4	51.9 ± 20.3	75.7 ± 21.2*
Non-CE/AF	23 males	65.5 ± 8.9	Right: 21 patients	28.9 ± 22.7	42.8 ± 16.1	1.2 ± 0.2	5.3 ± 1.3	54.9 ± 19	73.9 ± 22.7*
		$P = 0.95$		$P = 0.55$	$P = 0.74$	$P = 0.21$	$P = 0.86$	$P = 0.49$	$P = 0.72$

Data are expressed as mean ± SD. DD: disease duration, LOH: length of hospitalization, CIRS (SI): cumulative Illness Rating score (severity index), CIRS (CI): Cumulative Illness Rating score (comorbidity index), FIM: functional independence measures, *significant treatment (time) effect.

TABLE 2: Results of multiple linear regression.

Factor	Value	95% CI	P
time	21.35	15.05 to 27.65	<0.0001
age	−0.45	−0.81 to −0.09	0.014
sex	−5.67	−12.11 to 0.76	0.086
case	−0.64	−6.94 to 5.65	0.8418

NOTE: intercept was 85.8 (95% CI 62–110); F statistic for regression = 13,72 $P < 0.0001$, R-squared = 0.26.

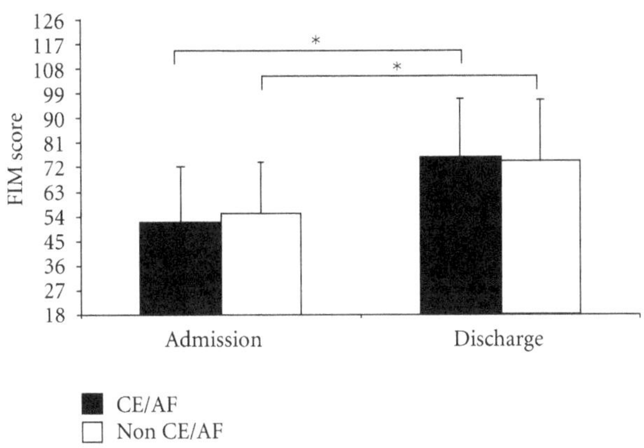

FIGURE 1: FIM score (means and SD) before and after a standard rehabilitative treatment in patients with (black column) and without (white column) CE/AF stroke. *significant treatment (time) effect.

Possible synergistic effects of factors were considered (case and time, sex and time, and age and time), but no significant interaction between factors was observed.

As it could be expected, the linear model used did not fully explain the individual differences in FIM before and after treatment. Indeed the R-squared value of 0.26 indicated that about 26% of the overall variability was explained. However, it illustrated and quantified the effects of treatment and of age, hinted at a possible systematic difference of FIM by sex, and corroborated the hypothesis that AF *per se* is not a significant factor in recovery.

4. Discussion

The main results of this study were that both groups of stroke patients—with and without CE/AF stroke—had similar FIM scores at admission and at the end of rehabilitative treatment. The similarity of FIM scores at admission reflects their homogeneity in terms of level of disability before the rehabilitative treatment. Moreover the lack of significant differences in CIRS (SI) and CIRS (CI) between the groups suggests an overall homogenous health status and comorbidity level. FIM and CIRS scores, along with the age and gender homogeneity between groups, rule out a bias in the assessment of their functional outcome after rehabilitation. As the improvement of FIM score after a rehabilitative treatment may be considered an index of functional outcome and therapeutic effectiveness, our results indicate that the short-term functional outcome is comparable in patients with CE/AF stroke and in patients with non-CE/AF stroke. Therefore, in a population homogeneous regarding age, gender, and initial level of disability and comorbidity, the presence of AF does not seem to be a significant factor in functional recovery of patients with ischemic stroke receiving inpatient rehabilitation. However, on the basis of the data of the present study, these considerations can be made only for patients with a moderate degree of disability that, in our study, is expressed by the FIM score at the admission of about 52–55 points. These data are consistent with those of Leys et al. [15], who reported that clinical outcome in young adults with ischemic stroke was independent from the cause of stroke.

These results seem to be at odds with other studies, according to which AF would play a negative prognostic role [7–9]. However in these studies patients with CE/AF stroke were mostly females, older, and have poorer prestroke functional status and more severe neurological deficits than patients with other types of ischemic stroke. It is likely that methodological differences may explain these discrepancies. The population-based studies cited above included the whole community of stroke patients, while our case-control study limited its observation to patients admitted for intensive rehabilitation. So, patients (presumably, more with AF) who died during the acute stage of disease or referred to an extensive rehabilitation department because of a more severe clinical state were not included. Similarly, those patients undergoing a rapid recovery from major neurological deficits (so called "spectacular shrinking deficit") due to reperfusion of brain with early lysis of the embolus were not studied.

Another factor that should be taken into account is the temporal window used. Unlike other studies [8], we have not followedup our patients after their discharge; therefore, we cannot exclude any possible effect of AF on the long-term functional outcome for sure. In such cases, as suggested by others, heart failure, but not the cerebral cardioembolism, is a predictor of dependency 1 year after a first-ever stroke [16].

Finally, the present study, consistently with data reported in literature, confirms that age plays a crucial role as a risk factor for dependency after a first-ever stroke [16]. Particularly, age explains an average loss of FIM of 4.5 per decade both before and after treatment. We should, however, be careful in the interpretation of this result, because our study was not designed to evaluate the effect of age on functional outcome after stroke rehabilitation; therefore, it is difficult to distinguish between age itself and age-associated factors (i.e., comorbidities, and lack of motivation...) as factors influencing the level of functional recovery after a stroke [17].

5. Conclusions

In summary, the short-term functional outcome is comparable in stroke patients with and without AF admitted to the poststroke rehabilitative treatment. Considering the expected ageing of population and the increasing incidence of AF and stroke, it is important to provide timely access to effective stroke rehabilitation programs for all stroke survivors, regardless of stroke pathogenesis.

Conflict of Interest

The authors declare that they have no conflict of interests.

References

[1] P. L. Kolominsky-Rabas, M. Weber, O. Gefeller, B. Neundoerfer, and P. U. Heuschmann, "Epidemiology of ischemic stroke subtypes according to TOAST criteria: incidence, recurrence, and long-term survival in ischemic stroke subtypes: a population-based study," *Stroke*, vol. 32, no. 12, pp. 2735–2740, 2001.

[2] S. M. Narayan, M. E. Cain, and J. M. Smith, "Atrial fibrillation," *The Lancet*, vol. 350, no. 9082, pp. 943–950, 1997.

[3] W. M. Feinberg, J. L. Blackshear, A. Laupacis, R. Kronmal, and R. G. Hart, "Prevalence, age distribution, and gender of patients with atrial fibrillation: analysis and implications," *Archives of Internal Medicine*, vol. 155, no. 5, pp. 469–473, 1995.

[4] A. S. Go, E. M. Hylek, K. A. Phillips et al., "Prevalence of diagnosed atrial fibrillation in adults: national implications for rhythm management and stroke prevention: the anticoagulation and risk factors in atrial fibrillation (ATRIA) study," *Journal of the American Medical Association*, vol. 285, no. 18, pp. 2370–2375, 2001.

[5] S. J. Phillips, "Is atrial fibrillation an independent risk factor for stroke?" *Canadian Journal of Neurological Sciences*, vol. 17, no. 2, pp. 163–168, 1990.

[6] T. S. M. Tsang, G. W. Petty, M. E. Barnes et al., "The prevalence of atrial fibrillation in incident stroke cases and matched population controls in Rochester, Minnesota: changes over three decades," *Journal of the American College of Cardiology*, vol. 42, no. 1, pp. 93–100, 2003.

[7] M. Lamassa, A. Di Carlo, G. Pracucci et al., "Characteristics, outcome, and care of stroke associated with atrial fibrillation in Europe: data from a multicenter multinational hospital-based registry (the European community stroke project)," *Stroke*, vol. 32, no. 2, pp. 392–398, 2001.

[8] G. W. Petty, R. D. Brown Jr., J. P. Whisnant, J. D. Sicks, W. M. O'Fallon, and D. O. Wiebers, "Ischemic stroke subtypes: a population-based study of functional outcome, survival, and recurrence," *Stroke*, vol. 31, no. 5, pp. 1062–1068, 2000.

[9] Y. Béjot, D. B. Salem, G. V. Osseby et al., "Epidemiology of ischemic stroke from atrial fibrillation in Dijon, France, from 1985 to 2006," *Neurology*, vol. 72, no. 4, pp. 346–353, 2009.

[10] A. Deutsch, S. Braun, and C. V. Granger, "The Functional Independence Measure (FIM Instrument)," *Journal of Rehabilitation Outcomes Measurement*, vol. 1, pp. 67–71, 1997.

[11] P. A. Parmelee, P. D. Thuras, I. R. Katz, and M. P. Lawton, "Validation of the cumulative illness rating scale in a geriatric residential population," *Journal of the American Geriatrics Society*, vol. 43, no. 2, pp. 130–137, 1995.

[12] F. Salvi, M. D. Miller, A. Grilli et al., "A manual of guidelines to score the modified Cumulative Illness Rating Scale and its validation in acute hospitalized elderly patients," *Journal of the American Geriatrics Society*, vol. 56, no. 10, pp. 1926–1931, 2008.

[13] C. V. Granger, B. B. Hamilton, M. Zielezny, and F. S. Sherwin, "Advances in functional assessment in medical rehabilitation," *Topics in Geriatric Rehabilitation*, vol. 1, pp. 59–74, 1994.

[14] B. B. Hamilton, J. A. Laughlin, R. C. Fiedler, and C. V. Granger, "Interrater reliability of the 7-level Functional Independence Measure (FIM)," *Scandinavian Journal of Rehabilitation Medicine*, vol. 26, no. 3, pp. 115–119, 1994.

[15] D. Leys, L. Bandu, H. Hénon et al., "Clinical outcome in 287 consecutive young adults (15 to 45 years) with ischemic stroke," *Neurology*, vol. 59, no. 1, pp. 26–33, 2002.

[16] P. Appelros, I. Nydevik, and M. Viitanen, "Poor outcome after first-ever stroke: predictors for death, dependency, and recurrent stroke within the first year," *Stroke*, vol. 34, no. 1, pp. 122–126, 2003.

[17] S. Bagg, A. P. Pombo, and W. Hopman, "Effect of age on functional outcomes after stroke rehabilitation," *Stroke*, vol. 33, no. 1, pp. 179–185, 2002.

Stroke Survivor and Caregiver Perspectives on Post-Stroke Visual Concerns and Long-Term Consequences

Theresa M. Smith,[1] Monique R. Pappadis,[2,3] Shilpa Krishnan,[4] and Timothy A. Reistetter[2,3,5]

[1]*Department of Occupational Therapy, Texas Woman's University, 6700 Fannin Street, Houston, TX 77030, USA*
[2]*Division of Rehabilitation Sciences, School of Health Professions, University of Texas Medical Branch, 301 University Blvd, Galveston, TX 77555, USA*
[3]*Sealy Center on Aging, University of Texas Medical Branch, 301 University Blvd, Galveston, TX 77555, USA*
[4]*Department of Rehabilitation Medicine, Division of Physical Therapy, Emory University, School of Medicine, 1462 Clifton Road, Atlanta, GA 30322, USA*
[5]*Department of Occupational Therapy, School of Health Professions, University of Texas Medical Branch, Galveston, 301 University Blvd, Galveston, TX 77555, USA*

Correspondence should be addressed to Timothy A. Reistetter; tareiste@utmb.edu

Academic Editor: Carolyn Baum

Approximately 800,000 people in the United States have a stroke annually. Up to two thirds of stroke survivors have some visual problems, which result in disability and can affect survivors' overall rehabilitation outcomes. Although some post-stroke visual impairments can be corrected and respond well to intervention, ocular signs can be subtle and may not be recognized or reported by the stroke survivor but rather by a vigilant caregiver. The purpose of this study was to explore the post-stroke visual concerns and consequences expressed by stroke survivors and caregivers. This study employed a qualitative design using semistructured interviews conducted with a convenience sample of stroke survivors and caregivers recruited from either a community support group or skilled nursing and long-term care facilities. Interviews were recorded and transcribed verbatim. Comparative content analysis was used to identify vision-related themes by two independent coders. All research team members completed quality checking of coding. Twenty participants (11 stroke survivors and 9 caregivers) expressed visual concerns or consequences following stroke: (1) eye movement problems, (2) perceptual issues, and (3) consequences of vision problems or issues, which affected their daily life/quality of life. Stroke survivors and caregivers reported receiving vision care from (1) eye doctors, (2) occupational therapists, and (3) other healthcare professionals. All vision care providers need to be observant of potential post-stroke visual concerns. Stroke survivors should have a thorough vision evaluation to optimize their independence in everyday activities and quality of life.

1. Introduction

Approximately 800,000 people in the United States have a stroke annually [1]. With the rising population of older adults, the incidence of stroke is expected to increase and survival rates of stroke continue to rise [2]. Up to two thirds of stroke survivors have some visual problems that result in disability [3]. A wide range of visual impairments can occur following stroke including low vision, eye movement and visual field abnormalities, and visual perceptual difficulties [4, 5]. These impairments invariably affect survivors' independence in daily living and quality of life, negatively influencing their ability to drive, work, and their confidence and familial relationships [6].

Stroke survivors reported low vision acuity for near and distance vision [4]. Nearly 20–60% of stroke survivors have permanent or resolving visual field deficits usually homonymous hemianopia or quadrantanopia, and 70% may be affected by eye movement disorders [7]. Eye movement disorders can result in a loss of depth perception, reduced eye-hand coordination, problems with scanning, and difficulties reading [7]. Strabismus, a misalignment of the eyes, can affect stroke survivors with resulting complaints of diplopia [8]. Visuospatial inattention, also termed visual neglect or hemispatial neglect, can occur following right hemisphere stroke [9]. Other post-stroke visual concerns pertain to eye-hand coordination deficits. These deficits have been shown to result in reduced independence and quality of life [10]. Other conditions that can lead to decreased visual acuity such as glaucoma, cataract, retinal diseases, macular degeneration, and refractive errors [10].

Visual impairments are not as evident as motor or speech impairment [11] and without thorough screening subtle visual complications may go undiagnosed. In the United States, visual acuity is commonly assessed with a Snellen chart [12, 13] and visual fields by the Humphrey visual field [14]. Visual field deficits may be screened using a confrontation test. Most eye movement disorders can be detected during a clinical evaluation [15]. Paper and pencil tasks are used routinely to assess visual perceptual symptoms of visual inattention even though they may not detect symptoms in a chronic stage [16].

Prior studies have identified patients with significant vision impairments, many of whom did not have proper corrective lens following a stroke. One study found that individuals admitted for rehabilitation following stroke usually do not have their glasses with them or have glasses that were not in acceptable condition [17]. Even among those with existing glasses, some still had impaired vision.

Ninety-two percent of stroke survivors with suspected visual problems have been determined to have low vision, eye movement deficit, visual field impairment, and/or visual perceptual deficits such as visual inattention [4]. It is important to treat visual problems that can adversely affect rehabilitation outcomes of stroke survivors [5, 17, 18]. Treatment for eye movement disorders could be restorative, compensative, substitutive, pharmacological, or assessment and screening interventions [19]. Visual fields deficits may improve, but maximal improvement generally occurs within a month [18]. Treatment for visual field deficits involves training in compensatory eye movements, and some patients have prisms in their glasses. Visual inattention is commonly treated by training the patient to scan to the neglected side. Increasing more complex tasks is completed to increase attention [20]. Other treatments for visual inattention include video feedback during treatment, training in visual imagery, diplopia, and vestibular, somatosensory, and optokinetic stimulation. Prisms may also be used [18]. With rehabilitation, partial to full recovery is possible for some visual disorders secondary to stroke [11, 18, 21].

Many of these visual impairments can be corrected and respond well to intervention [18]. However, some visual impairments can be subtle and may not be recognized or reported by the patient but rather by a vigilant caregiver [5]. Some visual problems resulting from stroke such as visual field deficits can be chronic [18] or resistant to treatment. The consensus in the literature is that a thorough vision evaluation in the rehabilitation setting and targeted rehabilitation are critical to maximize patient functional performance [4, 5, 11, 18, 21]. It is important for healthcare providers to understand how stroke survivors and their caregivers experience visual concerns after stroke to ensure that care is focused on areas that matter most to those affected by stroke. Hence, the purpose of this study was to identify the vision concerns of stroke survivors and the consequences of visual impairments as perceived by stroke survivors and caregivers.

2. Methods

2.1. Research Design. In the current qualitative study, interviews of stroke survivors and caregivers were only included if they discussed aspects related to vision. This cross-sectional study is a part of a larger patient-centered outcomes research study that collected data on stroke survivors and caregivers on their preferences and needs following stroke [22]. The University's Institutional Review Board approved this study.

2.2. Participants and Recruitment. Participants were recruited using convenience sampling techniques from local stroke support groups as well as skilled nursing and long-term care facilities in the Houston and Galveston area in Texas. The stroke survivors were included if they were 18 years and older, self-identified with a previous diagnosis of stroke, and communicated in English. The caregivers were recruited into the study if a survivor identified them as their primary caregiver. Not all caregivers agreed to participate, and in some cases, the caregivers identified by the stroke survivors participated even if the stroke survivors themselves did not participate. The eligible participants were identified and enrolled into this study by a research coordinator with a background in psychology.

2.3. Data Collection. After obtaining the participant's written consent to participate, semistructured, in-person interviews were conducted. Separate, independent interviews were conducted for stroke survivors and caregivers at their preferred location [23–25]. The interview guide was developed by a multidisciplinary team involving an occupational therapist (TR) with expertise in health services and outcomes research and a social scientist with over 30 years of experience in qualitative research [25, 26]. The semistructured interview guide included the following content: description of the stroke event and consequences following stroke, therapy and services received, goals in rehabilitation, and what was most important. The interview guide for caregivers included similar content, in addition to content related to their role in the decision-making process, need for information, and advice for other caregivers. All participants were probed for clarification and additional information [27]. The interview guide did not include specific vision-related questions; however, it did include general questions to identify all perceived stroke-related symptoms or concerns.

Male and female licensed occupational (TR) and physical therapists (SK) conducted the interviews. The interviewers had prior experience in conducting semistructured interviews, qualitative methods, and rehabilitating individuals with stroke. In addition, the interviewers had no current or previous connection with any participants recruited in this study. The interviewers revealed their existing affiliations and the purpose of the study to the participants. On an average, each interview lasted for 30 minutes (range: 20–60 minutes). These interviews were audio-recorded and transcribed using professional transcription services. The participants were compensated with a $25 gift card for their time and contribution to this study.

2.4. Data Analysis. We used a combination of thematic and content analysis approaches to code the transcripts (Bernard and Ryan [25]). We started with open coding (i.e., identifying initial codes and categories) and then continued with axial coding (i.e., identifying relationships between the initial codes), and then proceeding with selective coding (i.e., coding any data associated with our core vision-related themes). The transcripts of the stroke survivors were read and coded independently by MP and TR for themes and subthemes related to voluntarily disclosed vision concerns and quality-checked by SK and TS for relevance and consistency. The transcripts for the caregiver interviews were read and coded independently by SK and TR and quality-checked for consistency and relevance by MP and TS. Constant comparison was done within and across transcripts to enhance trustworthiness of the coding process.

For the current study, only themes related to vision were coded and discussed. Of the 65 interviews (41 stroke survivors and 24 caregivers) from the larger study, 20 participants (11 stroke survivors and 9 caregivers) expressed themes or concepts related to vision. Any disagreements in codes were resolved by discussion with the entire research team. The benefits of utilizing multiple coders with multidisciplinary backgrounds including occupational therapy, low vision rehabilitation, physical therapy, social work, expertise in qualitative methods and analyses, and expertise treating individuals with neurological impairments helped us refine our themes from multiple perspectives and limited specific biases [25, 28]. All members of the research team had their primary appointment in an academic university with a medical center during the time of this study.

The final codebook was created, and the refined themes and subthemes were entered into a qualitative analysis software, NVivo 10 [29]. We also performed text search queries in NVivo 10 with words and concepts related to vision, including but not limited to "see," "vision," "read," "eye," "glasses," and "perception" to make sure all concepts related to vision were coded from all interviews. Text queries also identified words with the same stem or synonyms. For example, when we queried *see*, we obtained text related to *seeing*, *read*, and *saw*. In addition, NVivo helped us organize and synthetize our themes.

The final set of themes and subthemes was formed after combining relevant subthemes and was agreed upon by all members in the research team. The themes were grouped into relevant categories to align in a consistent manner with the rehabilitation process along with supportive quotations. To ensure quality control of the data [30], we used triangulation methods for clarification and to better understand vision concerns if mentioned by both the caregiver and the stroke survivor. In addition, all members of the research team have been sufficiently engaged with stroke survivors and caregivers due to their clinical experience. Lastly, we maintained an audit trail by keeping records regarding code/theme development and team decisions regarding the analysis and interpretation of the data.

3. Results

During the qualitative interviews of a larger study including 65 participants, which included 40 stroke survivors and 25 caregivers, 11 stroke survivors and 9 caregivers reported visual concerns. There were four female and seven male survivors ranging in age from 42–74 years of age (mean age = 62.1, SD = 9.4). Five of the survivors were Caucasian, five were African-American, and one was Hispanic. Five survivors had inpatient rehabilitation, one of which also had home health, three had outpatient therapy, one survivor's rehabilitation was unknown, one had "other therapy," and one had no rehabilitation. The majority of stroke survivors were 1–2 years post-stroke ($n = 8$), while the others were 3–5 years post-stroke. There were eight female caregivers and one male caregiver who ranged in age from 24 to 89 years (mean age = 66.7, SD = 18.6). Eight of the caregivers were Caucasians, and one was African American. Half of the caregivers were caring for a stroke survivor who was 1–2 years post-stroke, whereas the others were 3–5 years post-stroke. A formal caregiver cared for a number of patients; therefore, it is unclear how long post-stroke they were.

The qualitative data results are presented below. The results are based on the two main themes derived from the data, which are the visual concerns and consequences mentioned by the stroke survivors and caregivers and the vision care providers to which they attributed their care.

3.1. Visual Concerns and Consequences. Three subthemes of visual concerns emerged from the data including eye movement problems, perceptual issues, and consequences of these problems or issues (see Table 1). Codes representing the eye movement problems subtheme included double vision, eyes cannot focus, eyes jumping around, and eyelid does not close. Codes demonstrating the perceptual issues subtheme consisted of trouble distinguishing colors, loss of depth perception and peripheral vision, left neglect, and impaired visual processing. The third subtheme of visual concerns and consequences encompassed the following codes: reading, impaired balance and falls, incapacity to drive, and inability to work.

3.2. Vision Care Providers. The stroke survivors and caregivers discussed which vision care providers they saw for these visual concerns and interventions they received from the different vision care providers (see Table 2). The three named vision care providers were eye doctors, occupational therapists, and other healthcare professionals. Participants related that eye doctors were seen for examination, magnifiers, glasses, and eye patch. Occupational therapists addressed visual concerns with scanning, gaming, and eye-hand coordination activities. Other healthcare professionals included

Table 1: Subthemes and codes for the theme: visual concerns and consequences.

Subthemes	Code frequency	Prototypical quotations
	Eye movement problems	
Double vision	1 ss; 3 c	"I got up to go to the bathroom and the double vision was so bad I could not make it from the bathroom to the bed." (ss24, 68, M, IRF) "She was now having real visual problems. She was seeing double and things were happening." (c17, 74, M, acute rehab only)
Eyes do not focus	1 ss	"Well, worse problem I have is with my eyes. They do not focus together." (ss5, 71,M, no rehab)
Eyes jumping around	1 c	"The one thing that I do regret is that I did not jump on them more about his eye and even Dr. *** and them ... I mean finally after we'd been there all through intensive care obviously they know his eyes are jumping around." (c1, 65, F, IRF)
Eyelid does not close	1 c	"...and the idea of his eye not staying shut is one big thing. And had I known more about it I would have insisted they get somebody in there to close that eye so that it would not get hurt, the cornea." (c1, 65, F, IRF)
	Perceptual issues	
Trouble distinguishing colors	1 ss	"I can see colors, all kinds of colors but if you have a pink and close to a pink, I can't distinguish, or a white and a yellow. Like, if it's a light yellow, I'm using that as a for instance. I can't distinguish that anymore." (ss23, 74, F, IRF)
Loss of depth perception	1 ss; 1 c	"My depth perception is real off." (ss7, 57, F, acute rehab) "We lay things out and his eyes still are a problem because he cannot see the depth perception." (c1, 65, F, IRF)
Lost peripheral vision	4 ss; 2 c	"It's my eyes. I can't see out of the peripheral..." (ss42, 67, F, IRF) "He did have peripheral vision on the right side was lost, and we noticed that weeks later we were driving down 610 and there's a Derek Hotel... he said, "What is a Derek Hot?" He didn't get the last part of it, the E-L, hotel." (c20, 76, F, outpatient rehab)
Left neglect	3 ss; 2 c	"I was determined to have left neglect as well. If you're not familiar with that, it's a pretty bizarre condition. Someone came from behind me and startled me. I kind of was spooked, so I, "Whoa," by the person coming around." (ss19, 55, M, acute care rehab only) "His perception is pretty off, he has left side of negligence." (c11, 73, F, home health)
Impaired visual processing	2 ss; 2 c	"I can see things all around me. No problem that way but when it comes to them together, I can put them together but I have to really concentrate." (ss23, 74, F, IRF) "And a problem she has today is that she can see something but it doesn't...it happened too quickly for her to digest." (c17,74, M, acute rehab only)
	Consequences of vision problems or issues	
Decreased eye-hand coordination	3 c	"But the hand-eye, those that have had visual issues and coordination issues" (c17,74, acute rehab only)
Difficulty reading	3 c	"He did teach himself to read, though. He worked about five hours a day on the computer and reading." (c20, 76, F, outpatient)
Impaired balance and falls	2 ss; 2 c	"Balance and vision? Yea...that's my main complaints." (ss7, 57, F, acute rehab only) "You are going to fall or something else is going to happen to you if we do not get you to the doctor and get your eyes examined." (c4, 76, F, NR)
Incapacity to drive	1 ss	"He said that I had lost peripheral vision in my left eye... I do not drive my car anymore." (ss37, 63, M, NR)
Inability to work	1 c	"For the longest time, all he wanted to do was go back to work and he began to realize that he couldn't read properly." (c11, 73, F, home health)

ss = stroke survivor; c = caregiver; IRF = inpatient rehabilitation facility; F = female; M = male; NR = not reported.

Table 2: Subthemes and codes for the theme: vision care providers.

Subthemes	Code frequency	Prototypical quotations
	Eye doctor	
Examination	2 c	"She's actually a[n] ophthalmologist. The exam that she performed was very thorough." (c17,74, M, home health)
Magnifiers	1 c	"The VA gave ** one of these magnifiers for reading, he used it for probably a year, and then... didn't need it anymore." (c11, 73, F, home health)
Glasses	3 ss; 1 c	"I also received prism glasses from a neuro ophthalmologist in California which was very helpful." (ss19, 55, M, outpatient) "*** can either come and have prism lenses or do some exercises for the eyes." (c2, 54, F, no rehab)
Eye patch	1 c	"An ophthalmologist...had us tape the eye shut...he did say if you were staying I think I would go ahead and stitch that eye up." (c1, 65, F, IRF)
	Occupational therapist	
Scanning	1 ss	"Occupational therapists showed me some techniques to ... to improve on my visual scanning." (ss36, 44, M, IRF)
Gaming	1 ss	"They [occupational therapists] gave me aids, such as apps and also games to play or something that will help with that." (ss36, 44, M, IRF)
Eye-hand coordination	2 c	"I guess the occupational therapy focused more on the hand-eye coordination kind of stuff." (c14, 24, F, IRF)
	Others	
Compensation	2 ss	"They had to turn my bed so I actually look to the left" (ss19, 55, M, outpatient)
Therapy	1 ss; 1 c	"A lot of therapies...for my vision." (ss41, 69, M, IRF & home health) "We didn't have occupational therapy because...vision comes out of our physical therapy budget, according to Medicare." (c17,74, M, home health)

ss = stroke survivors; C = caregivers; IRF = inpatient rehabilitation facility; M = male; F = female; rehab = rehabilitation.

unidentified professionals who provided compensation techniques and therapy.

4. Discussion

The purpose of this study was to explore voluntarily disclosed visual concerns from the perspectives of the stroke survivors and caregivers. Persons with stroke and caregivers expressed how the consequences of eye movement problems and perception issues led to a decrease in occupational performance of daily activities, such as eye-hand coordination, reading, maintaining balance, driving, and working. Conjugate eye deviations and neglect commonly occur together and reduce fast eye movements needed for reading, mobility, and visual exploration [11], and visual field deficits negatively affects one's ability to drive [31].

The emergence of visual concerns from survivors and caregivers within our study is substantiated by the findings of another research study that employed similar qualitative methodologies [7]. One of the top five priorities of stroke survivors and caregivers was to learn the best ways to treat visual problems after stroke [7]. Participants in our study described specific consequences of visual problems and perceptual issues, such as difficulty reading, impaired balance and falls, incapacity to drive, and inability to work. Other researchers have studied how visual problems can affect balance and contribute to fear of falling and falls [6]. Visuospatial neglect was associated with risk for falls, but the correlation of visual field deficit and falls is less clear [32]. Postural stability is also related among other factors to visual condition of stroke survivors, and decreased visual acuity increases the risk for falls [33]. Driving is a complicated occupation requiring many skills, but sufficient visual function is fundamental as it is for work.

Both stroke survivors and caregivers conveyed the importance of specialized care for visual concerns and named specific interventions used by vision care providers. Further, they expressed frustration when they were unable to access vision care providers or felt vision concerns were overlooked. Stroke survivors in a study by Rowe also communicated that visual concerns were overlooked by medical staff members as their attention was directed to other disabilities from the stroke [6]. Caregivers as well as survivors lamented that survivors were not referred for vision rehabilitation when it was needed following stroke.

I guess I am wishing and hoping something can be done about my eyesight ... I wish I would have pushed harder on my primary care doctor to look into the eye problem, but I didn't and we just kept passing that over.

Some participants discussed their issues with misdiagnosis of their visual impairments that resulted in them not receiving timely eye care. This misinformation frustrated the patients and their caregivers. For instance, a caregiver stated:

First we went to the Ophthalmology ... ... .and we saw doctor and he said this was probably a neurological issue for the visions so he sent us to the Neuro-Ophthalmologist doctor downtown ... [the] doctor was looking for horses before zebras, so he tested [him] for myasthenia gravis and thyroid malfunction cause he felt those could be an explanation for [his] vision problems, which also included some double vision, and of course, those test came back negative. [The] doctor wanted to see his CAT scan and everything from immediately after the stroke. Unbelievably, he just saw those on the last couple of weeks even though our report was back in July ... I just spoke from someone from their office today and [the doctor] said he can either come and have prism lenses and/or do some exercises for the eyes. It's taken from July 25th to literally today (December 4th) to find that out.

Accurate diagnosis for visual impairments must be conducted by utilizing reliable and valid outcome tools so that these individuals are referred to appropriate rehabilitation services. Healthcare providers must discuss these concerns in their multidisciplinary team meetings which can augment the diagnosis of vision-related impairments following stroke [34]. Our data suggest that stroke survivors who received inpatient rehabilitation (IRF) were more likely to be seen by occupational therapists. Prototypical quotations stating that occupational therapy was received were attributed to two caregivers and two stroke survivors. These stroke survivors received occupational therapy in an IRF.

The emerging themes from this study illuminate a number of implications for vision care providers. Stroke rehabilitation programs may not address stroke-related vision problems unless stroke survivors report difficulty and survivors thereby go untreated [35]. To date, no standardized vision screen to accurately assess all post-stroke visual impairment exists [36]. In a recent systematic review, the authors identify two vision screening tools purported to screen for vision problems post-stroke [36]. Due to varying levels of sensitivity when administered, we argue first that all stroke survivors should be screened using a standardized performance-based functional vision screen. At the Royal London Hospital, all stroke survivors are administered a functional vision screen by occupational therapists to assess convergence, smooth pursuits, saccades, visual field deficits, and visual inattention [5] before being referred to an orthoptist for a full evaluation, including acuity testing. When compared to orthoptist findings, outcomes of the occupational therapy functional vision screen of stroke survivors were 68% analogous [5]. Routine use of a standardized vision screening tool could lead to targeted referrals to other vision care specialists and for appropriate interventions [36].

Second, it is vital that persons post-stroke be evaluated for refractive error correction or prisms as needed. All stroke survivors and caregivers strongly suggest the need for more thorough assessment of eye movement problems (i.e., double vision, eyes do not focus, eyes jumping around, and eyelid does not close) as well as perceptual issues (i.e., trouble distinguishing colors, loss of depth perception, loss of peripheral vision, left neglect, and impaired visual processing). Studies have shown that a significant number of visual deficits from stroke are undetected [4, 18].

Third, it would be advantageous for stroke survivors and caregivers to understand the behaviors or signs and symptoms that may be indicative of a visual problem and/or visual concerns. Vision care providers at all levels of care should provide education on post-stroke visual concerns to stroke survivors and caregivers that may require treatment. If these visual concerns cannot be remediated, then stroke survivors and caregivers would benefit by education on coping strategies [11].

Fourth, a straightforward linkage of diagnosed visual impairment to targeted interventions is needed [37]. Vision care providers need to know how to use evidenced-based practice to assess and treat eye movement problems and perception issues at all levels on the continuum of care to prevent and/or lessen their consequences [38]. Barriers to use of evidence-based practice for visual inattention by occupational therapists have been shown to be their lack of basic knowledge in accessing and using the evidence [39]. It is the ethical responsibility of vision care providers to ensure timely referral to other providers as indicated such as ophthalmologists, neurologists, optometrists, orthoptists, physiatrists, occupational therapists, physical therapists, low vision therapists, orientation and mobility specialists, or social workers. Last, all providers need to advocate for stroke survivors and their caregivers to receive much needed services throughout the care continuum and not be limited to IRFs.

4.1. Limitations of the Study. There are a number of limitations in the study. The original interview guide in the larger study did not include any direct questions on vision problems. Rather, stroke survivors and caregivers were asked to describe their post-stroke experiences. Only 20 of them discussed noticeable vision changes following stroke. This could have resulted in selection bias occurring with those 20 reporting vision problems possibly being more sensitive to vision problems, and their concerns may not be representative of other stroke survivors and caregivers. Conversely, those who did not mention vision problems may have focused on other stroke sequelae, lacked awareness of vision-related changes, or did not ultimately have vision problems. Although participants were queried on post-stroke experiences, they may not have taken into consideration premorbid visual problems or other diagnoses, such as diabetes or thyroid dysfunction, adversely affecting vision. Although vision-related questions were not probed, a large number of participants discussed these consequences—justifying the importance of the analysis conducted for this study.

Further, we did not have participants' baseline visual function and there was no optometrist or ophthalmologist involved in this study or in the assessment of the stroke survivor's visual complains. However, the first author is a certified low-vision occupational therapist with extensive experience with stroke-related vision problems. Since the majority of our participants were recruited from the community, we did not have access to clinical indicators (e.g., stroke location, type, and severity), which may confound the results and conclusions of this study. Future research is needed to explore how such clinical factors influence the development of vision-related concerns following stroke. However, our sample was diverse, and the results may guide future research and programs to address the vision-related needs of persons following stroke.

5. Conclusion

Findings from this study indicate that visual concerns of stroke survivors and caregivers may not be addressed sufficiently, thereby adversely affecting survivors' independence in everyday activities and quality of life. All vision care providers need to be vigilant of these unmet visual concerns and complement their care accordingly, including referring to other appropriate eye care providers. A thorough post-stroke vision evaluation is imperative to assess visual acuity, eye motility, visual fields, and visual perception. Evidence-based assessments and targeted treatments to address visual concerns are needed across the continuum of care, not limited to IRFs. Future research should focus on barriers to adhering to best practice in detecting and treating post-stroke visual concerns.

Disclosure

The content is solely the responsibility of the authors and does not necessarily represent the official views of the AHRQ, NIA, or NIDILRR, and you should not assume endorsement by the Federal Government.

Conflicts of Interest

The authors confirm that there is no conflict of interest.

Acknowledgments

This work was supported by the Agency for Healthcare Research and Quality (AHRQ) (R24HS022134 and R01HS024711); National Institute on Disability, Independent Living, and Rehabilitation Research (NIDILRR) (90SFGE0002 and 90AR5009), a center within the Administration for Community Living, Department of Health and Human Services; UTMB Claude D. Pepper Older Americans Independence Center (5P30-AG024832) funded by the National Institute on Aging (NIA); and UTMB Institute for Translational Sciences supported by the National Institutes of Health (NIH) Clinical Translational Science Award (CTSA) (UL1TR001439, KL2TR000072). The content is solely the responsibility of the authors and does not necessarily represent the official views of the AHRQ, NIDILRR, NIA, or NIH, and you should not assume endorsement by the Federal Government.

References

[1] D. Mozaffarian, E. J. Benjamin, A. S. Go et al., "Heart disease and stroke statistics—2015 update: a report from the American Heart Association," *Circulation*, vol. 131, no. 4, pp. e29–e322, 2015.

[2] A. S. Go, D. Mozaffarian, V. L. Roger et al., "Executive summary: heart disease and stroke statistics—2014 update: a report from the American Heart Association," *Circulation*, vol. 129, no. 3, pp. 399–410, 2014.

[3] Stroke Association, *Visual Problems after Stroke*, Stroke Association, London, UK, 2012.

[4] F. Rowe, D. Brand, C. A. Jackson et al., "Visual impairment following stroke: do stroke patients require vision assessment?," *Age and Ageing*, vol. 38, no. 2, pp. 188–193, 2009.

[5] Z. Naeem, "The prevalence of visual problems in stroke patients and the effectiveness of the current screening tool used," *British and Irish Orthoptic Journal*, vol. 9, pp. 55–58, 2015.

[6] F. J. Rowe, "Stroke survivors' views and experiences on impact of visual impairment," *Brain and Behavior*, vol. 7, no. 9, article e00778, 2017.

[7] A. Pollock, B. St George, M. Fenton, and L. Firkins, "Top 10 research priorities relating to life after stroke - consensus from stroke survivors, caregivers, and health professionals," *International Journal of Stroke*, vol. 9, no. 3, pp. 313–320, 2014.

[8] F. Rowe and VIS group UK3, "The profile of strabismus in stroke survivors," *Eye*, vol. 24, no. 4, pp. 682–685, 2010.

[9] S. P. Stone, P. Patel, R. J. Greenwood, and P. W. Halligan, "Measuring visual neglect in acute stroke and predicting its recovery: the visual neglect recovery index," *Journal of Neurology, Neurosurgery & Psychiatry*, vol. 55, no. 6, pp. 431–436, 1992.

[10] Y. Shen, P. W. Gu, S. K. Ong, and A. Y. C. Nee, "A novel approach in rehabilitation of hand-eye coordination and finger dexterity," *Virtual Reality*, vol. 16, no. 2, pp. 161–171, 2012.

[11] K. M. Sand, A. Midelfart, L. Thomassen, A. Melms, H. Wilhelm, and J. M. Hoff, "Visual impairment in stroke patients - a review," *Acta Neurologica Scandinavica*, vol. 127, no. 196, pp. 52–56, 2013.

[12] J. H. Levenson and A. Kozarsky, "Visual acuity change," in *Clinical Methods: The History, Physical, and Laboratory Examinations*, H. K. Walker, W. D. Hall, and J. W. Hurst, Eds., pp. 553–555, Butterworths, Boston, MA, USA, 1990.

[13] S. Sue, "Test distance vision using a Snellen chart," *Community Eye Health*, vol. 20, no. 63, pp. 52–52, 2007.

[14] M. K. Birch, P. K. Wishart, and N. P. O'Donnell, "Determining progressive visual field loss in serial Humphrey visual fields," *Ophthalmology*, vol. 102, no. 8, pp. 1227–1235, 1995.

[15] C. Danchaivijitr and C. Kennard, "Diplopia and eye movement disorders," *Journal of Neurology, Neurosurgery & Psychiatry*, vol. 75, Supplement 4, pp. iv24–iv31, 2004.

[16] E. Pedroli, S. Serino, P. Cipresso, F. Pallavicini, and G. Riva, "Assessment and rehabilitation of neglect using virtual reality: a systematic review," *Frontiers in Behavioral Neuroscience*, vol. 9, p. 226, 2015.

[17] A. J. Lotery, M. I. Wiggam, A. J. Jackson et al., "Correctable visual impairment in stroke rehabilitation patients," *Age and Ageing*, vol. 29, no. 3, pp. 221-222, 2000.

[18] S. A. Jones and R. A. Shinton, "Improving outcome in stroke patients with visual problems," *Age and Ageing*, vol. 35, no. 6, pp. 560–565, 2006.

[19] A. Pollock, C. Hazelton, C. A. Henderson et al., "Interventions for disorders of eye movement in patients with stroke," *Cochrane Database of Systematic Reviews*, no. 10, article CD008389, 2011.

[20] P. T. Diamond, "Rehabilitative management of post-stroke visuospatial inattention," *Disability and Rehabilitation*, vol. 23, no. 10, pp. 407–412, 2001.

[21] K. M. Sand, G. Wilhelmsen, H. Naess, A. Midelfart, L. Thomassen, and J. M. Hoff, "Vision problems in ischaemic stroke patients: effects on life quality and disability," *European Journal of Neurology*, vol. 23, no. S1, pp. 1-7, 2016.

[22] S. Krishnan, M. R. Pappadis, S. C. Weller, S. R. Fisher, C. C. Hay, and T. A. Reistetter, "Patient-centered mobility outcome preferences according to individuals with stroke and caregivers: a qualitative analysis," *Disability and Rehabilitation*, vol. 40, no. 12, pp. 1401–1409, 2018.

[23] M. B. Miles, A. M. Huberman, and J. Saldaña, *Qualitative Data Analysis: a Methods Sourcebook*, SAGE Publications, Inc, 2013.

[24] S. J. Taylor, R. Bogdan, and M. DeVault, *Introduction to Qualitative Research Methods: A Guidebook and Resource*, John Wiley & Sons, 2015.

[25] H. R. Bernard and G. W. Ryan, *Analyzing Qualitative Data: Systematic Approaches*, SAGE Publications, Inc, 2009.

[26] W. C. Adams, "Conducting semi-structured interviews," in *Handbook of Practical Program Evaluation*, p. 365, Jossey-Bass, 2010.

[27] M. Brod, L. E. Tesler, and T. L. Christensen, "Qualitative research and content validity: developing best practices based on science and experience," *Quality of Life Research*, vol. 18, no. 9, pp. 1263–1278, 2009.

[28] L. Berends and J. Johnston, "Using multiple coders to enhance qualitative analysis: the case of interviews with consumers of drug treatment," *Addiction Research & Theory*, vol. 13, no. 4, pp. 373–381, 2005.

[29] QSR International Pty Ltd, *NVivo Qualitative Data Analysis Software (Version 10)*, QSR International Pty Ltd, Doncaster, VIC, Australia, 2012.

[30] D. K. Padgett, *Qualitative Methods in Social Work Research*, SAGE Publications, Inc, 2016.

[31] J. S. Gilhotra, P. Mitchell, P. R. Healey, R. G. Cumming, and J. Currie, "Homonymous visual field defects and stroke in an older population," *Stroke*, vol. 33, no. 10, pp. 2417–2420, 2002.

[32] G. B. Campbell and J. T. Matthews, "An integrative review of factors associated with falls during post-stroke rehabilitation," *Journal of Nursing Scholarship*, vol. 42, no. 4, pp. 395–404, 2010.

[33] H. Corriveau, R. Hébert, M. Raîche, and F. Prince, "Evaluation of postural stability in the elderly with stroke," *Archives of Physical Medicine and Rehabilitation*, vol. 85, no. 7, pp. 1095–1101, 2004.

[34] F. J. Rowe, "The importance of accurate visual assessment after stroke," *Expert Review of Ophthalmology*, vol. 6, no. 2, pp. 133–136, 2011.

[35] K. H. Siong, G. C. Woo, D. Y. L. Chan et al., "Prevalence of visual problems among stroke survivors in Hong Kong Chinese," *Clinical and Experimental Optometry*, vol. 97, no. 5, pp. 433–441, 2014.

[36] K. L. Hanna, L. R. Hepworth, and F. Rowe, "Screening methods for post-stroke visual impairment: a systematic review," *Disability and Rehabilitation*, vol. 39, no. 25, pp. 2531–2543, 2017.

[37] A. M. Barrett, L. J. Buxbaum, H. B. Coslett et al., "Cognitive rehabilitation interventions for neglect and related disorders: moving from bench to bedside in stroke patients," *Journal of Cognitive Neuroscience*, vol. 18, no. 7, pp. 1223–1236, 2006.

[38] S. Trauzettel-Klosinski, "Current methods of visual rehabilitation," *Deutsches Ärzteblatt International*, vol. 108, no. 51-52, pp. 871–878, 2011.

[39] A. Petzold, N. Korner-Bitensky, N. M. Salbach, S. Ahmed, A. Menon, and T. Ogourtsova, "Determining the barriers and facilitators to adopting best practices in the management of poststroke unilateral spatial neglect: results of a qualitative study," *Topics in Stroke Rehabilitation*, vol. 21, no. 3, pp. 228–236, 2014.

Intravenous Thrombolysis in Acute Ischemic Stroke with Active Cancer

Ki-Woong Nam,[1] Chi Kyung Kim,[2] Tae Jung Kim,[1] Sang Joon An,[1] Kyungmi Oh,[2] Sang-Bae Ko,[1] and Byung-Woo Yoon[1]

[1]*Department of Neurology, Seoul National University Hospital, Seoul, Republic of Korea*
[2]*Department of Neurology, Korea University Guro Hospital and Korea University College of Medicine, Seoul, Republic of Korea*

Correspondence should be addressed to Byung-Woo Yoon; bwyoon@snu.ac.kr

Academic Editor: Gelin Xu

Ischemic stroke patients with active cancer are known to have poor clinical outcomes. However, the efficacy and safety of intravenous alteplase (IV t-PA) in this group are still unclear. In this study, we aimed to evaluate whether stroke patients with cancer had poor clinical outcomes after use of IV t-PA. We reviewed ischemic stroke patients with active cancer treated with isolated IV t-PA between April 2010 and March 2015 at three national university hospitals from the registry for ischemic stroke in Korea. The clinical outcomes of early neurological deterioration (END), hemorrhagic transformation, in-hospital mortality, 3-month modified Rankin scale (mRS), the National Institutes of Health Stroke Scale (NIHSS) discharge score, and duration of hospitalization were compared. We enrolled a total of 12 patients, and the cohort showed poor outcomes including 4 (33%) END events, 7 (58%) hemorrhagic transformations, 3 (25%) in-hospital mortality cases, and 7 (58%) poor mRS (3–6) scores. Additionally, the cryptogenic stroke group ($n = 6$) more frequently had high mRS scores ($P = 0.043$) as well as tendencies for frequent END events, hemorrhagic transformations, in-hospital mortality cases, and higher discharge NIHSS scores without statistical significance. In conclusion, ischemic stroke patients with active cancer, especially those with a cryptogenic mechanism, showed poor clinical outcomes after use of IV t-PA.

1. Introduction

Ischemic stroke in cancer patients, with a frequent occurrence of up to 15%, has been recently studied [1]. These patients have complicated stroke mechanism by conventional stroke mechanisms (e.g., large-artery atherosclerosis, small-vessel disease, and cardioembolism) and cancer-specific mechanisms (e.g., hypercoagulability, tumor embolism, and nonbacterial thrombotic endocarditis) [2]. Previously, patients who experienced stroke with cryptogenic mechanism, who had no evidence of conventional mechanisms, were proven to be more closely related to those with stroke with cancer-specific mechanisms (especially hypercoagulability) and had poorer clinical outcomes [1, 3–9].

Intravenous alteplase (IV t-PA) is a well-known treatment option to recover from poststroke disability during the acute period. However, its efficacy and safety in patients with active cancer have not been well addressed due to its complex stroke mechanisms [6]. With longer life-expectancy due to improved cancer treatments, we needed to assess the exact prognosis and identify the high-risk subset after use of IV t-PA in ischemic stroke patients with active cancer.

In this study, we evaluated whether ischemic stroke patients with active cancer had poor clinical outcomes after use of IV t-PA. In addition, we also aimed to evaluate the impact of stroke mechanisms (e.g., conventional versus cryptogenic mechanisms) on the clinical outcomes after use of IV t-PA.

2. Methods

2.1. Study Population. We retrospectively reviewed medical records from the consecutively enrolled stroke registry for ischemic stroke patients with active cancer who visited three national university hospitals (Seoul National University

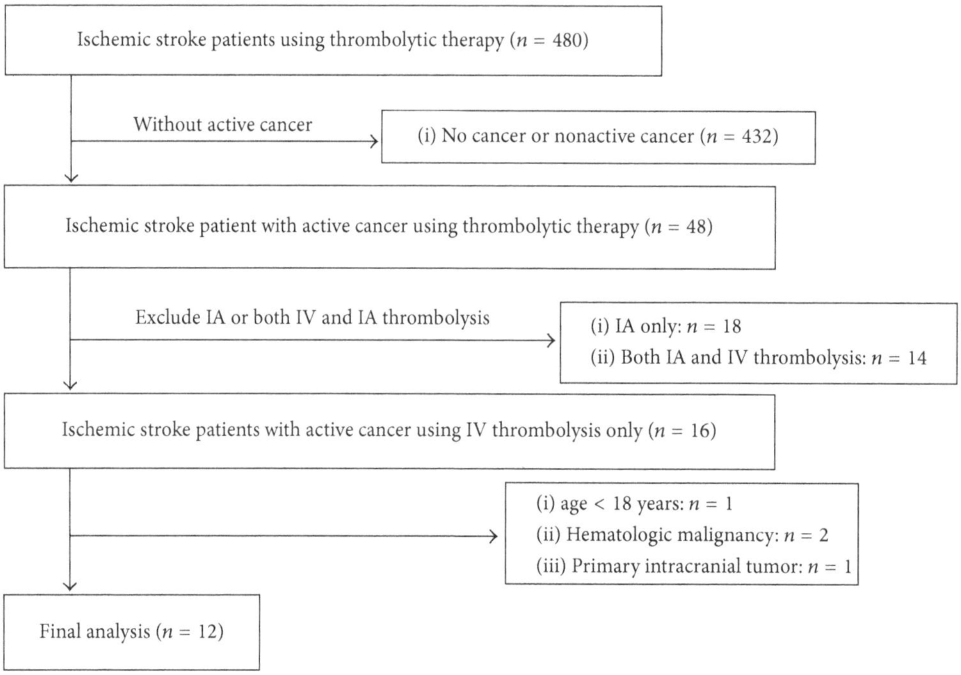

FIGURE 1: Patient selection for the study.

Hospital, Seoul National University Bundang Hospital, and Seoul Metropolitan Government-Seoul National University Boramae Medical Center) in Korea between April 2010 and March 2015. Active cancer was defined as any diagnosis, recurrence, metastasis, and progression of cancer within 6 months of enrollment [6]. Among the cases, we extracted the subpopulation that was treated with IV t-PA. Patients using both IV t-PA and intra-arterial thrombectomy were excluded as to evaluate the sole effects of IV t-PA for the study. In addition, we also excluded patients under the age of 18 years and those who had a hematologic malignancy or a primary intracranial tumor which are known to have different stroke mechanisms [6]. Finally, a total of 12 patients remained for the analysis (Figure 1). This study was approved by the institutional review board (IRB) of Seoul National University Hospital (H-1610-036-797) and designed according to the STrengthening the Reporting of OBservational studies in Epidemiology (STROBE) guidelines.

2.2. Clinical Assessment. We collected demographic, clinical, and cardiovascular risk factors, including the presence of hypertension, diabetes, hyperlipidemia, current smoking, use of alcohol, history of stroke, initial stroke severity, mechanisms of stroke, blood pressure (BP), initial antithrombotics taken, and dose of t-PA [3]. The initial stroke severity was assessed using the National Institutes of Health Stroke Scale (NIHSS) by well-trained neurologists. The mechanisms of stroke were classified using the Trial of Org 10172 in Acute Stroke Treatment (TOAST) classification. We, then, dichotomized the stroke mechanisms into conventional (large-artery atherosclerosis, small-vessel occlusion, and cardioembolism) and cryptogenic mechanisms [6]. BP was assessed for initial systolic BP and diastolic BP. Initial antithrombotics were divided into low-molecular weight heparin, warfarin, antiplatelet agent, and no treatment. Data regarding the patient's cancer were also assessed including cancer type, systemic or brain metastasis, and venous thromboembolism (e.g., deep-vein thrombosis, pulmonary embolism).

We assessed the clinical outcomes in variable aspects. We evaluated early neurological deterioration (END), hemorrhagic transformation, hospitalization duration, discharge NIHSS scores, in-hospital mortality events, and the 3-month modified Rankin scale (mRS) scores. END was defined as an increase of ≥1 in the motor NIHSS score or ≥2 in the total NIHSS score [3].

2.3. Radiological Assessment. All patients underwent brain magnetic resonance imaging (MRI) within 4 hours of admission using a 3.0-Tesla MR scanner (Achieva 3.0 T; Philips, Eindhoven, Netherlands). We dichotomized the initial diffusion-weighted image lesion into single territory lesions and multiple territory lesions [7]. Laboratory results, including C-reactive protein, D-dimer, prothrombin time, and activated partial thromboplastin time were assessed within 24 hours of admission.

2.4. Statistical Analysis. All statistical analyses were conducted using SPSS version 22 (IBM SPSS, Chicago, IL, USA). We presented continuous variables as the mean ± SD when data were normally distributed, while the others were presented as the median + interquartile range. Student's t-test or Mann–Whitney U test were used for continuous variables, and the chi-squared test or Fisher's exact test were

TABLE 1: Brief profile of participants in the study.

Number/sex/age, y	Cancer type	t-PA dose	Initial D-dimer	Mechanism	Initial NIHSS	END	3m mRS	Hemorrhagic transformation	Initial treatment
1/F/64	Lung	0.9	26.8	Cryptogenic	20	N	5	Y	Enoxaparin
2/M/61	Pancreas	0.9	5.11	Cryptogenic	7	Y	6	Y	Enoxaparin
3/F/74	Pancreas	0.9	3.7	Cryptogenic	13	Y	6	Y	No treatment
4/M/61	Lung	0.6	2.01	Cryptogenic	7	N	0	N	Enoxaparin
5/M/76	Lung	0.6	3.91	Cryptogenic	15	Y	6	Y	No treatment
6/M/82	Gastric	0.6	20	Cryptogenic	7	N	6	Y	Enoxaparin
7/M/70	Gastric	0.9	11.1	CE	7	N	1	Y	Warfarin
8/M/81	Colon	0.6	0.82	LAD	19	Y	3	Y	Antiplatelet
9/M/64	Colon	0.6	0.73	LAD	3	N	0	N	Antiplatelet
10/M/67	Lung	0.6	1.77	LAD	19	N	1	N	Antiplatelet
11/F/56	Cervical	0.6	0.16	LAD	5	N	1	N	Antiplatelet
12/F/76	Lung	0.9	8.28	CE	24	N	5	Y	Enoxaparin

used for categorical variables. All variables with $P < 0.05$ were considered significant in the statistical analyses.

3. Results

We enrolled a total of 12 ischemic stroke patients with active cancer who were treated with IV t-PA (mean age of 69 years, visit time 1 [0.5–1.75] hours, median NIHSS scores 10 [7–19], Table 1). Among them, 6 patients were classified as having a conventional stroke mechanism, and the remaining with a cryptogenic mechanism. In clinical outcomes, the cohort had 4 (33%) END events, 7 (58%) hemorrhagic transformations, 3 (25%) in-hospital mortalities, and 7 (58%) poor mRS (3–6) scores. The duration of hospitalization was 12 [9–25] days.

None of the demographic, clinical, cardiovascular, laboratory, or radiological variables were significantly different between the conventional and the cryptogenic groups (Table 2). However, in clinical outcomes, the cryptogenic group had higher 3-month mRS scores ($P = 0.043$, Figure 2). The cryptogenic group also had a tendency of more frequent END events, hemorrhagic transformations, in-hospital mortality cases, and higher discharge NIHSS scores without statistical significance. Three in-hospital mortality cases occurred only in the cryptogenic group, and the causes of death were pneumonia aggravation, myocardial infarction, and stroke recurrence.

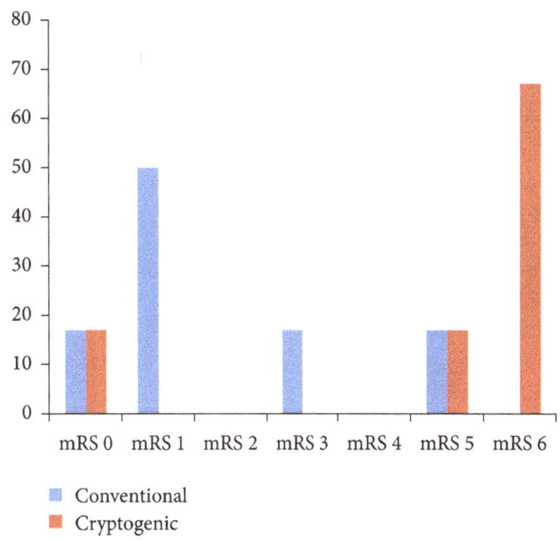

FIGURE 2: Distributions of 3-month mRS scores between patients that experienced stroke with conventional and cryptogenic mechanisms. P for trend < 0.043 in linear-by-linear association.

4. Discussion

In this study, ischemic stroke patients with active cancer showed poor outcomes after use of IV-tPA. Furthermore, cryptogenic stroke mechanisms seemed to be related to poor outcomes.

According to a previous study, ischemic stroke patients with cancer were proven to be as safe as noncancer patients in a large population study, showing 12% in-hospital mortality and 6% intracerebral hemorrhage cases [10]. However, this study included cancer-associated stroke with relatively heterogeneous traits (e.g., including hematologic malignancy, nonactive cancer with stably controlled states, treated by both IV-tPA and intra-arterial thrombectomy). Thus, the pure outcomes of cancer-associated stroke may be hard to interpret. Additionally, there have also been two case-series studies that reported on safety and hazardous events after use of t-PA in ischemic stroke with cancer [11, 12]. The cases that resulted in hazardous events occurred in patients with newly diagnosed cancer and high elevated D-dimer levels with nonbacterial thrombotic endocarditis, similar to our participants [11, 12]. In contrast, patients with fair outcomes were those with nonactive cancer status, defined as being stable after operation or in complete remission with regular treatment [12]. In this study, we attempted to collect data from patients with relatively homogenous cancer-related stroke, and these patients showed poorer outcomes than previous studies in variable clinical aspects (e.g., in-hospital mortality,

TABLE 2: Baseline characteristics and clinical outcomes between conventional and cryptogenic stroke mechanisms.

	Conventional (n = 6)	Cryptogenic (n = 6)	P value
Time delay to visit, h [IQR]	1 [1-2]	1 [0-1]	0.624
Age, y [SD]	69 ± 9	70 ± 9	0.899
Sex, male %	4 (67)	4 (67)	1.000
Hypertension, %	3 (50)	1 (17)	0.545
Diabetes, %	2 (33)	0 (0)	0.455
Hyperlipidemia, %	1 (17)	2 (33)	1.000
Current smoking, %	2 (33)	1 (17)	1.000
Alcohol, %	4 (67)	1 (17)	0.242
History of stroke, %	1 (17)	0 (0)	1.000
Venous thrombosis, %	0 (0)	2 (33)	0.455
Cancer type, %			0.688
Lung	2 (33)	3 (50)	
Gastric	1 (17)	1 (17)	
Colorectal	2 (33)	0 (0)	
Hepatobiliary	0 (0)	2 (33)	
Genitourinary	1 (17)	0 (0)	
Systemic metastasis, %	1 (17)	5 (83)	0.080
Brain metastasis, %	0 (0)	3 (50)	0.182
Initial NIHSS [IQR]	13 [5–19]	10 [7–15]	0.935
SBP, mmHg [SD]	130 ± 27	151 ± 28	0.213
DBP, mmHg [SD]	77 ± 23	84 ± 12	0.479
Initial antithrombotics, %			0.476
Low-molecular weight heparin	1 (17)	4 (67)	
Warfarin	1 (17)	0 (0)	
Antiplatelet agent	4 (67)	0 (0)	
No treatment	0 (0)	2 (33)	
Intravenous alteplase dose, %			1.000
0.6 mg/kg	4 (67)	3 (50)	
0.9 mg/kg	2 (33)	3 (50)	
Initial DWI lesion			0.061
Single territory	6 (100)	2 (33)	
Multiple territory	0 (0)	4 (67)	
D-dimer, μg/mL [IQR]	1.30 [0.73–8.28]	4.51 [3.70–20.0]	0.109
CRP, mg/dL [IQR]	0.03 [0.03–0.11]	2.79 [0.38–12.20]	0.085
PT, INR [SD]	1.09 ± 0.05	1.15 ± 0.20	0.497
aPTT, sec [SD]	34.1 ± 4.6	31.5 ± 9.8	0.578
Hospital stay, day [IQR]	16 [9–28]	12 [6–17]	0.420
Discharge NIHSS [IQR]	4 [2–7]	28 [8–42]	0.063
Early neurological deterioration, %	1 (17)	3 (50)	0.545
Hemorrhagic transformation, %	2 (33)	5 (83)	0.242
In-hospital mortality, %	0 (0)	3 (50)	0.182
3m mRS, %			0.043
0	1 (17)	1 (17)	
1	3 (50)	0 (0)	
2	0 (0)	0 (0)	

Table 2: Continued.

	Conventional ($n = 6$)	Cryptogenic ($n = 6$)	P value
3	1 (17)	0 (0)	
4	0 (0)	0 (0)	
5	1 (17)	1 (17)	
6	0 (0)	4 (67)	

We used Student's t-test or Mann–Whitney U test for continuous variables, while chi-square test or Fisher's exact test was used for categorical variables.

hemorrhagic transformation, and END), although the 3-month mRS scores were not significantly different [13].

Additionally, the mechanisms of stroke in this group seemed to play a role in the clinical outcomes. Those with cryptogenic stroke showed more frequent END events, hemorrhagic transformation, in-hospital mortality, and a higher number of discharge NIHSS scores and 3-month mRS scores despite these patients having the same initial NIHSS scores as the other group. We already knew that cryptogenic stroke in cancer patients had a worse outcome than conventional stroke in the clinical outcomes of stroke [14]. However, the result of having worse clinical outcomes with cryptogenic stroke after use of t-PA is interesting. We hypothesize that having a more advanced cancer and an impaired coagulation cascade might play a role.

This study is the first report on clinical outcomes after using t-PA in homogeneous cancer-related stroke and the impact of the stroke mechanisms on clinical outcomes. However, there are some caveats to this study. This study was designed as a three-center, uncontrolled, retrospective study. A small sample size limited the statistical power, despite considering the difficulty of collecting homogenous traits of this group. There was also a possibility of selection bias as a result of the retrospective.

In conclusion, ischemic stroke patients with active cancer showed poor clinical outcomes after use of IV t-PA. As the cryptogenic group showed worse outcomes, a more careful observation of this group should be recommended.

Conflicts of Interest

The authors declare that they have no conflicts of interest.

Authors' Contributions

Ki-Woong Nam and Chi Kyung Kim contributed equally in this work.

References

[1] K. Nam, C. K. Kim, T. J. Kim et al., "Predictors of 30-day mortality and the risk of recurrent systemic thromboembolism in cancer patients suffering acute ischemic stroke," *PLOS ONE*, vol. 12, no. 3, p. e0172793, 2017.

[2] A. Y. Lee, "Cancer and thromboembolic disease: pathogenic mechanisms," *Cancer Treatment Reviews*, vol. 28, no. 3, pp. 137–140, 2002.

[3] K. Nam, C. K. Kim, T. J. Kim et al., "D-dimer as a predictor of early neurologic deterioration in cryptogenic stroke with active cancer," *European Journal of Neurology*, vol. 24, no. 1, pp. 205–211, 2017.

[4] S. J. Kim, J. H. Park, M.-J. Lee, Y. G. Park, M.-J. Ahn, and O. Y. Bang, "Clues to occult cancer in patients with ischemic stroke," *PLoS ONE*, vol. 7, no. 9, p. e44959, 2012.

[5] C. J. Schwarzbach, A. Schaefer, and A. Ebert, "Stroke and cancer: the importance of cancer-associated hypercoagulation as a possible stroke etiology," *Stroke*, vol. 43, no. 11, pp. 3029–3034, 2012.

[6] S. G. Kim, J. M. Hong, H. Y. Kim et al., "Ischemic stroke in cancer patients with and without conventional mechanisms: a multicenter study in Korea," *Stroke*, vol. 41, no. 4, pp. 798–801, 2010.

[7] O. Y. Bang, J. M. Seok, S. G. Kim et al., "Ischemic stroke and cancer: stroke severely impacts cancer patients, while cancer increases the number of strokes," *Journal of Clinical Neurology*, vol. 7, no. 2, pp. 53–59, 2011.

[8] J. M. Seok, S. G. Kim, J. W. Kim et al., "Coagulopathy and embolic signal in cancer patients with ischemic stroke," *Annals of Neurology*, vol. 68, no. 2, pp. 213–219, 2010.

[9] M. J. Lee, J. Chung, M. Ahn et al., "Hypercoagulability and mortality of patients with stroke and active cancer: the OASIS-CANCER study," *Journal of Stroke*, vol. 19, no. 1, pp. 77–87, 2017.

[10] S. B. Murthy, S. Karanth, S. Shah et al., "Thrombolysis for acute ischemic stroke in patients with cancer: a population study," *Stroke*, vol. 44, no. 12, pp. 3573–3576, 2013.

[11] T. Yagi, K. Takahashi, M. Tanikawa, M. Seki, T. Abe, and N. Suzuki, "Fatal intracranial hemorrhage after intravenous thrombolytic therapy for acute ischemic stroke associated with cancer-related nonbacterial thrombotic endocarditis," *Journal of Stroke and Cerebrovascular Diseases*, vol. 23, no. 8, pp. e413–e416, 2014.

[12] I. Casado-Naranjo, M. L. Calle, A. Falcón et al., "Intravenous thrombolysis for acute stroke in patients with cancer," *Journal of Neurology, Neurosurgery & Psychiatry*, Article ID 207472, 2010.

[13] W. Hacke, G. Donnan, C. Fieschi et al., "Association of outcome with early stroke treatment: pooled analysis of ATLANTIS, ECASS, and NINDS rt-PA stroke trials," *The Lancet*, vol. 363, no. 9411, pp. 768–774, 2004.

[14] B. B. Navi, S. Singer, A. E. Merkler et al., "Cryptogenic subtype predicts reduced survival among cancer patients with ischemic stroke," *Stroke*, vol. 45, no. 8, pp. 2292–2297, 2014.

34

Benign Paroxysmal Positional Vertigo and the Increased Risk of Ischemic Stroke: A Nested Case-Control Study using a National Cohort Sample

Hyo Geun Choi[1] **and So Young Kim**[2]

[1]*Department of Otorhinolaryngology-Head & Neck Surgery, Hallym University College of Medicine, Anyang, Republic of Korea*
[2]*Department of Otorhinolaryngology-Head & Neck Surgery, CHA Bundang Medical Center, CHA University, Seongnam, Republic of Korea*

Correspondence should be addressed to So Young Kim; sossi81@hanmail.net

Academic Editor: Johan H.M. Frijns

A recent population cohort study reported that benign paroxysmal positional vertigo (BPPV) was a risk factor for ischemic stroke. This study investigated the risk of ischemic and hemorrhagic strokes in patients with BPPV. A nested case-control study used the data from the Korean National Health Insurance Service-National Sample Cohort between 2002 and 2013. We used data of patients aged ≥50 years obtained from the Korean National Health Insurance Service-National Sample Cohort between 2002 and 2013. A total of 15,610 patients with ischemic stroke and 4,923 patients with hemorrhagic stroke were matched for age, sex, income, residential location, hypertension, diabetes, and dyslipidemia with 62,440 and 19,692 controls, respectively. History of BPPV was evaluated in the stroke and control groups. Crude and adjusted odds ratios (ORs) for stroke in patients with BPPV were analyzed using stratified logistic regression analysis. Subgroup analyses were performed for age and sex. Notably, 3.7% (572/15,610) of patients with ischemic stroke and 2.7% (1,702/62,440) of the control subjects reported a history of BPPV ($P < 0.001$). The adjusted OR for BPPV in patients with ischemic stroke was 1.35 (95% confidence interval (CI) 1.22–1.49, $P < 0.001$). Patients with ischemic stroke showed higher ORs for BPPV in the subgroup of women. Patients with hemorrhagic stroke did not show a high OR for BPPV. Ischemic stroke patients demonstrated the increased OR for BPPV in subjects aged ≥50 years old.

1. Introduction

Benign paroxysmal positional vertigo (BPPV) is a common cause of vertigo. A study that investigated German patients reported that the prevalence of BPPV was 2.4%, and BPPV accounted for moderate-to-severe dizziness in 8% of the patients investigated [1]. Previous studies have reported that the prevalence of BPPV increases with age [2]. Dislodgement of otoconia from the macula of the utricle or saccule produces symptoms of vertigo causing BPPV, and this condition is typically aggravated by positional changes [3]. BPPV is a benign condition, and patients do not usually present with systemic issues [4, 5]. However, recent studies have reported a high prevalence of chronic diseases, including hypertension, coronary heart disease, and diabetes, in patients with BPPV [6–8]. Additionally, a few studies have suggested that vertebrobasilar ischemia can induce dizziness and inner ear disorders that include BPPV [9–11].

Strokes are a major cause of mortality and morbidity worldwide. Globally, approximately 6,500,000 deaths and 113,000,000 disability-adjusted life-years are attributable to strokes [12]. In South Korea, the stroke incidence rate is 216 per 100,000 person-years, and the stroke prevalence rate is 15.9 per 1,000 persons [13]. Early diagnosis and intervention are crucial for successful treatment in patients with acute ischemic stroke because prompt thrombolytic treatment improves outcomes [14]. Several chronic diseases including hypertension, dyslipidemia, diabetes, and depression serve as risk factors for stroke [15, 16]. A recent population cohort study reported that BPPV was a predictor of ischemic strokes [7]; however, patients with ischemic stroke included in the study showed a high prevalence of chronic diseases, which might serve as confounders. Although the potential confounders were adjusted in the study, only age and sex were matched between the ischemic stroke and control groups. Matching the control group for medical history is crucial because it may influence the association between independent and dependent variables [17].

We hypothesized that BPPV increases the risk of ischemic stroke even after matching and adjusting for past medical history, and we investigated a large population-based cohort of patients aged ≥50 years to address this hypothesis. Strokes are rare in young individuals and are usually associated with a specific underlying etiology. Therefore, we selected older patients for our study, although previous studies investigating BPPV used patients aged ≥20 years [7]. We performed subgroup analyses to investigate the age- and sex-specific risks of stroke in patients with BPPV. Because hemorrhagic stroke is one of the causes of vertigo attack and has common risk factors [18, 19], we also separately investigated the association between BPPV and hemorrhagic strokes.

2. Materials and Methods

2.1. Statement of Approval of the Institution's Ethics Committee. The Hallym University Ethics Committee approved the use of the study data (approval protocol number: 2017-I102). The Institutional Review Board waived the need for written informed consent for this study.

This national cohort study used data from the Korean National Health Insurance Service (NHIS)-National Sample Cohort. Details regarding this data have been described in our previous studies [20, 21].

Patients with ischemic and hemorrhagic stroke were matched in a ratio of 1 : 4 with control group subjects who were not diagnosed with a hemorrhagic or ischemic stroke between 2002 and 2013. The control groups were selected from the parent population ($n = 1{,}101{,}609$). The matches were processed for age, sex, income, residential location, and medical history (hypertension, diabetes, and dyslipidemia). To prevent a selection bias when matching subjects, control group subjects were sorted randomly and were selected from top to bottom. The control group subjects were matched with patients with stroke for the index date (diagnosed date of their matched stroke). Therefore, control group subjects who died before the index date were excluded. The following patients were excluded from the study: patients with cerebral or vertebral anomalies (Q28) ($N = 19$ with ischemic stroke and $N = 48$ with hemorrhagic stroke), patients with stroke for whom a sufficient number of matching subjects could not be identified ($N = 476$ for patients with ischemic stroke and $N = 8$ for patients with hemorrhagic stroke), and patients aged <50 years ($N = 1{,}453$ for patients with ischemic and $N = 1{,}545$ for patients with hemorrhagic stroke). Finally, 1 : 4 matching resulted in the inclusion of 15,610 patients with ischemic and 4,923 patients with hemorrhagic stroke and 62,440 subjects in control group I and 19,692 subjects in control group II (Figure 1). Notably, patients were not matched strictly for history of ischemic heart disease and depression because this would increase the drop-out rate secondary to the lack of an adequate number of subjects in the control group. After matching, we obtained information regarding a previous history of BPPV in both, the stroke and the control groups.

2.2. Selection of Participants. Among a total of 1,125,691 cases with 114,369,638 medical claim codes, we included patients with a diagnosis of hemorrhagic or ischemic strokes. Hemorrhagic (I60–I62) and ischemic (I63) strokes were diagnosed using the International Classification of Diseases, Tenth Revision, Clinical Modification (ICD-10) codes. We selected patients who had been treated for stroke at least once. This method has been used to evaluate the stroke incidence rate in previous South Korean studies [13, 22]. A total of 17,558 patients with ischemic and 6,524 patients with hemorrhagic stroke were identified between 2002 and 2013.

BPPV was diagnosed using the ICD-10 codes (H811) for cases recorded between 2002 and 2013. Among these cases, we only included patients who had been treated at least twice.

2.3. Variables. Patients were grouped by age at 5-year intervals into 8 groups as follows: 50–54, 55–59, 60–64, 65–69, 70–74, 75–79, 80–84, and ≥85 years. Patients were categorized into 41 income groups (1: health aid class, 20: self-employed health insurance class, and 20: employed health insurance class). These groups were recategorized into 5 subclasses, with class 1 = the lowest income and class 5 = the highest income. Residential locations were categorized into 16 regions based on their administrative center. These regions were recategorized as urban (Seoul, Busan, Daegu, Incheon, Gwangju, Daejeon, and Ulsan) and rural (Gyeonggi, Gangwon, Chungcheongbuk, Chungcheongnam, Jeollabuk, Jeollanam, Gyeongsangbuk, Gyeongsangnam, and Jeju) regions.

The past medical histories of patients were evaluated based on the ICD-10 codes. To ensure accurate diagnoses, patients with hypertension (I10 and I15), diabetes (E10–E14), and dyslipidemia (E78) were defined as those who were treated for these conditions at least twice. Patients with ischemic heart disease (I24 and I25), peripheral vascular disease (I71, I790, I739, R02, Z958, and Z959), and atrial fibrillation and flutter (I48) were defined as those who were treated at least once. Patients with depression were defined as those in whom depression was diagnosed by a psychiatrist on ≥2 occasions based on ICD-10 codes for bipolar affective disorder (F31) through unspecified mood disorder (F39). Patients with chronic obstructive pulmonary disease (COPD) were defined as those diagnosed with emphysema (J43) through other COPD (J44) and were treated with short- and long-acting beta2-agonists, long-acting muscarinic antagonists, and corticosteroids [23].

2.4. Statistical Analysis. Chi-squared tests were used to compare general characteristics between the stroke and control groups. Unconditional logistic regression analysis was performed to analyze the odds ratios (ORs) for BPPV in patients

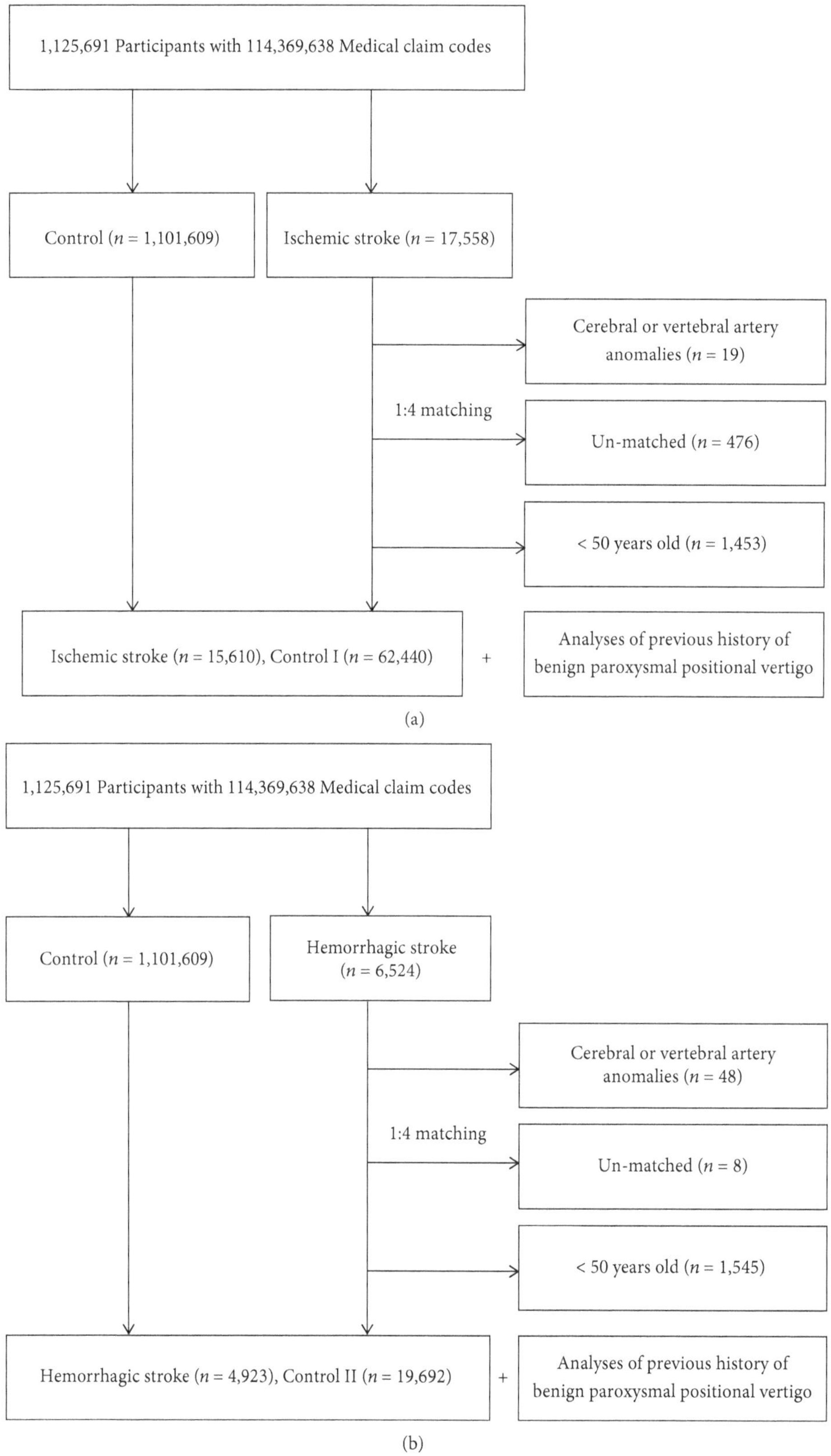

FIGURE 1: Schematic illustration of the participant selection process used in this study. (a) From a total of 1,125,691 participants, 15,610 ischemic stroke participants were matched with 62,440 control I participants for age, group, sex, income group, residential location, and past medical history. (b) From a total of 1,125,691 participants, 4,923 hemorrhagic stroke participants were matched with 19,692 control II participants for age, group, sex, income group, residential location, and past medical history.

TABLE 1: General characteristics of participants.

Characteristics	Ischemic stroke			Hemorrhagic stroke		
	Ischemic stroke (n, %)	Control I group (n, %)	P value	Hemorrhagic stroke (n, %)	Control II group (n, %)	P value
Age (years old)						
50-54	1,121 (7.2)	4,484 (7.2)		656 (13.3)	2,624 (13.3)	
55-59	1,390 (8.9)	5,560 (8.9)		619 (12.6)	2,476 (12.6)	
60-64	1,926 (12.3)	7,704 (12.3)		714 (14.5)	2,856 (14.5)	
65-69	2,537 (16.3)	10,148 (16.3)		771 (15.7)	3,084 (15.7)	
70-74	3,027 (19.4)	12,108 (19.4)		791 (16.1)	3,164 (16.1)	
75-79	2,795 (17.9)	11,180 (17.9)		674 (13.7)	2,696 (13.7)	
80-84	1,765 (11.3)	7,060 (11.3)		402 (8.2)	1,608 (8.2)	
85+	1,049 (6.7)	4,196 (6.7)		296 (6.0)	1,184 (6.0)	
Sex						
Male	7,653 (49.0)	30,612 (49.0)		2,379 (48.3)	9,516 (48.3)	
Female	7,957 (51.0)	31,828 (51.0)		2,544 (51.7)	10,176 (51.7)	
Income						
1 (lowest)	3,295 (21.1)	13,180 (21.1)		1,005 (20.4)	4,020 (20.4)	
2	1,935 (12.4)	7,740 (12.4)		654 (13.3)	2,616 (13.3)	
3	2,342 (15.0)	9,368 (15.0)		781 (15.9)	3,124 (15.9)	
4	3,019 (19.3)	12,076 (19.3)		996 (20.2)	3,984 (20.2)	
5 (highest)	5,019 (32.2)	20,076 (32.2)		1,487 (30.2)	5,948 (30.2)	
Region of residence						
Urban	6,251 (40.0)	25,004 (40.0)		2,045 (41.5)	8,180 (41.5)	
Rural	9,359 (60.0)	37,436 (60.0)		2,878 (58.5)	11,512 (58.5)	
Hypertension	12,559 (80.5)	50,236 (80.5)		3,534 (71.8)	14,136 (71.8)	
Diabetes	6,429 (41.2)	25,716 (41.2)		1,367 (27.8)	5,468 (27.8)	
Dyslipidemia	5,791 (37.1)	23,164 (37.1)		1,259 (25.6)	5,036 (25.6)	1.000
Ischemic heart disease	2,555 (16.4)	8,456 (13.5)	<0.001*	530 (10.8)	2,181 (11.1)	0.535
Depression	2,058 (13.2)	6,968 (11.2)	<0.001*	537 (10.9)	2,144 (10.9)	0.967
Peripheral vascular disease	4,791 (30.7)	19,805 (31.7)	0.012*	1,078 (21.9)	5,607 (28.5)	<0.001*
Atrial fibrillation and flutter	1,652 (10.6)	3,004 (4.8)	<0.001*	336 (6.8)	785 (4.0)	<0.001*
COPD	2,742 (17.6)	10,921 (17.5)	0.825	179 (15.2)	3,667 (15.7)	0.687
BPPV	572 (3.7)	1,702 (2.7)	<0.001*	132 (2.7)	473 (2.4)	0.258

*Chi-square test. Significance at $P < 0.05$. COPD: chronic obstructive pulmonary disease; BPPV: benign paroxysmal positional vertigo.

with stroke. A crude (simple) model and a model adjusted for ischemic heart disease, peripheral vascular disease, atrial fibrillation and flutter, depression, and COPD were used for analysis. Age, sex, income, and residential location were stratified. Additionally, 95% confidence intervals (CIs) were calculated. Additionally, we analyzed the interaction of age ∗ sex in the logistic regression model (Table S1). As the age ∗ sex were statistically significant variables, we added subgroup analyses according to age and sex. For subgroup analyses, patients were categorized on the basis of age and sex (<70 years, ≥70 years, men, and women). Two-tailed tests were used, and a P value < 0.05 was considered statistically significant. All data were analyzed using the SPSS software, ver. 22.0 (IBM, Armonk, NY, USA).

3. Results

We observed that 3.7% (572/15,610) of the patients with ischemic stroke reported a history of BPPV, which was higher than that observed in the control I group (2.7% (1,702/62,440); $P < 0.001$, Table 1), and of the patients with hemorrhagic stroke, 2.7% (132/4,923) of the stroke group and 2.4% (473/19,692) of the control II groups reported a history of BPPV ($P = 0.258$). The 25.2% (95%CI = 23.4 – 27.0) and 19.9% (95%CI = 19.6 – 20.1) of BPPV and non-BPPV participants had ischemic stroke ($P < 0.001$, Table S2). The 21.8% (95%CI = 18.6 – 25.3) and 20.0% (95%CI = 19.5 – 20.5) of BPPV and non-BPPV participants had hemorrhagic stroke ($P = 0.258$, Table S2). The stroke and control groups were

Table 2: Crude and adjusted odds ratios (95% confidence interval) of stroke for BPPV.

Characteristics	BPPV			
	Crude†	P value	Adjusted†‡	P value
Ischemic stroke	1.36 (1.24-1.50)	<0.001*	1.35 (1.22-1.49)	<0.001*
Control I	1.00		1.00	
Hemorrhagic stroke	1.12 (0.92-1.37)	0.254	1.18 (0.84-1.66)	0.343
Control II	1.00		1.00	

*Conditional logistic regression analyses, significance at $P < 0.05$. †Stratified for age, sex, income, region of residence, hypertension, diabetes, and dyslipidemia. ‡Adjusted model for chronic obstructive pulmonary disease, ischemic heart disease, peripheral vascular disease, atrial fibrillation and flutter, and depression.

matched for age, sex, income, residential location, and medical history of hypertension, diabetes, and dyslipidemia. Ischemic heart disease, depression, and atrial fibrillation and flutter were more prevalent in the ischemic stroke group than in the control I group (both $P < 0.001$). However, the prevalence rates of ischemic heart disease and depression were comparable with the control II group in the hemorrhagic stroke group. The prevalence of atrial fibrillation and flutter was higher in the hemorrhagic stroke group ($P < 0.001$). The prevalence of peripheral vascular disease was lower in the ischemic stroke and hemorrhagic stroke groups compared to those of control groups.

The crude OR for BPPV was higher in the ischemic stroke group than in the control I group (OR 1.36, 95% CI 1.24–1.50, $P < 0.001$, Table 2). The OR for BPPV remained higher in the ischemic stroke group than in the control I group even after adjusting for ischemic heart disease, peripheral vascular disease, and atrial fibrillation and flutter, depression, and COPD (adjusted OR 1.35, 95% CI 1.22–1.49, $P < 0.001$). In the age/sex subgroup analyses, the group comprising women aged <70 years showed higher ORs for BPPV in the ischemic stroke group (adjusted OR 1.83, 95% CI 1.47–2.26, $P < 0.001$, Table 3). The group comprising women aged ≥70 years showed an OR of 1.29 for BPPV in the ischemic stroke group (95% CI 1.11–1.49, $P < 0.001$).

Patients with hemorrhagic stroke only show a high OR for BPPV in ≥70 years old women (adjusted OR 1.34, 95% CI 1.00-1.79, $P = 0.048$).

4. Discussion

The risk of ischemic stroke was higher in patients with BPPV than in the control group subjects matched and adjusted for age, sex, income, residential location, and past medical history. The women's subgroup showed a higher OR for BPPV in patients with ischemic stroke. In contrast, the OR for BPPV was not high in patients with hemorrhagic stroke. This study was an extension of previous studies and included a large population cohort and matched control groups. Additionally, few previous studies have evaluated and differentiated between the risks of ischemic and hemorrhagic stroke in patients with BPPV.

Previous studies investigating the association between BPPV and stroke have reported conflicting results. A previous study reported a higher risk of ischemic stroke in patients with BPPV [7], which concurs with our study. The risk of ischemic stroke was 1.42-fold higher in patients with BPPV than in the control group after adjusting for age, sex, and past medical history (95% CI 1.16–1.73, $P = 0.001$) [7]. However, another population-based study reported that only 0.7% (9/1,297) of patients with an isolated episode of dizziness developed a stroke or transient ischemic attack [24]. This particular study did not compare between patients with dizziness and a control group nor did it stratify patients with dizziness based on their diseases. No previous studies have investigated the association between hemorrhagic stroke and BPPV.

Physical inactivity following BPPV might increase the risk of an ischemic stroke. Episodes of vertigo tend to recur, and anxiety may be associated with dizziness; therefore, patients with BPPV may be less physically active following an episode of BPPV. Notably, physical activity scores were lower in patients with BPPV than in control subjects, particularly in those aged >60 years [25]. Physical inactivity can increase the risk of stroke. A previous study has reported that physical inactivity increased the risk of stroke in middle-aged and older adults (OR 1.74, 95% CI 1.16–2.59) [26]. Previous studies have shown indirect associations between these factors in that a sedentary lifestyle increased the risk of obesity, cardiovascular disease, and diabetes [27, 28], and these chronic diseases are known to contribute to stroke onset [29]. Although this study matched and adjusted control subjects with respect to these chronic diseases, indirect effects could alter the risk of ischemic stroke in patients with BPPV.

Ischemic changes affecting the vestibular artery in patients with BPPV could precede a full-blown ischemic stroke. Several previous studies have suggested that ischemic vascular changes may contribute to the pathophysiology of BPPV [7, 30]. The vascular supply to the vestibular system originates from the anterior inferior cerebellar artery, which branches into the anterior vestibular artery. Owing to the limited collateral supply to the vestibular system, it is vulnerable to ischemic obstruction. Therefore, ischemic changes affecting the vertebrobasilar system could initially produce vestibular symptoms, such as BPPV. A few retrospective studies have reported that the prevalence of cardiovascular diseases, including hypertension, was higher in patients with BPPV than in control groups [6, 7]. Moreover, the carotid artery intima-media thickness is known to be greater in patients with BPPV than in patients with other peripheral vestibular disorders [31]. In addition to the mechanical pathophysiology explained by displacement of otoconia, the aforementioned atherosclerotic changes observed in patients

TABLE 3: Subgroup analyses of crude and adjusted odds ratios (95% confidence interval) of stroke for BPPV according to age and sex.

Characteristics	BPPV			
	Crude†	*P* value	Adjusted†‡	*P* value
Age < 70 years old, men (n = 21,100)				
Ischemic stroke	1.34 (1.04-1.73)	0.026*	1.29 (0.99-1.67)	0.057
Control I	1.00		1.00	
Age < 70 years old, women (n = 13,770)				
Ischemic stroke	1.87 (1.51-2.31)	<0.001*	1.83 (1.47-2.26)	<0.001*
Control I	1.00		1.00	
Age ≥ 70 years old, men (n = 17,165)				
Ischemic stroke	1.15 (0.92-1.44)	0.227	1.15 (0.92-1.44)	0.222
Control I	1.00		1.00	
Age ≥ 70 years old, women (n = 26,015)				
Ischemic stroke	1.28 (1.11-1.48)	<0.001*	1.29 (1.11-1.49)	<0.001*
Control I	1.00		1.00	
Age < 70 years old, men (n = 7,665)				
Hemorrhagic stroke	1.13 (0.64-1.97)	0. 679	1.13 (0.64-1.99)	0.672
Control II	1.00		1.00	
Age < 70 years old, women (n = 6,135)				
Hemorrhagic stroke	0.85 (0.56-1.29)	0.443	0.91 (0.60-1.38)	0.660
Control II	1.00		1.00	
Age ≥ 70 years old, men (n = 4,230)				
Hemorrhagic stroke	1.20 (0.75-1.94)	0.445	1.24 (0.77-2.00)	0.383
Control II	1.00		1.00	
Age ≥ 70 years old, women (n = 6,585)				
Hemorrhagic stroke	1.27 (0.95-1.68)	0.108	1.34 (1.00-1.79)	0.048*
Control II	1.00		1.00	

*Conditional logistic regression analyses, significance at $P < 0.05$. †Stratified for age, sex, income, region of residence, hypertension, diabetes, and dyslipidemia. ‡Adjusted model for chronic obstructive pulmonary disease, ischemic heart disease, peripheral vascular disease, atrial fibrillation and flutter, and depression.

with BPPV indicate the role of a vascular etiology in patients with BPPV.

Common risk factors associated with both, BPPV and ischemic stroke, contribute to the increased risk of ischemic stroke in patients with BPPV. Although we matched and adjusted for several potential confounders in this study, an unknown factor could increase the risk of both, ischemic stroke and BPPV. For example, previous research has indicated that osteoporosis increased the risks of both, stroke and BPPV [32, 33].

In this study, age/sex subgroup analyses showed that the risk of ischemic stroke was higher in the subgroup of women with BPPV. The higher prevalence of BPPV in women might affect the statistical likelihood of a higher risk of ischemic stroke in these patients with BPPV [34]. Additionally, other risk factors associated with ischemic stroke, such as smoking habits and alcohol consumption, are more commonly associated with men than women. The ORs for ischemic stroke in patients with BPPV were higher in subgroups with patients aged <70 years than in subgroups with patients aged ≥70 years. Other comorbidities might affect the risk of ischemic stroke in older patients secondary to the higher prevalence of these comorbidities in older patients. A previous study reported that labyrinthine hemorrhage could induce BPPV via the action of residual debris from the blood in the endolymphatic fluid [35]. However, hemorrhagic stroke was not associated with BPPV in this study. The small percentage of hemorrhagic stroke observed might explain the lack of association between BPPV and hemorrhagic stroke. However, the prevalence rates of different types of stroke differ across countries in that approximately 80% of strokes were reportedly ischemic strokes, per an Asian survey [36].

This study is based on nationwide representative data that were validated using a previous study [37]. Because the NHIS data include all citizens of the nation without exception, no patients were missing in the study cohort. The control group was randomly selected and matched for age, sex, income, residential location, and past medical history of hypertension, diabetes, and dyslipidemia. Income levels and residential location are important determinants of access to medical care; therefore, these variables were matched and adjusted using the NHIS data. The BPPV classification was based on physicians' diagnoses and a history of receiving treatments on ≥2 occasions. However, it is possible that positional nystagmus of central origin can also manifest as BPPV [38]. Approximately 97.5% of central nystagmus reportedly occurs in an atypical direction during the Dix-Hallpike maneuver; however, if central nystagmus is caused by cerebellar or brainstem pathology, it may be misinterpreted as BPPV [38]. The potential misinterpretation of cerebellar or brainstem pathology as BPPV might overestimate the association of BPPV with stroke in the present study. However, this was attenuated by excluding the participants with cerebral or vertebral artery anomalies and adjusted ischemic/hemorrhagic stroke and peripheral vascular diseases.

Additional limitations of this study are as follows: although we adjusted for several confounders, we did not consider a few variables, including body mass index, smoking status, and alcohol consumption. Reportedly, smoking shows a negative association with BPPV [39]. To attenuate the possible confounding effect of smoking habits, COPD was added and adjusted as a variable for analysis in this study. The study drop-out rate increased with the number of matching variables; thus, these variables were limited to ensure that the study population was representative of the South Korean population. In this study, stroke groups were diagnosed using ICD-10 codes. However, the Health Insurance Review and Assessment Service National Patient Sample data did not include information on the severity and radiological confirmation regarding the site of each stroke. For example, anterior vs. posterior circulation strokes were not differentiated. Similarly, details of the semicircular canals affected by BPPV and information regarding patient recovery were unavailable.

5. Conclusion

Ischemic stroke increased the OR of BPPV in patients aged ≥50 years. The OR for BPPV in patients with ischemic stroke was higher in subgroups comprising women. Hemorrhagic stroke did not increase the OR for BPPV.

Disclosure

The funders have no role in the design and conduct of the study; collection, management, analysis, and interpretation of the data; preparation, review, or approval of the manuscript; and decision to submit the manuscript for publication.

Conflicts of Interest

The authors declare that they have no conflicts of interest relevant to this study.

Authors' Contributions

HGC designed the study. HGC acquired the data. HGC and SYK analyzed and interpreted the data. HGC and SYK drafted the manuscript. HGC and SYK critically revised the manuscript for intellectual content. HGC and SYK acquired funding.

Acknowledgments

This work was supported in part by a research grant (NRF-2018-R1D1A1A02085328 and 2020R1A2C4002594) from the National Research Foundation (NRF) of Korea.

References

[1] M. von Brevern, A. Radtke, F. Lezius et al., "Epidemiology of benign paroxysmal positional vertigo: a population based study," *Journal of Neurology, Neurosurgery and Psychiatry*, vol. 78, no. 7, pp. 710–715, 2006.

[2] K. Parham and G. A. Kuchel, "A geriatric perspective on benign paroxysmal positional vertigo," *Journal of the American Geriatrics Society*, vol. 64, no. 2, pp. 378–385, 2016.

[3] J. M. Epley, "New dimensions of benign paroxysmal positional vertigo," *Otolaryngology and Head and Neck Surgery*, vol. 88, no. 5, pp. 599–605, 1980.

[4] T. Brandt and R. B. Daroff, "Physical therapy for benign paroxysmal positional vertigo," *Archives of Otolaryngology - Head and Neck Surgery*, vol. 106, no. 8, pp. 484-485, 1980.

[5] V. Pisani, S. Mazzone, R. Di Mauro, P. G. Giacomini, and S. Di Girolamo, "A survey of the nature of trauma of post-traumatic benign paroxysmal positional vertigo," *International Journal of Audiology*, vol. 54, no. 5, pp. 329–333, 2015.

[6] L. J. D'Silva, H. Staecker, J. Lin et al., "Retrospective data suggests that the higher prevalence of benign paroxysmal positional vertigo in individuals with type 2 diabetes is mediated by hypertension," *Journal of Vestibular Research: Equilibrium & Orientation*, vol. 25, no. 5-6, pp. 233–239, 2016.

[7] C. L. Kao, Y. Y. Cheng, H. B. Leu et al., "Increased risk of ischemic stroke in patients with benign paroxysmal positional vertigo: a 9-year follow-up nationwide population study in Taiwan," *Frontiers in Aging Neuroscience*, vol. 6, p. 108, 2014.

[8] P. M. Picciotti, D. Lucidi, E. De Corso, D. Meucci, B. Sergi, and G. Paludetti, "Comorbidities and recurrence of benign paroxysmal positional vertigo: personal experience," *International Journal of Audiology*, vol. 55, no. 5, pp. 279–284, 2016.

[9] D. Zhang, S. Zhang, H. Zhang et al., "Evaluation of vertebrobasilar artery changes in patients with benign paroxysmal positional vertigo," *Neuroreport*, vol. 24, no. 13, pp. 741–745, 2013.

[10] J. S. Kim and H. Lee, "Inner ear dysfunction due to vertebrobasilar ischemic stroke," *Seminars in Neurology*, vol. 29, no. 5, pp. 534–540, 2009.

[11] E. S. Mohamed, W. A. Kaf, T. A. Rageh, N. F. Kamel, and A. M. Elattar, "Evaluation of patients with vertigo of vertebrobasilar insufficiency origin using auditory brainstem response, electronystagmography, and transcranial Doppler," *International Journal of Audiology*, vol. 51, no. 5, pp. 379–388, 2012.

[12] V. L. Feigin, R. V. Krishnamurthi, P. Parmar et al., "Update on the global burden of ischemic and hemorrhagic stroke in 1990-2013: the GBD 2013 study," *Neuroepidemiology*, vol. 45, no. 3, pp. 161–176, 2015.

[13] K. S. Hong, O. Y. Bang, D. W. Kang et al., "Stroke statistics in Korea: part I. Epidemiology and risk factors: a report from the Korean Stroke Society and clinical research center for stroke," *Journal of Stroke*, vol. 15, no. 1, pp. 2–20, 2013.

[14] K. Sauser, D. A. Levine, A. V. Nickles, and M. J. Reeves, "Hospital variation in thrombolysis times among patients with acute ischemic stroke: the contributions of door-to-imaging time and imaging-to-needle time," *JAMA Neurology*, vol. 71, no. 9, pp. 1155–1161, 2014.

[15] T. E. Madsen, V. J. Howard, M. Jiménez et al., "Impact of conventional stroke risk factors on stroke in women: an update," *Stroke*, vol. 49, no. 3, pp. 536–542, 2018.

[16] F. Zhao, Y. Yue, H. Jiang, and Y. Yuan, "Shared genetic risk

factors for depression and stroke," *Progress in neuro-psychopharmacology & biological psychiatry.*, vol. 93, pp. 55–70, 2019.

[17] S. Y. Kim, S. Sim, H. J. Kim, and H. G. Choi, "Sudden sensory neural hearing loss is not predictive of myocardial infarction: a longitudinal follow-up study using a national sample cohort," *Scientific Reports*, vol. 8, no. 1, p. 946, 2018.

[18] A. K. Boehme, C. Esenwa, and M. S. Elkind, "Stroke risk factors, genetics, and prevention," *Circulation Research*, vol. 120, no. 3, pp. 472–495, 2017.

[19] R. Doijiri, H. Uno, K. Miyashita, M. Ihara, and K. Nagatsuka, "How commonly is stroke found in patients with isolated vertigo or dizziness attack?," *Journal of Stroke and Cerebrovascular Diseases*, vol. 25, no. 10, pp. 2549–2552, 2016.

[20] S. Y. Kim, H. J. Kim, H. Lim, I. G. Kong, M. Kim, and H. G. Choi, "Bidirectional association between gastroesophageal reflux disease and depression: two different nested case-control studies using a national sample cohort," *Scientific Reports*, vol. 8, no. 1, article 11748, 2018.

[21] S. Y. Kim, J. S. Lim, I. G. Kong, and H. G. Choi, "Hearing impairment and the risk of neurodegenerative dementia: a longitudinal follow-up study using a national sample cohort," *Scientific Reports*, vol. 8, no. 1, article 15266, 2018.

[22] R. B. Kim, B. G. Kim, Y. M. Kim et al., "Trends in the incidence of hospitalized acute myocardial infarction and stroke in Korea, 2006-2010," *Journal of Korean Medical Science*, vol. 28, no. 1, pp. 16–24, 2013.

[23] diseases TKAoTaR, "Clinical guideline for chronic obstructive lung disease," https://www.lungkorea.org/bbs/?code=guide.

[24] K. A. Kerber, D. L. Brown, L. D. Lisabeth, M. A. Smith, and L. B. Morgenstern, "Stroke among patients with dizziness, vertigo, and imbalance in the emergency department: a population-based study," *Stroke*, vol. 37, no. 10, pp. 2484–2487, 2006.

[25] L. Pollak, M. Kushnir, and H. S. Goldberg, "Physical inactivity as a contributing factor for onset of idiopathic benign paroxysmal positional vertigo," *Acta Oto-Laryngologica*, vol. 131, no. 6, pp. 624–627, 2010.

[26] Y. Gan, J. Wu, S. Zhang et al., "Prevalence and risk factors associated with stroke in middle-aged and older Chinese: a community-based cross-sectional study," *Scientific Reports*, vol. 7, no. 1, p. 9501, 2017.

[27] J. R. Pharr, C. A. Coughenour, and T. J. Bungum, "An assessment of the relationship of physical activity, obesity, and chronic diseases/conditions between active/obese and sedentary/ normal weight American women in a national sample," *Public Health*, vol. 156, pp. 117–123, 2018.

[28] A. R. Weinstein, H. D. Sesso, I. M. Lee et al., "Relationship of physical activity vs body mass index with type 2 diabetes in women," *Journal of the American Medical Association*, vol. 292, no. 10, pp. 1188–1194, 2004.

[29] Y. Chen, W. K. Copeland, R. Vedanthan et al., "Association between body mass index and cardiovascular disease mortality in east Asians and south Asians: pooled analysis of prospective data from the Asia Cohort Consortium," *BMJ*, vol. 347, no. -oct01 1, p. f5446, 2013.

[30] A. Yazici and Y. Inanc, "Evaluation of BPPV with vertebral artery values," *Neuropsychiatric Disease and Treatment*, vol. 14, pp. 1975–1979, 2018.

[31] M. Wada, H. Naganuma, K. Tokumasu, S. Hashimoto, A. Ito, and M. Okamoto, "Arteriosclerotic changes as background factors in patients with peripheral vestibular disorders," *The International Tinnitus Journal*, vol. 14, no. 2, pp. 131–134, 2008.

[32] M. Laroche, V. Pécourneau, H. Blain et al., "Osteoporosis and ischemic cardiovascular disease," *Joint, Bone, Spine*, vol. 84, no. 4, pp. 427–432, 2017.

[33] K. C. Chan, Y. T. Tsai, Y. H. Yang, P. C. Chen, and P. H. Chang, "Osteoporosis is associated with increased risk for benign paroxysmal positional vertigo: a nationwide population-based study," *Archives of Osteoporosis*, vol. 12, no. 1, p. 106, 2017.

[34] C. Silva, A. M. Amorim, and A. Paiva, "Benign paroxysmal positional vertigo–a review of 101 cases," *Acta Otorrinolaringologica Espanola*, vol. 66, no. 4, pp. 205–209, 2015.

[35] C. H. Kim, J. E. Shin, H. J. Park, J. W. Koo, and J. H. Lee, "Concurrent posterior semicircular canal benign paroxysmal positional vertigo in patients with ipsilateral sudden sensorineural hearing loss: is it caused by otolith particles?," *Medical Hypotheses*, vol. 82, no. 4, pp. 424–427, 2014.

[36] N. Venketasubramanian, B. W. Yoon, J. Pandian, and J. C. Navarro, "Stroke epidemiology in south, east, and South-East Asia: a review," *Journal of Stroke*, vol. 19, no. 3, pp. 286–294, 2017.

[37] J. Lee, J. S. Lee, S. H. Park, S. A. Shin, and K. Kim, "Cohort profile: the National Health Insurance Service-National Sample Cohort (NHIS-NSC), South Korea," *International Journal of Epidemiology.*, vol. 46, no. 2, article e15, 2016.

[38] N. K. Macdonald, D. Kaski, Y. Saman, A. Al-Shaikh Sulaiman, A. Anwer, and D. E. Bamiou, "Central positional nystagmus: a systematic literature review," *Frontiers in Neurology*, vol. 8, p. 141, 2017.

[39] K. Sunami, R. Tochino, Y. Tokuhara et al., "Effects of cigarettes and alcohol consumption in benign paroxysmal positioning vertigo," *Acta Oto-Laryngologica*, vol. 126, no. 8, pp. 834–838, 2009.

35

Amino Acid Biosignature in Plasma among Ischemic Stroke Subtypes

Vânia A. M. Goulart,[1,2] Marcelo M. Sena,[2,3] Thiago O. Mendes,[4] Helvécio C. Menezes,[2] Zenilda L. Cardeal,[2] Maria J. N. Paiva,[2] Valéria C. Sandrim,[4] Mauro C. X. Pinto,[5] and Rodrigo R. Resende[1]

[1]*Department of Biochemistry and Immunology, Federal University of Minas Gerais, Belo Horizonte-MG, Brazil*
[2]*Department of Chemistry, Federal University of Minas Gerais, Belo Horizonte-MG, Brazil*
[3]*National Institute of Science and Technology in Bioanalytics, Campinas-SP, Brazil*
[4]*Institute of Learning and Research Santa Casa de BH, Belo Horizonte-MG, Brazil*
[5]*Department of Pharmacology, Federal University of Goiás, Goiânia-GO, Brazil*

Correspondence should be addressed to Mauro C. X. Pinto; pintomcx@gmail.com

Academic Editor: Carl Muroi

Ischemic stroke is a neurovascular disorder caused by reduced or blockage of blood flow to the brain, which may permanently affect motor and cognitive abilities. The diagnostic of stroke is performed using imaging technologies, clinical evaluation, and neuropsychological protocols, but no blood test is available yet. In this work, we analyzed amino acid concentrations in blood plasma from poststroke patients in order to identify differences that could characterize the stroke etiology. Plasma concentrations of sixteen amino acids from patients with chronic ischemic stroke (n = 73) and the control group (n = 16) were determined using gas chromatography coupled to mass spectrometry (GC-MS). The concentration data was processed by Partial Least Squares-Discriminant Analysis (PLS-DA) to classify patients with stroke and control. The amino acid analysis generated a first model able to discriminate ischemic stroke patients from control group. Proline was the most important amino acid for classification of the stroke samples in PLS-DA, followed by lysine, phenylalanine, leucine, and glycine, and while higher levels of methionine and alanine were mostly related to the control samples. The second model was able to discriminate the stroke subtypes like atherothrombotic etiology from cardioembolic and lacunar etiologies, with lysine, leucine, and cysteine plasmatic concentrations being the most important metabolites. Our results suggest an amino acid biosignature for patients with chronic stroke in plasma samples, which can be helpful in diagnosis, prognosis, and therapeutics of these patients.

1. Introduction

Stroke is a complex neurological syndrome, which involves a sudden abnormality in brain function by interruption of cerebral circulation or bleeding. Each year, approximately 795,000 people in the United States are affected by stroke [1]. About 610,000 of these cases are first attacks and 185,000 are recurrent attacks [1, 2]. Stroke caused by ischemia contributes to 87% of the cases and is triggered by a vascular occlusion, leading to an interruption in oxygen and glucose supply to the brain that affects metabolic processes of the involved region [3, 4]. According to Trial of Org 10172 in Acute Stroke Treatment (TOAST) diagnostic classification system, ischemic stroke can be classified into five subtypes based on its etiology: atherothrombotic, cardioembolic, lacunar, undetermined, and other specific etiologies [5, 6].

Immediately after the ischemic stroke, a cascade of biochemical events promotes the death of brain tissue and subsequent activation of the immune response to area affected [7]. The severity of stroke is directly related to the volume of the lesion, the brain area involved, and the time of the start of treatment[8]. Recognizing the specific cause of strokes, which are etiologically heterogeneous,

Table 1: Demographic data of the study group.

Subjects	Controls	Stroke Atherothrombotic	Cardioembolic	Lacunar	Undetermined
Male	7	13	7	10	8
Female	9	7	11	10	7
Age (years, mean±SD)	54.75 (±12.34)	68.70 (±8.09)	62.50 (±12.15)	64.20 (±11.28)	54.93 (±14.50)
Risk factors					
Hypertension (%)	68.8	80	83.3	85	67
Diabetes mellitus (%)	0	30	5.6	30	6.7
Alcoholism (%)	18.8	35	27.8	45	26.7
Previous stroke (%)	0	40	33.3	20	26.7
Smoking (%)	31.3	55	44.4	50	33.3
Obesity (%)	18.8	15	11.11	5	13.3
[a]**mRS ≥ 2 (%)**	-	20	44.4	35	26.6

[a]mRS: modified Rankin Scale.

has important clinical implications [9]. The prognosis and administration of early and long-term strategies to prevent relapse can vary considerably for the different stroke subtypes [10]. For recovery, patients should be treated with specific restorative therapies. Most patients show some improvement, usually during the first 3 to 6 months after the ischemia [11].

The most understanding of how manifestations of neuroplasticity are related to stroke recovery is obtained through multimodal techniques in brain imaging [12]. Currently, the standard techniques for a diagnosis and prognosis of stroke are based on clinical observations and evaluation of neuroimaging [13]. Just as neuroimaging, cardiac evaluation and arterial imaging are used in the diagnosis of stroke, determining its causes and mechanisms of recovery, in the same way molecular features in the form of proteins, RNA, metabolites, lipids, and other biomarkers may also have utility [14].

The metabolomics approach focuses on measurement of the relative concentrations of endogenous small molecules in biofluids, cells, and tissues that characterize changes in metabolism, thus helping to unravel the metabolic state of biological systems [15]. Advances in analytical chemistry together with multivariate statistical methods can allow for the investigation of metabolites as potential biomarkers of various diseases [16–19].

In this study, we compared the amino acid profiles of patients after stroke with healthy subjects and studied different ischemic stroke subtypes. We developed a model to characterize and classify plasma samples of patients from healthy individuals and four stroke subtypes using GC-MS associated with a multivariate method of supervised classification, PLS-DA. Our model determined the amino acid profile that differentiates between healthy individuals from ischemic stroke patients and the amino acids that most contribute to discrimination of each stroke subtypes and controls.

2. Methods

2.1. Subjects. Human plasma samples were provided by Institute of Education and Research Santa Casa Belo Horizonte, Laboratory of Biomarker. Seventy-three plasma samples from patients diagnosed with one of the ischemic stroke subtypes by magnetic resonance imaging (MRI), based on the TOAST classification system, and being in the chronic phase of the disease (after 7 days of the onset of ischemic stroke diagnostic) were analyzed. We also analyzed 16 plasma samples from healthy subjects (individuals without history of ischemic or hemorrhagic stroke), which were considered the control group. Demographic data are presented in Table 1.

The modified Rankin Scale (mRS) indicates degree of disability of stroke patients (index ranged from 0 to 6). Score 2 designates slight disability or individuals able to look after own affairs without assistance. Score 3 designates moderate disability that will worsen with the increasing of the score value, and the maximum score 6 indicates death. This study was approved by the Ethics Committee in Research of Universidade Federal de Minas Gerais under number 312.840. It was also approved by the Ethics Committee in Research of Santa Casa Misericórdia of Belo Horizonte under number 315.034.

2.2. Sample Preparation. The amino acid extraction protocol was adapted from Pinto et al. [20]. Briefly, in order to precipitate proteins, 100μL of plasma samples were dissolved in 900μL of methanol at -10°C. Subsequently, samples were vortexed for 2 minutes followed by centrifugation at 10,000g for 10 minutes at 25°C. The supernatant (100μL) was transferred from each sample into a glass vial and evaporated at room temperature.

Sample derivatization process was performed as described by de Paiva et al. [21]. To each vial containing dried sample was added 15μL of methoxamine solution diluted with 20mg/mL pyridine (Fluka, St. Louis, MO, USA), followed by 35μL N,O-bis (trimethylsilyl) trifluoroacetamide (BSTFA) + Trimethylchlorosilane (TMCS; Fluka, St. Louis, MO, USA). Then, each vial was vortexed for 30s and subjected to 700W of microwave irradiation (Philco, São Paulo, SP, Brazil) for 3 min. After derivatization, the vial was vortexed for 10s. Finally, 1μL of sample was removed with a glass microsyringe (Hamilton, Bonaduz, GR, Switzerland) and manually injected into the chromatograph.

2.3. Gas Chromatography Coupled to Mass Spectrometry (GC-MS). The analyses were performed on a Shimadzu chromatograph, GC-2010/QP-2010 model (Kyoto, Japan), with a high-performance mass analyzer quadrupole. The mass spectrometer was operated in the electron impact mode at 70eV. A fused silica, nonpolar, capillary column (Restek, Bellefont, PA, USA), RTX-5MS model 30m x 0.25mm, id. x 0.25μm), was employed. The temperature program used for oven column was as follows: 80°C for 2min, gradient up to 120°C at a rate of 3°C/min, gradient to 190°C at 8°C/min, gradient up to 300°C at 30°C/min, and then constant 300°C for 3min. The injector was operated at 280°C in the splitless mode for 3min and then at a 1:20 split ratio. Helium gas (99.999%) was used as the carrier gas at a flow rate of 1mL/min. The ion source temperature was 200°C, and the GC-MS interface was kept at 260°C. The analyses were performed in full scan mode, monitoring the mass range of 45-300 m/z, and in the single ion monitoring (SIM) mode for the selection, identification, and quantification of specific ions. Signal acquisition and data processing were performed using the LabSolutions software (Shimadzu, Kyoto, Japan).

2.4. Identification and Quantification of Amino Acids. For the method validation, commercial standards of 16 amino acids were used (see Supplementary Materials, Table S1). Standard solutions of each amino acid were prepared and analyzed for construction of calibration curves. Amino acid identification was performed by analyzing the m/z fragments and retention time of specific abundance in the derivatized standard solution, followed by the similarity analysis of the mass spectra with the spectral library. The retention time obtained for each amino acid and the fragments used for quantification are listed in Table S1 (see Supplementary Materials).

2.5. Conversion of Peak Areas to Concentration. Calibration curves for each amino acid were built using Excel (Microsoft, USA). For each curve construction, five different concentrations of each standard solution were used. The peak area related to the chosen ions for the measurements was recorded for each concentration and used to build each curve. Through a linear regression, the straight-line equation $y = a + bx$ was estimated, obtaining the slope b and the intercept a. The amino acid concentrations present in the samples were determined in μmol/L using the following equation: peak area+b/a∗(1000/molar mass of amino acid)∗sample dilution. The correlation coefficients, r, were calculated for each analytical curve, so that all curves showed values greater than 0.99.

2.6. Statistical Analysis. The Kruskal-Wallis test followed by Dunn's multiple comparison test was used to compare each IS subtype of samples group and control group. To complement the visualization of differences in metabolic profiles, a heatmap was constructed based on the mean amino acid concentration in each subtype of ischemic stroke and controls (see Supplementary Materials).

For supervised classification of IS subtypes and identification of potential biomarkers from 16 amino acids, the multivariate supervised classification method, PLS- DA, was employed [22, 23]. Data were handled with MetaboAnalyst 3.0 web server (https://www.metaboanalyst.ca/) and PLS Toolbox, version 6.5 (Eigenvector Technologies, Manson, WA, USA). For PLS-DA analysis the data were previously autoscaled and leave-one-out cross-validation (LOOCV) was used.

The samples were split into the training and test sets using the Kennard-Stone algorithm[24]. The amino acids with most positive/negative regression coefficients and largest variable importance in the projection (VIP) scores were candidate biomarkers [25]. More details about PLS-DA models and their analytical validation are presented in Supplementary Materials.

3. Results

3.1. Amino Acid Analysis Distinguishes Patients with Stroke and Control Group. Plasma amino acid concentrations are kept relatively constant in postabsorptive state of a healthy human; however, circulating amino acid levels change during disease. There is a subtle, but important, change in plasma amino acid concentrations of ischemic stroke patients. The concentrations of 16 amino acids were compared for each subtype of stroke with the control group using the Kruskal-Wallis test followed by Dunn's multiple comparison test to identify statistical differences (Figure 1). Atherothrombotic subtype samples had higher concentrations of Leu and lower concentrations of Met when compared to control. Lacunar subtype samples had lower concentration of Ala when compared to health control. Interestingly, the undetermined subtype samples presented higher concentrations of Leu and Pro than control samples. This fluctuation in amino acid concentration between subtypes and controls can be seen in the heatmap, Figure S1 (see Supplementary Materials).

Based on the plasma concentration of amino acids, we analyzed the biomarker potential of these molecules to discriminate between stroke patients and healthy volunteers by PLS-DA. We built different PLS1-DA models for classifying the plasma samples (see more in Supplementary Materials). The first model was used to classify plasma samples in only two classes, as healthy/control or stroke (independent of the subtype). The other models were developed in order to classify specifically each stroke subtype.

The first model (#model 1) was defined considering only two classes, stroke (class 1) and control (class 0) (Figure 2(a)). To obtain a robust model, the data for an independent validation was separated from the external test set. A systematic approach was adopted using the Kennard-Stone algorithm (see Supplementary Materials) to select representative

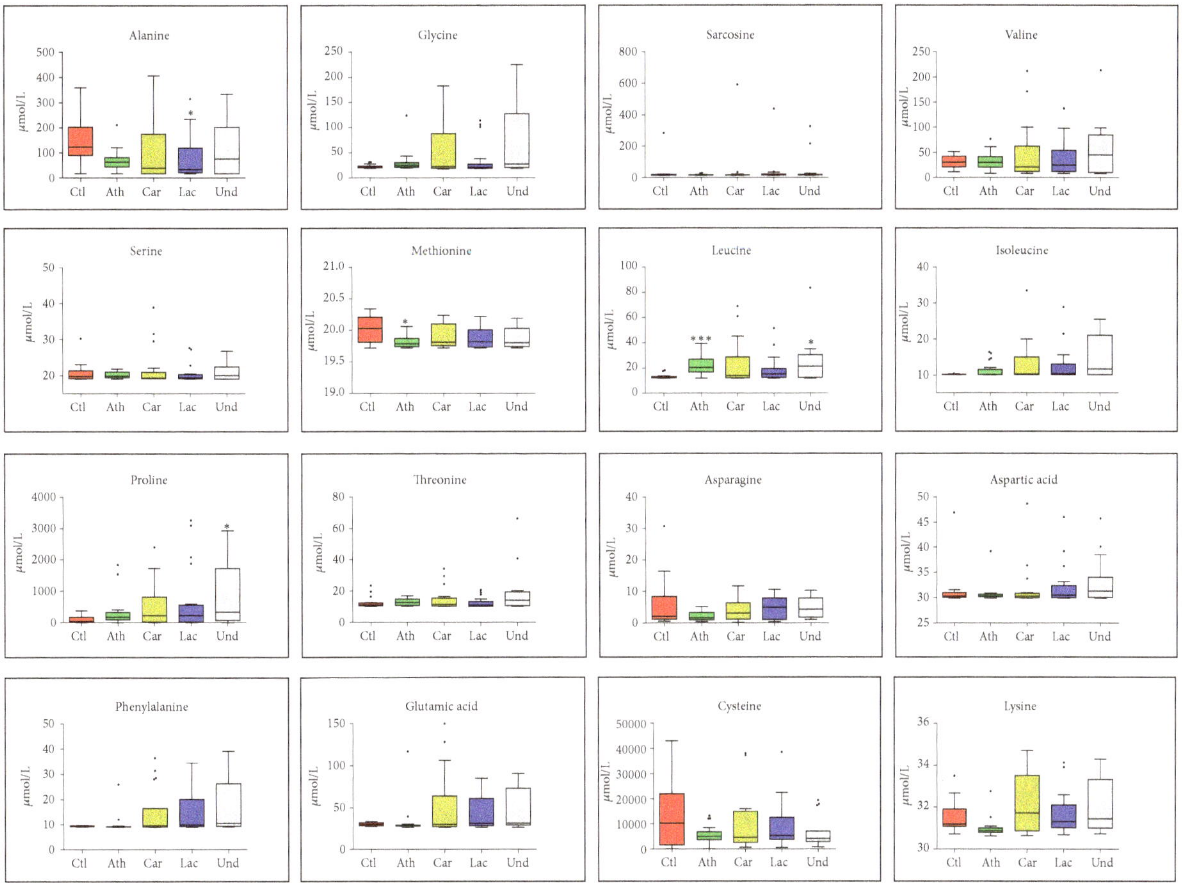

FIGURE 1: Differences in the amino acid concentrations between stroke subtypes and control individuals. Control individuals (Ctl), atherothrombotic stroke (Ath), cardioembolic stroke (Car), lacunar stroke (Lac), and undetermined stroke (Und). Kruskal-Wallis test followed by Dunn's multiple comparison test: * $p \leq 0.05$, ** $p \leq 0.01$, and ***$p \leq 0.0001$.

training samples inside each class. Thus, the data were divided into 62 samples for the training set and 27 samples for test set. The best PLS-DA model was selected by LOOCV based on the minimum cross-validation classification error (CVCE).

The best model was built with three latent variables (LV). Model quality can be evaluated through the estimate of figures of merit, such as sensitivity, i.e., the rate of true positives (correct ischemic stroke predictions), and specificity, i.e., the rate of true negatives (correct control predictions). Other parameters used for evaluating the models were cross-validation Q^2 and area under the receiver operator characteristic (AUROC). For training set, sensitivity was 0.961, and the specificity was 0.909 (Table 2). Nevertheless, only two control samples were incorrectly predicted as ischemic stroke cases, 54 and 88 (circled in red in Figure 2(b)), which can be identified as outliers in a plot of studentized residuals at the 99.7% confidence level. Thus, a global figure of merit can be estimated for the quality of this model, the efficiency rate (EFR) (see Supplementary Materials). The EFR for training and test sets of the developed model was 96.1% and 95.5%, respectively, upon elimination of the two outliers.

Once the reliability of this PLS-DA model was confirmed, the variable statistics (informative vectors) can be used to search for the most discriminant amino acids. The amino acids Met, Ala, Asp, Pro, and Cys presented the most significant VIP scores (Figure 2(c)). The most positive and most negative regression coefficients are the most discriminant ones, directly related to the power of the variables for the classification of classes 1 (ischemic stroke) and 0 (control), respectively. Pro was the most important amino acid for ischemic stroke sample classification, while Met and Ala were the most discriminant ones to classify control samples (Figure 2(d)). Thus, the joint analysis of VIP scores and regression coefficients indicated that Pro, Met, and Ala were the most discriminating amino acids for this model.

Based on these results, a variable selection was performed, and these three most important amino acids (Met, Ala, and Pro) were chosen as potential biomarkers, in order to build a new PLS-DA model (#model 2). This reduced model was somewhat worse than the full model (Figure 3; Table 2). The regression equation for the reduced model was - 0.20Ala - 0.44Met + 0.53Pro; the negative signs on Ala and Met indicate that plasma samples of healthy individuals have higher levels of these amino acids than ischemic stroke samples. In contrast, the positive sign of Pro indicates that ischemic stroke samples have higher levels of Pro.

3.2. Amino Acid Analysis Distinguishes Different Types of Chronic Stroke. To understand the most discriminant amino acids between ischemic stroke subtypes, we tried

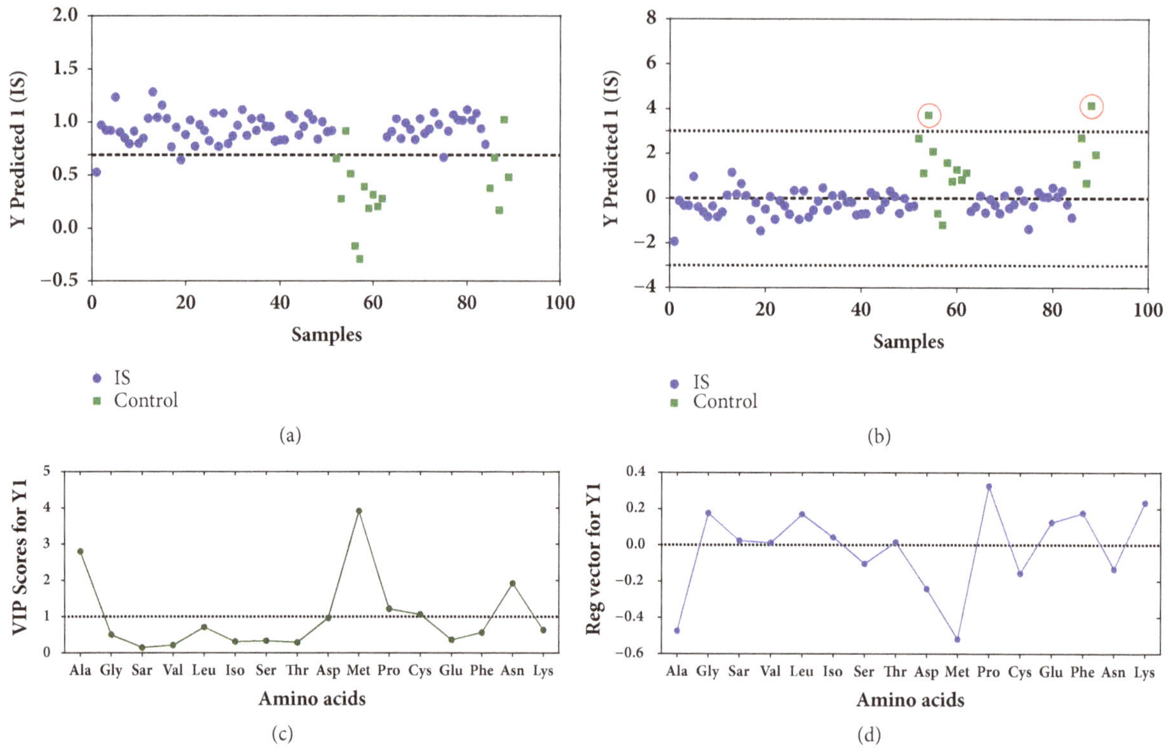

FIGURE 2: PLS-DA predictions to classify ischemic stroke and control samples (a); studentized residuals for this model at the 99.7% confidence level (b); two samples (red circles) being detected as outliers. Variable importance in the projection (VIP scores) (c) and regression coefficients (d).

TABLE 2: Figures of merit for PLS-DA models to discriminate chronic ischemic stroke from control/healthy plasma samples.

Parameters	Model #1	Model #2
Sensitivity (training set)	0.961	0.902
Specificity (training set)	0.909	0.818
EFR (training set)	0.870∗	0.870
Sensitivity (test set)	0.955	0.955
Specificity (test set)	0.800	0.800
EFR (test set)	0.755∗	0.720
N° of LV	3	2
Variance in X	66.02%	79.64%
Variance in Y	63.63%	31.62%
Q^2	0.478	0.176
AUROC	0.800	0.800

∗ Considering the detection of two control samples as outliers by the studentized y residuals at 95% confidence level, the EFR is 0.961 and 0.955 for the training and test sets, respectively.

to develop specific PLS1-DA models (one class against all the other classes) for discriminating each of the four classes: atherothrombotic, cardioembolic, lacunar, and undetermined. Undetermined ischemic stroke was the poorest modeled class, with 36.4% of sensitivity (data not shown). This is coherent with the fact that this is a nonhomogeneous class in terms of etiology causes.

The best-modeled class was atherothrombotic ischemic stroke (Figure 4(a) and Table 3) presenting only two false negatives (out of 14) in the training set and no false negative in the test set. Particularly, cardioembolic and lacunar ischemic stroke samples were poorly discriminated between them, since many samples of one class were predicted as false positive in the other. The regression coefficients for predicting these two classes presented a strong correlation (r=0.9987), indicating their very similar amino acid profiles. Thus, to verify the separation of these two classes compared to others, another model was built including cardioembolic and lacunar ischemic stroke samples in a combined single class. This model showed better results with a sensitivity of 0.833 and a specificity of 0.909 for the test set (Figure 4(b) and Table 3).

TABLE 3: Figures of merit for PLS-DA models for classifying atherothrombotic and cardioembolic plus lacunar ischemic stroke subtypes.

Parameters	Athe*	Card+Lac*
Sensitivity (training set)	0.857	0.769
Specificity (training set)	0.811	0.760
EFR (training set)	0.668	0.529
Sensitivity (test set)	1.000	0.833
Specificity (test set)	0.541	0.909
EFR (test set)	0.541	0.742
N° of LV	4	3
Variance in X	74.77%	63.82%
Variance in Y	27.80%	33.62%
Q^2	0.359	0.396
AUROC	0.882	0.883

* Athe: atherothrombotic; Card: cardioembolic; Lac: lacunar

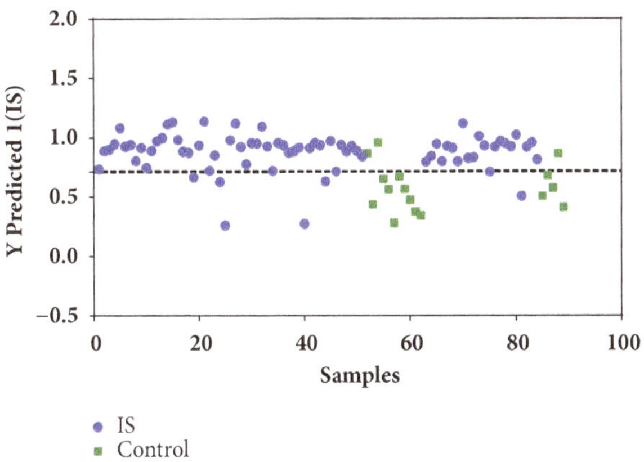

FIGURE 3: PLS-DA predictions for discriminating ischemic stroke from control samples. This PLS-DA model was built with reduced dataset, containing only the three most discriminant amino acids: Met, Ala, and Pro.

The joint analysis of regression coefficients and VIP scores for atherothrombotic ischemic stroke samples (Figures 4(a) and 4(c)) indicated that the most discriminating amino acids were related to the contrast between Leu versus Cys and Lys; i.e., the samples of this subtype were discriminated mainly by higher contents of Leu and lower contents of Cys and Lys. Similarly, by observing the same parameters for the class formed by cardioembolic and lacunar ischemic stroke samples (Figures 4(b) and 4(d)), the main discrimination was related to the contrast between Lys versus Ala and Met.

Using the two first developed PLS models (model #1 and model #2), we can suggest a biosignature for ischemic stroke dependent on Pro, Met, and Ala concentrations. Of the three ischemic stroke subtypes, the best classification was observed for the atherothrombotic subtype, while cardioembolic and lacunar ischemic stroke subtypes were more difficult to distinguish and were modeled together in a single class. This observed similarity may be related to the cardioembolic and lacunar subtypes etiology; both can be caused by thrombosis, besides other possibilities. The lacunar ischemic stroke is related to thrombosis of small arteries, while the cardioembolic one is related to the obstructions of large arteries [26, 27]. We were not able to model undetermined IS subtype due to its intrinsic heterogeneity. Samples of this subtype were predominantly classified in other subtypes, likely because this subtype does not have a common etiology, and its samples may belong to other subtypes [28].

4. Discussion

In our study, we observed that amino acids from TCA cycle (Pro, Lys, Ala, and Leu) and the Folate cycle (Met and Cys) are the most important to distinguish chronic ischemic stroke and its subtypes from health volunteers. These amino acids are involved in energy metabolism, in methyl groups generation and DNA synthesis (Figure 5). Recently, Wang and collaborators have demonstrated that tyrosine, lactate, and tryptophan were jointly enabling a high precision (91.7%) to diagnose acute ischemic stroke, within seven days of stroke symptoms [29]. Szpetnar et al. 2017 demonstrated a decrease of proline and a simultaneous increase of glutamate serum level as a marker of acute ischemic stroke; here, we demonstrated an increase in proline as a marker of chronic ischemic stroke [30]. Kimberly et al. 2013 demonstrated that valine, leucine, and isoleucine are reduced in acute ischemic stroke, and here, we observed that leucine is increased in chronic ischemic stroke [31]. Amino acids fluctuations are present in acute and chronic ischemic stroke and it can be used as markers for this pathology.

We highlight the role of Pro as an example: Proline, once oxidized to pyrroline-5-carboxylate (P5C) or its tautomer glutamic-γ-semialdehyde, can be interconverted to many other substrates and it is source for carbon exchange between TCA cycle and urea cycle. Furthermore, Pro can be stored in collagen, the most abundant protein by weight in body. As nearly 25% of the residues in collagen are incorporated as Pro, collagen can be a dump as well as a reservoir for Pro. In this context, Pro concentrations may be elevated in plasma from stroke patients as a product of extracellular matrix degradation (mostly collagen) by metalloproteinases activation during brain ischemia (Figure 5(a)). In these low energy-supply cases, Pro metabolic pathway is activated as a cell survival strategy. During nutritional stress, Pro is easily released by extracellular matrix degradation, and this degradation can

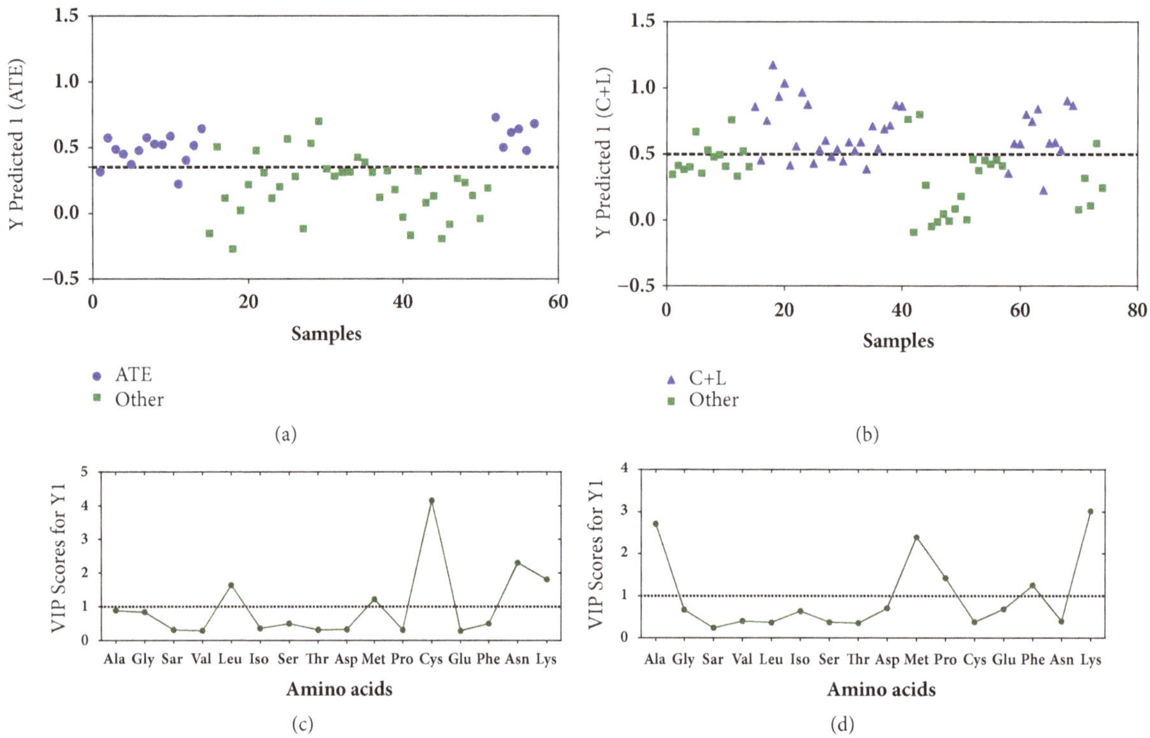

FIGURE 4: PLS-DA models built with 16 amino acids for classifying ischemic stroke subtypes. Models for discriminating atherothrombotic ischemic stroke from other samples (a) and for cardioembolic plus lacunar ischemic stroke (b). VIP scores (c) for atherothrombotic ischemic stroke. VIP scores (d) for cardioembolic plus lacunar ischemic stroke.

result in adenosine triphosphate (ATP) production. Proline oxidase (POX), an inner mitochondrial membrane enzyme, catalyzes the released proline to P5C; this process generates electrons that are donated to electron transport chain in mitochondria and generate ATP [32]. There are no reports that indicate how long Pro concentration remains high after a stroke in humans. The use of plasminogen activator (tPA) for the stroke patient treatment can also contribute to the mobilization of Pro from the extracellular matrix. The tPA is an enzyme capable of converting plasminogen to plasmin. Plasmin can degrade several extracellular matrix molecules directly, as well as activating and increasing the metalloproteinases production [33].

The ischemic brain damage is associated with acute and prolonged inflammatory response characterized by activation of the inflammatory resident glial cells as well as the infiltration of leukocytes [34]. In subacute and chronic phases of stroke, infiltrating leukocytes release cytokines and chemokines, and excessive production of reactive oxygen species (ROS) leads to induction/activation of matrix metalloproteinases (especially MMP-9) amplifying the inflammatory response in brain. This process can lead to disruption of the blood brain barrier, cerebral edema, neuronal death, and hemorrhagic transformation [35]. However, many proinflammatory factors play a dual role in early and late stages of stroke. For example, it has been demonstrated that MMP-9 at the beginning of ischemic brain injury operates in a deleterious manner contributing to the enlargement of the lesion, but can promote the regeneration of the brain and neurovascular remodeling at later stages of repair [36]. Activation of matrix metalloproteinases in injury process and repair results in amino acid release, including lysine and proline[32].

Lys is negatively associated with atherothrombotic ischemic stroke and it showed a lower concentration in the samples of this subtype. On the other hand, Lys is positively associated with cardioembolic and lacunar stroke. The role of Lys in stroke has not yet been elucidated, but some studies have shown an important role of this amino acid in reducing ischemic injury and its contribution to angiogenesis process [37]. Based on our results, Lys can be pointed out as an amino acid that can specifically discriminate atherothrombotic ischemic stroke patients from cardioembolic and lacunar ones.

Our results also demonstrated a general decrease in Ala in stroke patient plasma. Karkela and coworkers have analyzed the alanine concentration in cerebrospinal fluid of patients after acute ischemic stroke and found that alanine levels gradually increased within the first four hours, and then, there was a rapid decline [38]. Waagepetersen and coworkers have demonstrated that alanine has an important role as a carrier of nitrogen glutamatergic neurons to astrocytes [39]. It has been found that there is synthesis and release of alanine by glutamatergic neurons while astrocytes are responsible for alanine reuptake. Thus, it has been proposed that this transport through alanine can operate via supplying ammonia to glutamine synthesis in astrocytes and then releasing ammonia through glutaminase reaction inside glutamatergic

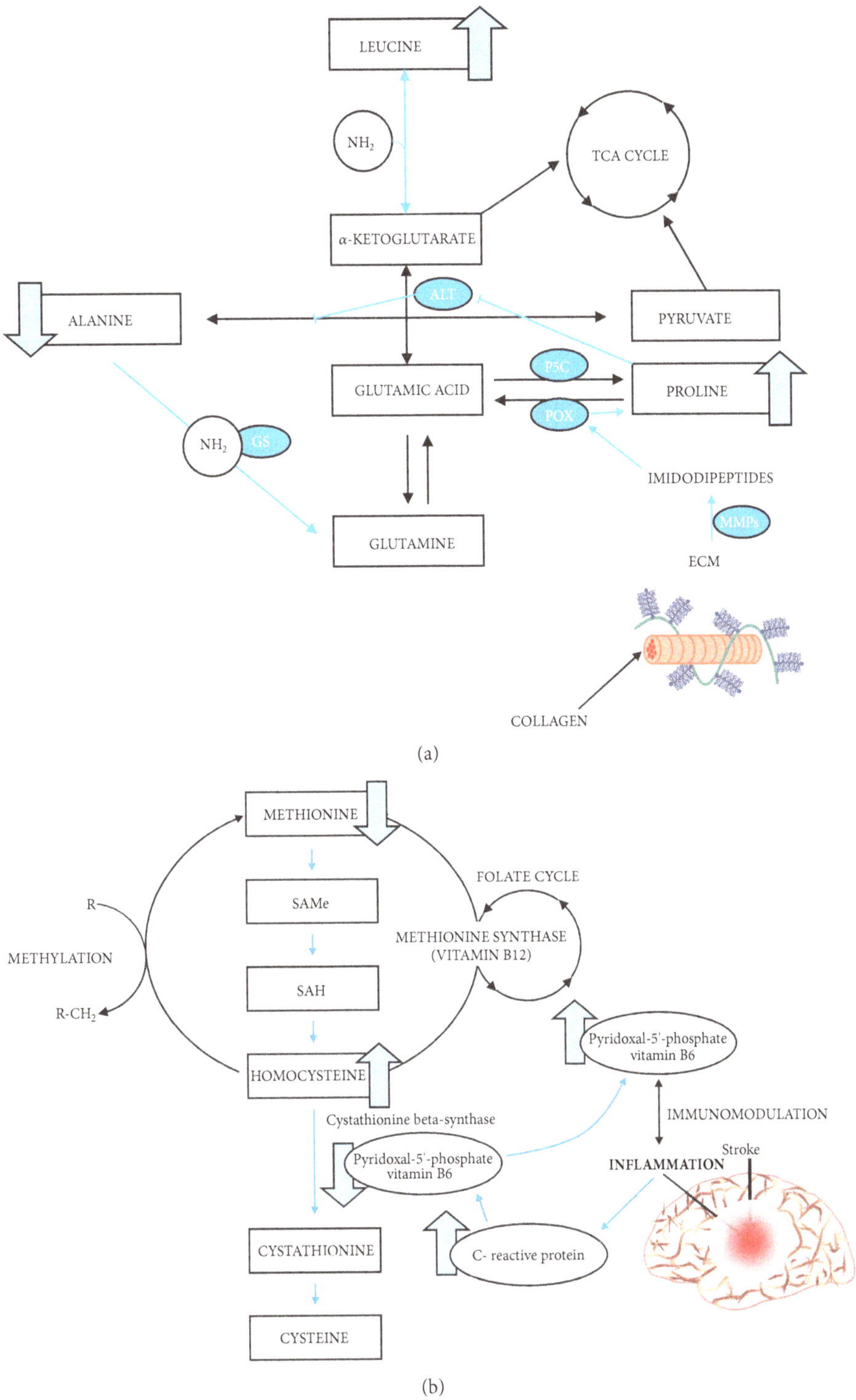

Figure 5: Metabolic pathways activated in chronic ischemic stroke. (a) The increase of proline is promoted by activation of extracellular matrix degradation. High levels of proline can inhibit ALT enzyme and cause alanine concentration reduction. The reduction in alanine concentration can also be related to donation of this amino group for glutamine synthesis, which can be converted to glutamic acid in the neurons and, then, it can be used to increase the levels of leucine. (b) Decrease of methionine concentration due to its conversion to homocysteine; homocysteine increases as a result of the cofactor pyridoxal 5′-phosphate inhibition by inflammatory mediators (C-reactive protein); decrease of pyridoxal 5′-phosphate due to its migration to inflammatory sites. Blue arrows: activated pathways. ECM: extracellular matrix. MMPs: matrix metalloproteinases.

neurons, thus forming a cycle. In case of ischemic stroke, there is a dysregulation of brain cell processes, so we can infer that the alanine synthesis by glutamatergic neurons is not possible, since adequate concentrations of derivative lactate pyruvate or glucose in neurons are necessary for this synthesis to occur. Another possible explanation for decrease in alanine concentrations in the plasma of stroke patients may be related to proline increase. Furthermore, Shanti et al. have demonstrated that chronic administration of Pro subcutaneously in rats resulted in the inhibition of the activity of enzyme alanine aminotransferase (ALT), cytosolic and mitochondrial, in brain tissues (Figure 5(a)) [40].

Leu concentration also keeps high plasma after stroke, especially in the atherothrombotic subtype. Branched chain amino acids, particularly Leu, play an important role as amino group donors in glutamic acid synthesis in the brain [41]. These amino acids readily cross the blood brain barrier, and Leu can penetrate more rapidly than any other amino acid [42]. In astrocytes, Leu donates the amino group to α-ketoglutarate, converting glutamic acid into glutamine in the glial cells (Figure 5(a)). The Leu carbon skeleton is converted to α-ketoisocaproate, which, like glutamine, is released into the extracellular medium. The α-ketoisocaproate is captured again by neurons through a reverse transaminase reaction, regenerating Leu in a process using glutamate. The newly formed Leu is released to extracellular medium, where it can again be used by astrocytes, completing the Glu-Leu cycle. In neurons, this cycle provides a "buffer" mechanism for glutamate, especially when there is an excess, as is the case during the ischemic cascade in ischemic stroke. This mechanism may explain the increase in Leu concentration in the plasma of patients with ischemic stroke [43].

In our study, we observed that Met concentration was higher in the control group than in all stroke subtypes. The decrease of Met concentrations in stroke patients may reflect the conversion of Met to homocysteine. Methionine is a substrate for the enzyme methionine adenosyltransferase (MAT) being converted to S-adenosylmethionine (SAMe), which is the major donor of methyl groups to coenzymes in the body. The SAMe methylation is a critical step in many proteins stabilization, including myelin [44]. Among other functions, methylation is also important for protection and stabilization of DNA molecules and influences gene transcription. Furthermore, SAMe is involved in polyamines formation, and serotonin and niacinamide metabolism [44, 45]. Methionine also can be used as a precursor of homocysteine (Figure 5(b)). When SAMe transfers its methyl group to an acceptor, S-adenosylhomocysteine is formed. Hydrolysis of S-adenosylhomocysteine by S-adenosylhomocysteine hydrolase (SAH) leads to the formation of homocysteine and adenosine [45]. Although this study did not determine homocysteine levels, an increase of plasmatic homocysteine concentration from patients with occlusive vascular disease or atherothrombotic and lacunar stoke is well-documented[46]. Lindgren and colleagues have found that patients with stroke present increased levels of homocysteine in relation to acute phase of the disease when compared to control group [47].

We found that Cys, a nonessential amino acid, is negatively associated with atherothrombotic stroke. Inflammation process may be related to plasma level decrease of Cys in patients after stroke. Kelly et al. have found high levels of C-reactive protein, which is the primary biomarker of inflammation, in the plasma of patients after ischemic stroke [48]. The contents of this protein were inversely proportional to the levels of pyridoxal $5'$-phosphate (PLP), the active form of vitamin B6. PLP acts as a cofactor for a variety of enzymes, including cystathionine β-synthase which is responsible for homocysteine conversion into Cys. Low levels of coenzyme PLP in plasma have been associated with their recruitment to inflammatory sites for degradation of tryptophan via the kynurenine pathway, metabolism of sphingolipids, immunomodulatory, and proliferation of immune cells [49]. The decrease in plasma PLP results in decreased Cys and then contributes to the increase of homocysteine levels (Figure 5(b)) [48].

5. Conclusion

In this work, we identified amino acid biosignatures in plasma from stroke patients using a GC/MS analysis. The most important amino acids for stroke patient's determination were Pro, Met, and Ala. Although patients are submitted to different environmental factors (e.g., medication use, diet, and risk factors), these amino acids were detected as comprehensive separation between stroke patients and healthy individuals. Other amino acids, Lys, Leu, and Cys, are important to discriminate atherothrombotic subtype from cardioembolic and lacunar stroke. Our results suggest a biosignature for patients with stroke and these amino acids may be considered as biomarkers with great predictive potential.

Abbreviations

Ala: Alanine
ALT: Alanine aminotransferase
Asp: Asparagine
ATP: Adenosine triphosphate
AUROC: Area under the receiver operator characteristic
Cys: Cysteine
CVCE: Cross-validation classification error
ERF: Efficiency rate
Glu: Glutamic acid
IS: Ischemic stroke
Leu: Leucine
Lys: Lysine
LOOCV: Leave-one-out cross-validation
MAT: Methionine adenosyltransferase
Met: Methionine
MMP-9: Matrix metalloproteinase 9
MRI: Magnetic resonance imaging
mRS: Modified Rankin Scale
P5C: Pyrroline-5-carboxylate
PLP: Pyridoxal $5'$-phosphate
Phe: Phenylalanine
Pro: Proline
RNA: Ribonucleic acid
ROS: Reactive oxygen species

SAMe: S-adenosylmethionine
SAH: S-adenosylhomocysteine hydrolase
TOAST: Trial of Org 10172 in Acute Stroke Treatment
Thr: Threonine
tPA: Plasminogen activator
VIP: Variable importance in the projection.

Conflicts of Interest

The authors declare that they have no conflicts of interest.

Acknowledgments

This work was supported by Foundation for Research Support of Minas Gerais (FAPEMIG, Brazil), National Council for Scientific and Technological Development (CNPq, Brazil), and Coordination for the Improvement of Higher Education Personnel (CAPES, Brazil).

Supplementary Materials

Table S1. Retention time, ions (m/z), and specific abundance for each amino acid. Figure S1. Heatmap of the ischemic stroke amino acid dataset. The colors represent the concentration of metabolites. The subtypes of ischemic stroke and controls are represented in horizontal axis and amino acids in vertical axis and are separated using hierarchical clustering (Ward's algorithm), with the dendrogram being scaled to represent the distance between each branch (distance measure: Euclidean). The contrast in the average concentrations of metabolites between the group of patients with stroke and healthy individuals is presented. *(Supplementary Materials)*

References

[1] D. Mozaffarian, E. J. Benjamin, A. S. Go et al., "Heart disease and stroke statistics—2016 update: a report from the American Heart Association," *Circulation*, vol. 133, no. 4, pp. e38–e60, 2016.

[2] D. Mozaffarian, E. J. Benjamin, A. S. Go et al., "Heart disease and stroke statistics—2015 update: a report from the American Heart Association," *Circulation*, vol. 131, no. 4, pp. e29–e322, 2015.

[3] S. E. Lakhan, A. Kirchgessner, and M. Hofer, "Inflammatory mechanisms in ischemic stroke: therapeutic approaches," *Journal of Translational Medicine*, vol. 7, article 97, 2009.

[4] P. Deb, S. Sharma, and K. M. Hassan, "Pathophysiologic mechanisms of acute ischemic stroke: an overview with emphasis on therapeutic significance beyond thrombolysis," *Pathophysiology*, vol. 17, no. 3, pp. 197–218, 2010.

[5] H. P. Adams Jr., B. H. Bendixen, L. J. Kappelle et al., "Classification of subtype of acute ischemic stroke: definitions for use in a multicenter clinical trial," *Stroke*, vol. 24, no. 1, pp. 35–41, 1993.

[6] P.-H. Chen, S. Gao, Y.-J. Wang, A.-D. Xu, Y.-S. Li, and D. Wang, "Classifying Ischemic Stroke, from TOAST to CISS," *CNS Neuroscience & Therapeutics*, vol. 18, no. 6, pp. 452–456, 2012.

[7] C. Xing, K. Arai, E. H. Lo, and M. Hommel, "Pathophysiologic cascades in ischemic stroke," *International Journal of Stroke*, vol. 7, no. 5, pp. 378–385, 2012.

[8] N. Kodumuri, R. Sebastian, C. Davis et al., "The association of insular stroke with lesion volume," *NeuroImage: Clinical*, vol. 11, pp. 41–45, 2016.

[9] R. Mikulik and N. Wahlgren, "Treatment of acute stroke: an update," *Journal of Internal Medicine*, vol. 278, no. 2, pp. 145–165, 2015.

[10] J. Montaner, M. Perea-Gainza, P. Delgado et al., "Etiologic diagnosis of ischemic stroke subtypes with plasma biomarkers," *Stroke*, vol. 39, no. 8, pp. 2280–2287, 2008.

[11] J. B. Green, "Brain Reorganization after Stroke," *Topics in Stroke Rehabilitation*, vol. 10, no. 3, pp. 1–20, 2003.

[12] C. Grefkes and N. S. Ward, "Cortical reorganization after stroke: how much and how functional?" *The Neuroscientist*, vol. 20, no. 1, pp. 56–70, 2014.

[13] K. S. Yew and E. Cheng, "Acute stroke diagnosis," *American Family Physician*, vol. 80, no. 1, pp. 33–40, 2009.

[14] Y. Miao and J. K. Liao, "Potential serum biomarkers in the pathophysiological processes of stroke," *Expert Review of Neurotherapeutics*, vol. 14, no. 2, pp. 173–185, 2014.

[15] C. H. Johnson, J. Ivanisevic, and G. Siuzdak, "Metabolomics: Beyond biomarkers and towards mechanisms," *Nature Reviews Molecular Cell Biology*, vol. 17, no. 7, pp. 451–459, 2016.

[16] A. Alonso, S. Marsal, and A. Julià, "Analytical methods in untargeted metabolomics: State of the art in 2015," *Frontiers in Bioengineering and Biotechnology*, vol. 3, p. 23, 2015.

[17] F. Farshidfar, A. M. Weljie, K. A. Kopciuk et al., "A validated metabolomic signature for colorectal cancer: Exploration of the clinical value of metabolomics," *British Journal of Cancer*, vol. 115, no. 7, pp. 848–857, 2016.

[18] D. S. Wishart, "Emerging applications of metabolomics in drug discovery and precision medicine," *Nature Reviews Drug Discovery*, vol. 15, no. 7, pp. 473–484, 2016.

[19] S. J. Kim, G. J. Moon, and O. Y. Bang, "Biomarkers for Stroke," *Journal of Stroke*, vol. 15, no. 1, pp. 27–30, 2013.

[20] M. C. X. Pinto, M. J. N. de Paiva, O. C. Oliveira-Lima et al., "Neurochemical study of amino acids in rodent brain structures using an improved gas chromatography-mass spectrometry method," *Journal of Chemical Neuroanatomy*, vol. 55, pp. 24–37, 2014.

[21] M. J. N. de Paiva, H. C. Menezes, P. P. Christo, R. R. Resende, and Z. D. L. Cardeal, "An alternative derivatization method for the analysis of amino acids in cerebrospinal fluid by gas chromatography-mass spectrometry," *Journal of Chromatography. B, Analytical Technologies in The Biomedical And Life Sciences*, vol. 931, pp. 97–102, 2013.

[22] M. Barker and W. Rayens, "Partial least squares for discrimination," *Journal of Chemometrics*, vol. 17, no. 3, pp. 166–173, 2003.

[23] R. G. Brereton and G. R. Lloyd, "Partial least squares discriminant analysis: Taking the magic away," *Journal of Chemometrics*, vol. 28, no. 4, pp. 213–225, 2014.

[24] R. W. Kennard and L. A. Stone, "Computer aided design of experiments," *Technometrics*, vol. 11, no. 1, pp. 137–148, 1969.

[25] I.-G. Chong and C.-H. Jun, "Performance of some variable selection methods when multicollinearity is present," *Chemometrics and Intelligent Laboratory Systems*, vol. 78, no. 1-2, pp. 103–112, 2005.

[26] A. Arboix and J. Alió, "Cardioembolic stroke: clinical features, specific cardiac disorders and prognosis," *Current Cardiology Reviews*, vol. 6, no. 3, pp. 150–161, 2010.

[27] T. Wessels, C. Röttger, M. Jauss, M. Kaps, H. Traupe, and E. Stol, "Identification of embolic stroke patterns by diffusion-weighted MRI in clinically defined lacunar stroke syndromes," *Stroke*, vol. 36, no. 4, pp. 757–761, 2005.

[28] M. Altieri, P. Troisi, I. Maestrini, and G. L. Lenzi, "Cryptogenic stroke: Cryptic definition?" *Stroke*, vol. 40, no. 8, p. e530, 2009.

[29] D. Wang, J. Kong, J. Wu, X. Wang, and M. Lai, "GC–MS-based metabolomics identifies an amino acid signature of acute ischemic stroke," *Neuroscience Letters*, vol. 642, pp. 7–13, 2017.

[30] M. Szpetnar, A. Hordyjewska, I. Malinowska, P. Golab, and J. Kurzepa, "The fluctuation of free amino acids in serum during acute ischemic stroke," *Current Issues in Pharmacy and Medical Sciences*, vol. 29, no. 4, pp. 151–154, 2016.

[31] W. T. Kimberly, Y. Wang, L. Pham, K. L. Furie, and R. E. Gerszten, "Metabolite profiling identifies a branched chain amino acid signature in acute cardioembolic stroke," *Stroke*, vol. 44, no. 5, pp. 1389–1395, 2013.

[32] J. M. Phang, S. P. Donald, J. Pandhare, and Y. Liu, "The metabolism of proline, a stress substrate, modulates carcinogenic pathways," *Amino Acids*, vol. 35, no. 4, pp. 681–690, 2008.

[33] D. M. Hermann and C. M. Matter, "Tissue plasminogen activator-induced reperfusion injury after stroke revisited," *Circulation*, vol. 116, no. 4, pp. 363–365, 2007.

[34] J. Kriz and M. Lalancette-Hébert, "Inflammation, plasticity and real-time imaging after cerebral ischemia," *Acta Neuropathologica*, vol. 117, no. 5, pp. 497–509, 2009.

[35] R. Jin, G. Yang, and G. Li, "Molecular insights and therapeutic targets for blood-brain barrier disruption in ischemic stroke: critical role of matrix metalloproteinases and tissue-type plasminogen activator," *Neurobiology of Disease*, vol. 38, no. 3, pp. 376–385, 2010.

[36] D. Amantea, G. Nappi, G. Bernardi, G. Bagetta, and M. T. Corasaniti, "Post-ischemic brain damage: pathophysiology and role of inflammatory mediators," *FEBS Journal*, vol. 276, no. 1, pp. 13–26, 2009.

[37] T. Kondoh, M. Kameishi, H. N. Mallick, T. Ono, and K. Torii, "Lysine and arginine reduce the effects of cerebral ischemic insults and inhibit glutamate-induced neuronal activity in rats," *Frontiers in Integrative Neuroscience*, vol. 4, no. 18, pp. 1–10, 2010.

[38] J. Kärkelä, K.-M. Marnela, J. Odink, T. Koivula, and S. Kaukinen, "Amino acids and glucose in human cerebrospinal fluid after acute ischaemic brain damage," *Resuscitation*, vol. 23, no. 2, pp. 145–156, 1992.

[39] H. S. Waagepetersen, U. Sonnewald, O. M. Larsson, and A. Schousboe, "A possible role of alanine for ammonia transfer between astrocytes and glutamatergic neurons," *Journal of Neurochemistry*, vol. 75, no. 2, pp. 471–479, 2000.

[40] N. Desai Shanti, K. C. Shashikumar, and P. V. Desai, "Influence of proline on rat brain activities of alanine aminotransferase, aspartate aminotransferase and acid phosphatase," *Neurochemical Research*, vol. 29, no. 12, pp. 2197–2206, 2004.

[41] M. Ruiz-Canela, E. Toledo, C. B. Clish et al., "Plasma branched-chain amino acids and incident cardiovascular disease in the PREDIMED Trial," *Clinical Chemistry*, vol. 62, no. 4, pp. 582–592, 2016.

[42] Q. R. Smith, S. Momma, M. Aoyagi, and S. I. Rapoport, "Kinetics of neutral amino acid transport across the blood-brain barrier," *Journal of Neurochemistry*, vol. 49, no. 5, pp. 1651–1658, 1987.

[43] Y. Daikhin and M. Yudkoff, "Compartmentation of brain glutamate metabolism in neurons and glia," *Journal of Nutrition*, vol. 130, no. 4, pp. 1026S–1031S, 2000.

[44] M. Varela-Rey, M. Iruarrizaga-Lejarreta, J. J. Lozano et al., "S-adenosylmethionine levels regulate the schwann cell DNA methylome," *Neuron*, vol. 81, no. 5, pp. 1024–1039, 2014.

[45] H. Tomitori, T. Usui, N. Saeki et al., "Polyamine oxidase and acrolein as novel biochemical markers for diagnosis of cerebral stroke," *Stroke*, vol. 36, no. 12, pp. 2609–2613, 2005.

[46] L. Brattström, A. Lindgren, B. Israelsson et al., "Hyperhomocysteinaemia in stroke: prevalence, cause, and relationships to type of stroke and stroke risk factors," *European Journal of Clinical Investigation*, vol. 22, no. 3, pp. 214–221, 1992.

[47] A. Lindgren, L. Brattstrom, B. Norrving, B. Hultberg, A. Andersson, and B. B. Johansson, "Plasma homocysteine in the acute and convalescent phases after stroke," *Stroke*, vol. 26, no. 5, pp. 795–800, 1995.

[48] P. J. Kelly, J. P. Kistler, V. E. Shih et al., "Inflammation, homocysteine, and vitamin B6 status after ischemic stroke," *Stroke*, vol. 35, no. 1, pp. 12–15, 2004.

[49] L. Paul, P. M. Ueland, and J. Selhub, "Mechanistic perspective on the relationship between pyridoxal 5'-phosphate and inflammation," *Nutrition Reviews*, vol. 71, no. 4, pp. 239–244, 2013.

36

Effect of Acupuncture on Neuroplasticity of Stroke Patients with Motor Dysfunction: A Meta-Analysis of fMRI Studies

Qiuyi Lv,[1] Guixing Xu,[2] Yuxin Pan,[3] Tongtong Liu,[4] Xiaodong Liu,[5] Linqing Miao,[6] Xing Chen,[1] Lan Jiang,[1] Jie Chen,[7] Yingjia He,[5] Rong Zhang,[5] and Yihuai Zou[1]

[1]*Department of Neurology and Stroke Center, Dongzhimen Hospital, The First Affiliated Hospital of Beijing University of Chinese Medicine, Beijing, China*
[2]*The Acupuncture and Tuina School/The 3rd Teaching Hospital, Chengdu University of Traditional Chinese Medicine, Chengdu, China*
[3]*Institute of Neuroscience, Chinese Academy of Sciences, Shanghai, China*
[4]*Guang'anmen Hospital, China Academy of Chinese Medical Sciences, Beijing, China*
[5]*Beijing University of Chinese Medicine, Beijing, China*
[6]*Beijing Institute of Technology, Beijing, China*
[7]*School of Life Science, Peking University, Beijing, China*

Correspondence should be addressed to Yihuai Zou; zouyihuai2004@163.com

Academic Editor: Yasuo Terao

Importance. Acupuncture is an effective treatment for stroke, especially in the aspect of motor deficit. Many brain imaging studies of acupuncture have found significant changes in brain function after acupuncture treatment in order to reveal its underlying mechanisms in regulating neural plasticity. However, no definite consensus has been reached. *Objective.* To analyze the pattern of intrinsic brain activity variability that is altered by acupuncture compared with conventional treatment in stroke patients with motor dysfunction, thus providing the mechanism of stroke treatment by acupuncture. *Methods.* Chinese and English articles published up to May 2020 were searched in the PubMed, Web of Science, EMBASE, and Cochrane Library databases, China National Knowledge Infrastructure, Chongqing VIP, and Wanfang Database. We only included randomized controlled trials (RCTs) using resting-state fMRI to observe the effect of acupuncture on stroke patients with motor dysfunction. R software was used to analyze the continuous variables, and Seed-based d Mapping with Permutation of Subject Images (SDM-PSI) was used to perform an analysis of fMRI data. *Findings.* A total of 7 studies comprising 143 patients in the treatment group and 138 in the control group were included in the meta-analysis. The results suggest that acupuncture treatment helps the healing process of motor dysfunction in stroke patients and exhibits hyperactivation in the bilateral basal ganglia and insula and hypoactivation in motor-related areas (especially bilateral BA6 and left BA4). *Conclusion.* Acupuncture plays a role in promoting neuroplasticity in subcortical regions that are commonly affected by stroke and cortical motor areas that may compensate for motor deficits, which may provide a possible mechanism underlying the therapeutic effect of acupuncture.

1. Introduction

Stroke is a syndrome characterized by an acute onset of neurologic deficit resulted from ischemia or hemorrhage. It became the leading cause of death and years of life lost (YLLs) at the national level in China [1]. Patients with stroke are susceptible to several complications, including pain, dysphagia, pneumonias, incontinence, depression, and somatic dyskinesia, which usually impede clinical recovery and require specific intervention [2, 3]. In this review, we mainly focus on the motor dysfunction after stroke. As a common and severe complication of stroke, motor dysfunction recovery requires multidisciplinary treatment and still remains a clinical challenge [4]. Seeking an effective and safe alternative therapy meets the requirement of the Healthy China 2030 plan [5].

Acupuncture, a key modality of Traditional Chinese Medicine (TCM) therapy, is recommended by the World Health Organization (WHO) as an alternative and complementary strategy for poststroke treatment [6, 7]. Acupuncture has been widely used to relieve pain and improve motor or neurological function [8, 9]. Sufficient previous studies including animal experiments, clinical trials, and systematic reviews have proven that acupuncture was beneficial for stroke rehabilitation [10]. Although the application of acupuncture has shown good clinical efficacy, the mechanisms of acupuncture remain unknown. One hypothesis suggests that acupuncture may induce neuroplasticity to exert therapeutic effects [11–13].

Neuroplasticity refers to the capability of the nervous system to modify and reorganize the brain structure and function in response to impairment or experience; various behavioral, neurophysiological, and neuroimaging studies can document changes in the nervous system [14, 15]. One of the recommended modalities used to measure neuroplasticity in humans is resting-state functional magnetic resonance imaging (rs-fMRI), which is often used to assess resting-state networks in participants [16, 17]. The main analysis approaches of rs-fMRI are regional homogeneity (ReHo) and amplitude of low-frequency fluctuations (ALFFs). The former evaluates the temporal homogeneity of the regional blood oxygen level-dependent (BOLD) signal, and the latter reflects intrinsic brain low frequency [18, 19]. Aimed at a better understanding of the cerebral characters of acupuncture treatment, more and more acupuncture studies have applied rs-fMRI in the clinical trials. However, no consensus has been reached, possibly due to the small sample size or distinctions of experimental design between studies. For example, Schaechter et al. [20] have reported that acupuncture would activate the ipsilateral lesional motor cortex to improve motor function in patients with hemiparetic stroke, while others suggested that the basal ganglia would be predominantly activated by acupuncture [21].

Therefore, in order to elucidate which brain area plays a crucial role in the therapeutic effect of acupuncture, this review synthesized corresponding studies and introduced coordinate-based meta-analysis (CBMA) to quantitatively integrate the results of individual neuroimaging studies [22, 23]. The feature of CBMA is the use of effect sizes, which allows combination of peak coordinates with statistical parametric maps and it has been fully validated in many studies [24–28]. In the present study, we applied the Seed-based d Mapping with Permutation of Subject Images (SDM-PSI), which is a new generation algorithm for CBMA meta-analysis, to analyze the rs-fMRI data of included studies [29, 30]. The results would determine whether acupuncture has a differential effect on brain activity as compared to regular or conventional treatment. The apprehension of neuroplasticity mechanisms induced by acupuncture can not only elucidate the central mechanism of acupuncture but also possibly provide novel ideas for applying acupuncture to the treatment of other neurodegenerative diseases.

2. Methods

We conducted the meta-analysis in line with the *Cochrane Handbook for Systematic Reviews of Interventions*. All procedure followed the Preferred Reporting Items for Systematic Reviews and Meta-Analyses guidelines (PRISMA guidelines). The study was registered in the PROSPERO International prospective register of systematic reviews (registration number: CRD 42020185421).

2.1. Literature Search. Studies that examined the neuroprotective effect of acupuncture in stroke patients were included in the present study. The PubMed, EMBASE, and Cochrane Library databases, Web of Science, China National Knowledge Infrastructure (CNKI), Chongqing VIP (VIP), and the Wanfang Database (WF) were searched from inception until May 2020 by two independent researchers. The following English search terms were used: (stroke OR Poststroke OR Cerebrovascular Accident OR Cerebrovascular Apoplexy OR Apoplexy OR Brain Vascular Accident OR Cerebrovasc∗ OR brain∗ OR brain vasc∗ OR hemipleg∗ OR apoplex∗ OR CVA OR TIA) AND (acupuncture OR acupuncture therapy OR acupuncture treatment OR electroacupuncture OR electro-acupuncture OR acupuncture, ear OR ear acupuncture OR auriculotherapy OR scalp acupuncture) AND (RCT OR randomized controlled trial OR controlled clinical trial OR randomized OR clinical trial OR randomly OR RCT OR trial) AND (fMRI OR functional MRI OR functional magnetic resonance imaging OR neuroimaging). The languages of the trials were restricted to English or Chinese, and the search strategy for each database was based on its own unique characteristics.

2.2. Inclusion/Exclusion Criteria. Two researchers independently conducted the search and screened the titles, abstracts, and full texts of the papers. Studies were included based on the following criteria: (1) an RCT conducted in patients with stroke sequelae at any-stroke stage, of any age and gender; (2) manual acupuncture or electroacupuncture with or without other therapies in the treatment group, while other therapies including conventional rehabilitation or sham acupuncture in the control group; (3) involved whole-brain functional imaging (ReHo or ALFFs) in resting state; (4) three-dimensional coordinates (x, y, z) reported in standard stereotactic space Talairach or Montreal Neurological Institute (MNI); (5) if one study involved two or more comparable datasets, all samples were included; and (6) used secondary outcomes to assess clinical efficacy. The exclusion criteria were as follows: (1) the study only used region of interest (ROI) method; (2) the sample size in each group was less than 5; (3) if separate papers used the same or similar datasets, only the largest sample was included.

2.3. Data Extraction and Quality Assessment. Data were extracted from the included studies into a standard form with respect to publishing year, name of the first author, sample size, participants' condition, intervention design, fMRI method, and secondary outcome measures. Missing or unclear data for the meta-analysis were obtained after corresponding with the original authors by email or telephone.

Two independent researchers carried out the data extraction; any disagreements were resolved by a third reviewer. This information is showed in Table 1. Quality assessment was based on Cochrane Risk of Bias Tool and carried out by two researchers independently. All the reports were evaluated according to the following seven criteria: random sequence generation, allocation concealment, blinding of participants and personnel, blinding of outcome assessment, incomplete outcome data, selective reporting, and other sources of bias. For each criterion, studies were judged to be at low, high, or unclear risk of bias.

2.4. Data Synthesis and Meta-Analysis. ReHo results: the differences of brain activity between the treatment group and the control group were analyzed by SDM-PSI (version 6.21, https://www.sdmproject.com/). A step-by-step tutorial is provided on this website. First, reported peak coordinates and effect sizes (t value, or equivalently from z-scores or P values) were extracted to prepare the peaks' text files. In the step of preprocessing, software will use those files to recreate the lower and upper bounds of the possible effect-size values of the studies. Second, the meta-analysis consisted in calculating the random-effects mean of the ReHo values and the mean map was weighted by the sample size and variance of each study. We reported results using family-wise error (FWE) correction ($P < 0.05$ and voxel extent ≥ 10) with the threshold-free cluster enhancement approach (TFCE) and 5000 permutations. The heterogeneity analyses were also assessed. The peak MNI coordinate would be extracted to derive standard heterogeneity statistics I^2, and an $I^2 < 50\%$ indicates low heterogeneity. Funnel plots were not performed because the amount of included studies ($n = 7$) was less than 10, but the Egger test was used to assess the publication bias. Finally, a metaregression analysis was carried out to figure out the relationship between ReHo changes and clinical variables. All results would be reported using the TFCE-based FWE corrected threshold ($P < 0.05$ and voxel extent ≥ 10).

Clinical variables: statistical analyses of continuous data were performed with R software, version 3.6.2 (R Foundation for Statistical Computing, Vienna, Austria), using the Meta and Metafor meta-analysis packages. Weighted mean difference (WMD) with 95% CIs was used. Heterogeneity was tested by the I^2 statistic. We selected fixed or random-effects model to pool the data depending on whether the trials had good homogeneity ($P > 0.10$, $I^2 < 50\%$) or not. A forest plot was adopted to show the hypothesis test results, and if necessary, a sensitivity analysis or subgroup analysis would be performed to find sources of heterogeneity.

3. Results

3.1. Included Studies. The database search yielded 1195 articles. 272 duplicates were removed, and 883 articles were excluded after screening titles and abstracted. Of the 40 potentially relevant reports, 6 articles [31–36] and 7 studies (Chen et al. [35] conducted two trials at the same time) proved eligible after full-text screening (Figure 1).

Trials were published after 2000, and each study enrolled 10 to 100 patients (140 individuals in the treatment group and 138 in the control group). All studied recruited ischemic stroke patients. There were no significant differences in demographic baseline characteristics, including age, gender, disease status including symptom duration, or secondary outcome measures between the two groups. Three studies reported the patient limb dysfunction of the right side and the most lesions of brain regions had the left laterality (especially in the left basal ganglia) [32, 35, 36]. All patients in both groups received conventional treatment and, on this basis, participants in the treatment group underwent two or four courses (weeks) of manual acupuncture therapy, one study combined with sham acupuncture as comparison [32]. The manual acupuncture methods include lifting yang to dredging du meridian needling method (LYDDM) and Xingnao Kaiqiao needling method (XNKQ) and empirical acupoints. The LYDDM and XNKQ needling methods are based on long-term clinical experiments and were developed in by Professor Peilin Zhang and Xuemin Shi, respectively. And the application of empirical acupoints means that doctors manipulate the acupuncture based on their clinical experience. All studies reported rs-fMRI data by using ReHo variations to compare differences before and after treatment in patients from both groups. Clinical efficacy was examined by Fugl-Meyer assessment (FMA; $n = 7$), nervous functional deficiency scale (NDS; $n = 3$), Barthel index (BI; $n = 4$), or modified Barthel index (MBI; $n = 3$). The details and features of the studies are shown in Table 1.

3.2. Quality Assessment. The quality assessment was based on Cochrane Risk of Bias Tool. Among 7 RCTs, all the studies reported the methods of random sequence generation but only three studies of two articles employed allocation concealment [31, 36]. Only two studies reported the methods of patient blinding [32, 35], while Zhou et al. [34] admitted that it was at high risk. Methods of blinding of outcome assessment were only applied in two studies [34, 35]. Evaluation of incomplete outcome data depended on whether the clear descriptions of baseline data were shown. According to this standard, all studies were at low risk. None of the studies have published study protocols before, so it was difficult to evaluate selective reporting. We tended to believe a study was at low risk only if it reported all the three secondary outcome measures (FMA, NDS, BI, or MBI). Thus, low risk of bias in the domain of selective reporting was given to four studies [31, 33–35]. In addition, we did not find any other sources of bias. Overall, these studies were not of high quality, mainly in terms of allocation concealment, patient blinding, and outcome blinding. Figure 2 presents the quality assessment of these 7 included studies.

3.3. Meta-Analysis of ReHo Changes

3.3.1. Mean Analysis. Patients in the treatment group showed hyperactivation in the right basal ganglia ($P < 0.05$, $z = 6.622$) and left insula ($P < 0.05$, $z = 5.232$) after acupuncture therapy and the decreased activity of the left precentral gyrus (PG; $P < 0.05$, $z = -4.477$) and right superior frontal gyrus (SFG; $P < 0.05$, $z = -4.723$). Patients in the control group showed hyperactivation in the right middle frontal gyrus

Table 1: Clinical characteristics of subjects in the included studies.

Study	Cases (T/C)	Participant: Condition	Lesion location	Duration (days)	Age (years)	Gender (male/female)	Comparison: T	C	Intervention: Acupoints	Regimen	Outcome measures: Analysis of fMRI	Coordinate	Secondary outcomes
Zhengfei Ye 2018	84 (42/42)	Poststroke limb motion dysfunction	Unclear	Not reported	T: 55.67 ± 8.38 C: 57.01 ± 6.97	T: 22/20 C: 24/18	Acu +Conv	Conv	LYDDM	7/week for 2 weeks	ReHo	MNI	FMA, BI
Zhihong Chen 2016	60 (30/30)	Poststroke limb motion dysfunction	Unclear	T: 29.83 ± 7.27 C: 30.17 ± 7.55	T: 62.67 ± 3.79 C: 65.50 ± 6.43	T: 17/13 C: 16/14	Acu +Conv	Conv	LYDDM	7/week for 2 weeks	ReHo	MNI	IFMA, BI
Zhihong Chen 2016	60 (30/30)	Poststroke limb motion dysfunction	Unclear	T: 23.33 ± 5.92 C: 30.17 ± 7.55	T: 65.33 ± 5.31 C: 65.50 ± 6.43	T: 18/12 C: 16/14	Acu +Conv	Conv	XNKQ	7/week for 2 weeks	ReHo	MNI	FMA, BI
Nana Chen 2017	12 (6/6)	R limb motion dysfunction	L basal ganglia or corona radiata	T: 14.83 ± 13.848 C: 12.83 ± 14.566	T: 62.00 ± 8.485 C: 67.33 ± 8.779	T: 2/4 C: 4/2	Acu +Conv	Sham acu +Conv	Empirical acupoints	7/week for 2 weeks	ReHo	MNI	FMA, MBI
Ping Wu 2017	21 (11/10)	Poststroke limb motion dysfunction	Unclear	T: 52.818 ± 45.31 C: 52.200 ± 47.852	T: 69.364 ± 12.075 C: 61.300 ± 11.107	T: 7/4 C: 5/5	Acu +Conv	Conv	Empirical acupoints	5/week for 4 weeks	ReHo	Tal	NSD, FMA, MBI
Ximei Xie 2012	20 (10/10)	R limb motion dysfunction	Pons or thalamus or L basal ganglia	T: 19.50 ± 1.66 C: 19.10 ± 1.18	T: 67.70 ± 3.82 C: 64.80 ± 3.72	T: 6/4 C: 5/5	Acu +Conv	Conv	Empirical acupoints	5/week for 4 weeks	ReHo	Tal	NDS, FMA, BI
Yumei Zhou 2015	21 (11/10)	R limb motion dysfunction	L basal ganglia	T: 52.20 ± 34.20 C: 52.80 ± 30.47	T: 69.36 ± 4.06 C: 61.30 ± 7.94	T: 7/4 C: 4/6	Acu +Conv	Conv	Empirical acupoints	5/week for 4 weeks	ReHo	MNI	NSD, FMA, MBI

Abbreviations: Acu: acupuncture treatment; BA: Brodmann area; BI: Barthel index; C: control group; Conv: conventional treatment; FMA: Fugl-Meyer assessment; BMI: modified Barthel index; LYDDM: lifting yang to dredging du meridian needling method; MNI: Montreal Neurological Institute; R: right; ReHo: regional homogeneity; S: sensitivity; SDM: signed differential mapping; T: treatment group; XNKQ: Xingnao Kaiqiao needling method.

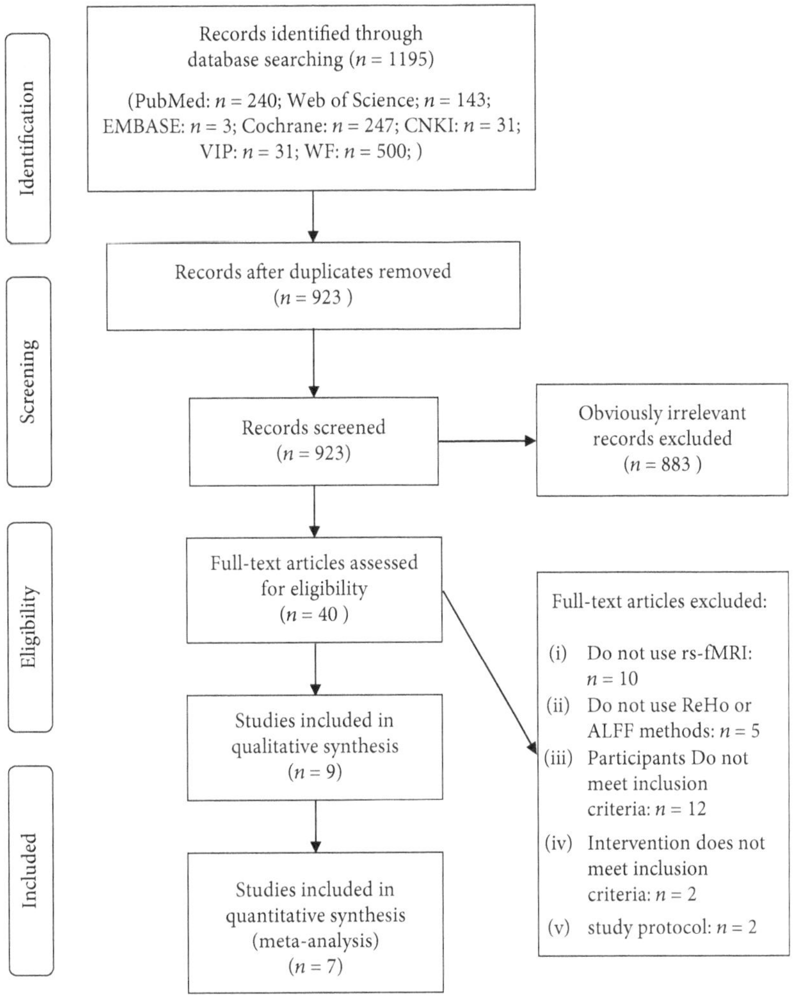

FIGURE 1: Flowchart for study inclusion and exclusion process.

(MFG; $P < 0.05$, $z = 5.457$) and left supplementary motor area (SMA; $P < 0.05$, $z = 4.867$) after conventional treatment and a decrease of activity in the left striatum ($P < 0.05$, $z = -4.876$) and left inferior frontal gyrus (IFG; $P \leq 0.05$, $z = -5.547$). Peak coordinates and cluster breakdowns are shown in Table 2. Differences in the brain regions between conventional treatment and acupuncture treatment have been visualized in Figure 3.

3.3.2. Heterogeneity Analysis and Publication Bias. In the treatment group, the ganglia, insula, left PG, and right SFG showed low between-study heterogeneity of effect size differences in peak coordinates ($I^2 = 0.88\% - 7.40\%$) and low between-study heterogeneity for each significant peak in the control group ($I^2 = 0.09\% - 1.29\%$). The heterogeneity results are shown in Table 2. The Egger tests were insignificant in the treatment group ($P = 0.464$) and the control group ($P = 0.501$).

3.3.3. Metaregression Analysis. Metaregression was used to search for potential correlation between FMA scores, mean age, and disease duration in the treatment group. The FMA scores are associated with the left insula (Table S1A). The analysis of mean age shows significance in the brain regions of the left cerebellum (Table S1B). The disease duration is associated with many regions, including the left cerebellum, arcuate network and right SMG, and SFG (Table S1C).

3.4. Meta-Analysis of Secondary Outcomes. Compared with conventional treatment, manual acupuncture therapy was associated with a decrease of NDS score (−4.40; 95% CI, 3.79 to 5.01; $I^2 = 0$), indicating that acupuncture could mitigate the impairment of nervous function. The change in BI score was 3.47 (3.47; 95% CI, 0.99 to 5.95; $I^2 = 87\%$) and that in MBI score was 7.49 (7.49; 95% CI, 5.38 to 9.59; $I^2 = 0$). The increase of BI or MBI suggested that patients had better daily living ability after acupuncture. A greater increase of FMA score (5.73; 95% CI, 4.35 to 7.11; $I^2 = 77\%$) also demonstrated that acupuncture could improve motor function of the upper and lower limb. The forest plots are shown in Figures S1A–S1D.

4. Discussion

4.1. Main Findings. It is suggested that acupuncture therapy could relieve neurological deficiency (NDS) and improve

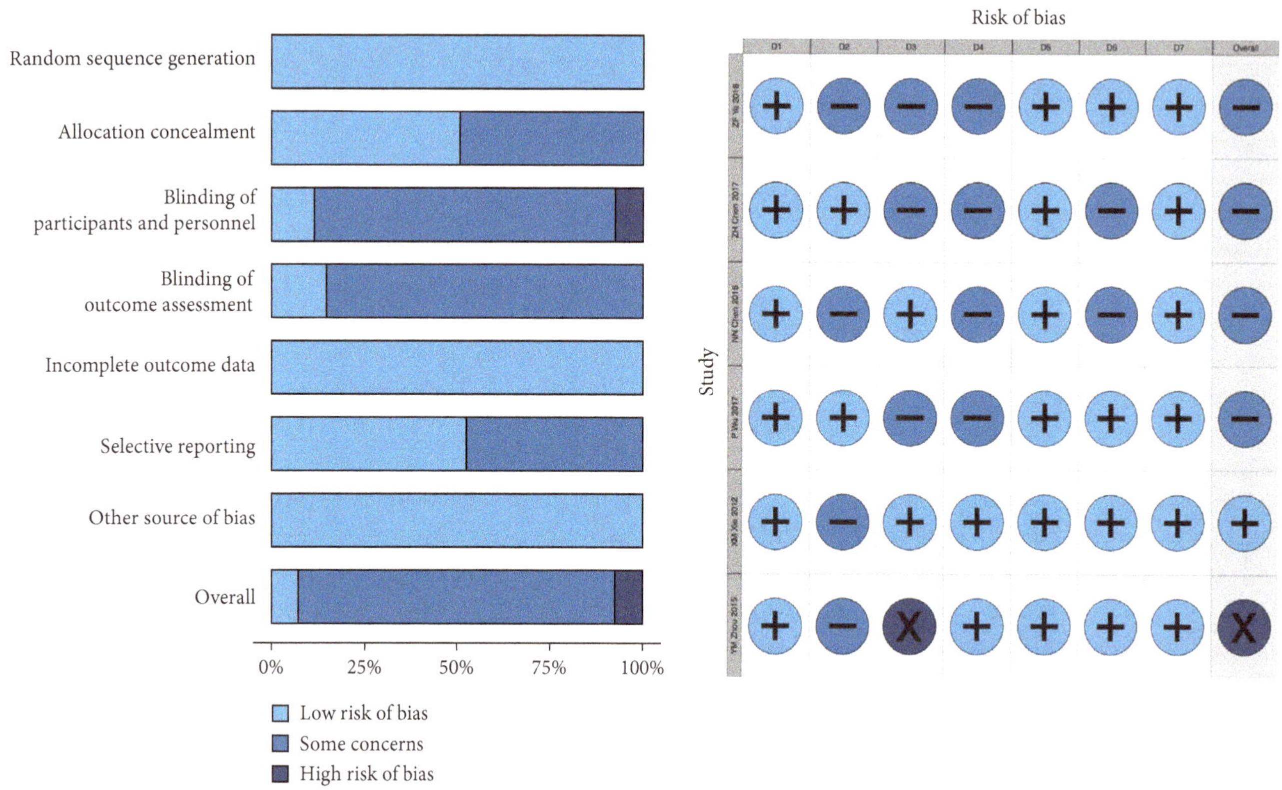

FIGURE 2: Risk of bias summary. Each color represents a level of risk of bias: light blue, low risk of bias; medium blue, unclear risk of bias; dark blue, high risk of bias. D1: random sequence generation; D2: allocation concealment; D3: blinding of participants and personnel; D4: blinding of outcome data; D5: incomplete outcome data; D6: selective reporting; D7: other sources of bias.

TABLE 2: Brain activity changes in patients after treatment compared to baseline.

	MNI coordinates			SDM z -score[a]	P value[b]	Voxels[c]	Cluster breakdown	I^2
	x	y	z					
Treatment group								
R basal ganglia	34	-12	8	6.622	<0.05	1244	R lenticular nucleus, putamen, striatum, insula, rolandic operculum, BA48	0.88%
L insula	-32	-14	10	5.232	<0.05	887	L insula, lenticular nucleus, putamen, rolandic operculum, BA48	1.02%
L precentral gyrus	-28	-24	66	-4.477	<0.05	337	L precentral gyrus, corpus callosum, superior frontal gyrus, dorsolateral, BA6	5.83%
R superior frontal gyrus	22	2	62	-4.723	<0.05	20	Right superior frontal gyrus, dorsolateral, BA6	7.40%
Control group								
R middle frontal gyrus	38	-6	56	5.457	<0.05	575	R middle frontal gyrus, superior frontal gyrus, dorsolateral, BA6	0.42%
L supplementary motor area	-6	4	66	4.867	<0.05	83	L supplementary motor area, BA6	1.29%
L basal ganglia	-24	0	-6	-4.876	<0.05	249	L lenticular nucleus, putamen, striatum, insula, BA48	0.09%
L inferior frontal gyrus	-32	32	-14	-5.547	<0.05	166	L inferior frontal gyrus, orbital part, BA47	0.52%

[a]Peak height threshold: $z > 1$. [b]Voxel probability threshold: $P < 0.005$ uncorrected and remained after correcting threshold (TFCE) of $P < 0.05$. [c]Cluster extent threshold: number ≥ 10 voxels. Abbreviations: BA: Brodmann area; I^2: heterogeneity I^2; MNI: Montreal Neurological Institute; R: right; ReHo: regional homogeneity; SDM: signed differential mapping.

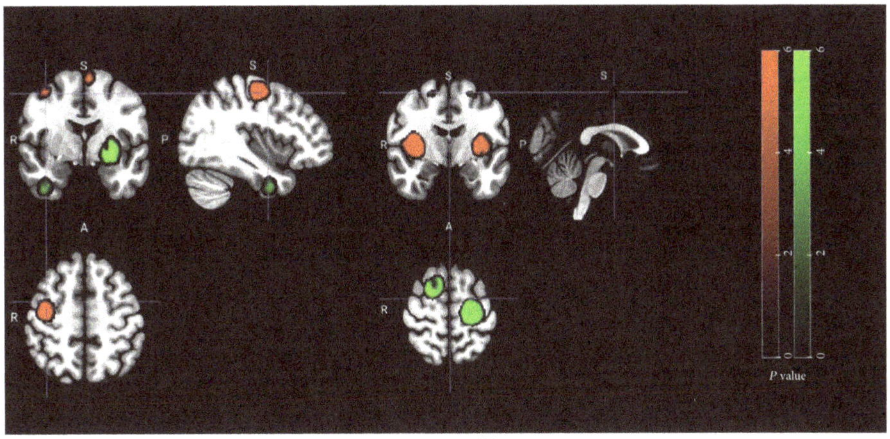

(a) (b)

FIGURE 3: SDM-PSI meta-analysis for (a) ReHo change in poststroke patients after conventional treatment and (b) ReHo change in poststroke patients after acupuncture treatment. Red color refers to hyperactivation, and green color refers to hypoactivation.

motor function (FMA) and daily living ability (MBI). These findings are discussed in many previous meta-analysis studies, so we will not discuss further here [10, 37, 38]. In this paper, we mainly focus on the meta-analysis of ReHo changes. In the treatment group, stroke patients showed hyperactivation in the bilateral basal ganglia and insula. In the control group, patients showed that brain activities were increased in the bilateral frontal gyrus (BA6). However, the decreased activity of the bilateral frontal gyrus (BA6) and left precentral gyrus (BA4) was found in the treatment group. Additionally, the ReHo index of the left insula significantly correlated with FMA scores across all stroke patients after acupuncture therapy.

4.2. The Involvement of the Basal Ganglia and Insula in Neuroplasticity Induced by Acupuncture. The results showed that resting-state spontaneous brain activity was obviously increased in the bilateral basal ganglia and insula after acupuncture treatment. Hyperactivation in the basal ganglia comprised mostly the striatum. The basal ganglia play an important integrative role in motor regulation [39]. It is implicated in human dystonia and motor control [40]. Wang et al. have compared ischemic stroke patients to healthy participants, and they found that stroke patients showed low ReHo values in the basal ganglia, which is consistent with previous conclusions that the basal ganglia are vulnerable to ischemia [41, 42]. Regarding motor function, the extent of damage to the basal ganglia seems to be a neural correlate for motor deficit. Three studies included in this review reported that the lesion locations were primarily in the basal ganglia [32, 34, 35], which is in line with the theory that a common ischemic stroke in deep brain regions featured by high disability rate is basal ganglia lacunar stroke [43]. Thus, it can be speculated that limb motor dysfunction of included ischemic stroke patients was mainly related to basal ganglia impairment. The results revealed that acupuncture therapy was also associated with hyperactivation in the insula. The insula integrates different functional systems including sensory motor and cognition and plays a part in motor programing and control [44, 45]. Existing evidence suggests that the anterior insula is commonly affected by acute middle cerebral artery stroke [46]. It seems that the damage of the insula is responsible for the motor dysfunction in stroke patients and acupuncture can activate it to exert therapeutic effect. The metaregression analysis also found that the ReHo increases of the insula are positively correlated to the increase in FMA scores, suggesting that acupuncture could improve ability of daily life via the activation of the insula. Here, our results show an increased spontaneous activity in the basal ganglia and insula after acupuncture treatment, indicating that acupuncture could remodel neuronal function of these areas.

4.3. The Involvement of Motor-Related Areas in Neuroplasticity Induced by Acupuncture. In both the treatment and control groups, our results showed significant alterations of brain activation in most parts of motor-related areas, including the bilateral superior frontal gyrus (especially BA6) and left precentral gyrus (especially BA4). BA4 and BA6 are traditional motor areas, consisting of the "classical" motor network. BA4 is the location of the primary motor cortex (M1), responsible for planning and controlling voluntary motor movement on the body's contralateral side. BA6 includes the premotor cortex (PMC) and supplementary motor area (SMA), where neurons have projections to M1 as well as the corticospinal tract (CST) [47]. It bridges prefrontal and primary motor cortices and is engaged in planning of complex and coordinated movements [48, 49]. Evidence from animal and clinical studies suggests that those areas associate with movement preparation and execution and the activation of these areas contributes to reorganization after stroke [50–52]. Therefore, the functional plasticity of BA6 and BA4 might explain the mechanism of motor recovery.

In this meta-analysis, the ReHo value of bilateral BA6 is significantly increased in the control group but decreased in the treatment group. Here, we speculate that the difference between two groups is in connection with the compensatory activity. Compensation at the neuronal level is characterized by activation in alternative brain areas not normally observed in nondisabled individuals [53]. Previous animal studies have demonstrated that reorganization of residual motor cortex contributes to the restoration of movement dysfunction after stroke, which indicates that increased fMRI signal within a given brain area can not only reflect neural recovery but also compensation [54, 55]. Thus, the increased activation of BA6 in the control group should be interpreted as being associated with compensation, which is in accordance with theories that the increased activity of BA6 is a form of compensation for motor deficit after stroke [56]. A longitudinal fMRI study observed, in the early phase of poststroke recovery (less than 6 months), hyperactivation in bilateral SMA and PMC [57]. Another study with similar results identified a positive correlation, involving increased signals in SMA, cingulate, and other motor areas of both hemispheres with good recovery process (from 2 to 7 weeks up to 6 months), suggesting that compensatory network may be the substrates of rehabilitation strategies [58]. All the 7 studies in this review were similar in the duration of symptoms, ranging from 9-14 days up to 6 months, at which status the activation of BA6 would be increased according to the conclusions above. Interestingly, after receiving acupuncture treatment, the activation level of bilateral BA6 is induced to reduce. The decreased activity of BA6 may implicate the reduced dependence on its compensation, indicating the recovery of motor network, thus helping the ipsilateral limb to recover. Similarly, the results revealed that acupuncture therapy was also associated with hypoactivation in left BA4. Evidence from meta-analysis describes that an increased activation in contralesional M1 (BA4) is a highly consistent finding across different impairment levels and times poststroke [59]. This is in accordance with theories that the increased activity of sound side hemisphere is a form of compensation for dysfunction of other damaged cerebral cortex [56]. From this perspective, if most brain lesions of included patients had the right laterality, we would expect to see a weakened compensation of contralesional BA4 by acupuncture. Considering that 4 studies in this review did not report the locations of infarcted lesions, this assumption warrants further experiments and opens a way for investigation of the relationship between acupuncture treatment and compensatory activity of BA4.

4.4. Strengths and Limitations. This review is unique and innovative. To our knowledge, we are the first to have SDM-PSI analysis of rs-fMRI used in RCTs of acupuncture. Altered cerebral activity in ischemic stroke patients with motor dysfunction provides a new insight into brain mechanism and clinical application, and this review is intended to serve as both a challenge and an encouragement. Also, strict inclusion criteria were made to minimize selection bias, and 7 studies were synthesized in the final analysis. These trials generally consisted of similar target participants and study designs, thus making results comparable.

As an innovative study, this systematic review still has certain limitations. The main limitation of this review is the small sample size. Only 7 trials and 278 participants met the inclusion criteria so that publication bias and subgroup analysis of secondary outcomes measures were not performed. The results of quality assessments indicated that some studies were of low quality, especially in terms of blinding. The lack of high-quality RCTs made it hard to perform an accurate analysis of the interaction between acupuncture efficacy and neuroplasticity. Thus, to better figure out the potential influence of acupuncture on neuroplasticity after stroke, it is time to organize large-scale and elaborate-designed RCTs for further investigations. Moreover, it is supposed that different acupuncture parameters (referring to different acupoints, duration, frequency, and operation methods) may cause fine distinctions of altered cerebral activity. Therefore, there may exist heterogeneity in the acupuncture therapy protocol between included studies. Considering the particularity of acupuncture treatment, it is significant to synthesize the studies focusing on specific manipulation of acupuncture.

5. Conclusion

The meta-analyses of clinical outcome measures (FMA, NDS, BI, or MBI) show that acupuncture treatment is effective for motor function recovery in ischemic stroke patients. The ReHo meta-analysis reveals that acupuncture could induce extensive changes of cerebral activity, which suggests that the alterations of the basal ganglia, insula, and motor-related areas are involved in neuroplasticity of acupuncture. These findings provide a new insight into the mechanisms underlying effectiveness of acupuncture and also lead to the articulation of a more general hypothesis that acupuncture plays a role in facilitating neuroplasticity.

Conflicts of Interest

The authors declare that there is no conflict of interest regarding the publication of this paper.

Acknowledgments

We thank Prof. Ying Zhang for the assistance. The study was supported by the National Natural Resources Fund (grant number 81873257) and Beijing Municipal Commission of Planning and Natural Resources (grant number 7182104).

Supplementary Materials

The supplementary material for this article can be found in the supplementary file. Figure S1A | Forest plot presenting the study meta-analysis for the living quality (nervous deficiency scale). Figure S1B | Forest plot presenting the study meta-analysis for the activity of daily living (Barthel index), Figure S1C | Forest plot presenting the study meta-analysis for the activity of daily living (modified Barthel index), Figure S1D | Forest plot presenting the study meta-analysis for the limb function (Fugl-Meyer assessment), Table S1A Meta-regression analysis of FMA scores in treatment group, Table S1B Meta-regression analysis of age in treatment group. Table S1C Meta-regression analysis of duration in treatment group. *(Supplementary Materials)*

References

[1] M. Zhou, H. Wang, X. Zeng et al., "Mortality, morbidity, and risk factors in China and its provinces, 1990-2017: a systematic analysis for the Global Burden of Disease Study 2017," *The Lancet*, vol. 394, no. 10204, pp. 1145–1158, 2019.

[2] J. SUN and W. CHEN, "Correlation studies of barium on pulmonary infection under the assessment of VFSS," *Experimental and Therapeutic Medicine*, vol. 11, no. 2, pp. 435–438, 2016.

[3] S. Kumar, M. H. Selim, and L. R. Caplan, "Medical complications after stroke," *The Lancet Neurology*, vol. 9, no. 1, pp. 105–118, 2010.

[4] S. Li, Y.-T. Chen, G. E. Francisco, P. Zhou, and W. Z. Rymer, "A unifying pathophysiological account for post-stroke spasticity and disordered motor control," *Frontiers in Neurology*, vol. 10, p. 468, 2019.

[5] X. Tan, X. Liu, and H. Shao, "Healthy China 2030: a vision for health care," *Value in Health Regional Issues*, vol. 12, pp. 112–114, 2017.

[6] J. Wang, J. Pei, D. Khiati et al., "Acupuncture treatment on the motor area of the scalp for motor dysfunction in patients with ischemic stroke: study protocol for a randomized controlled trial," *Trials*, vol. 18, no. 1, p. 287, 2017.

[7] M. Bonafede, A. Dick, K. Noyes, J. D. Klein, and T. Brown, "The effect of acupuncture utilization on healthcare utilization," *Medical Care*, vol. 46, no. 1, pp. 41–48, 2008.

[8] A. J. Vickers and K. Linde, "Acupuncture for chronic pain," *Journal of the American Medical Association*, vol. 311, no. 9, pp. 955-956, 2014.

[9] J. Wang, W. Shi, D. Khiati et al., *Scalp acupuncture treatment for motor dysfunction in children with cerebral palsy: study protocol for a multicenter randomized controlled trial*, vol. 21, no. 1, 2019, TRIALS, England, 2019.

[10] Z. Yang, J. Xie, and D. Liu, "Xingnao Kaiqiao needling method for acute ischemic stroke: a meta-analysis of safety and efficacy," *Neural Regeneration Research*, vol. 12, no. 8, pp. 1308–1314, 2017.

[11] X. He, Q. Sun, H. Liu, X. Guo, C. Chen, and L. Chen, "Timing of acupuncture during LTP-like plasticity induced by paired-associative stimulation," *Behavioural Neurology*, vol. 2019, 10 pages, 2019.

[12] Y. Maeda, H. Kim, N. Kettner et al., "Rewiring the primary somatosensory cortex in carpal tunnel syndrome with acupuncture," *Deutsche Zeitschrift für Akupunktur*, vol. 60, no. 3, pp. 23-24, 2017.

[13] Y. Ning, K. Li, C. Fu et al., "Enhanced functional connectivity between the bilateral primary motor cortices after acupuncture at Yanglingquan (GB34) in right-hemispheric subcortical stroke patients: a resting-state fMRI study," *Frontiers in Human Neuroscience*, vol. 11, 2017.

[14] G. Jiang, X. Yin, C. Li et al., "The plasticity of brain gray matter and white matter following lower limb amputation," *Neural Plasticity*, vol. 2015, 10 pages, 2015.

[15] B. Dan, "Neuroscience underlying rehabilitation: what is neuroplasticity?," *Developmental Medicine & Child Neurology*, vol. 61, no. 11, pp. 1240–1240, 2019.

[16] L. B. Reid, R. N. Boyd, R. Cunnington, and S. E. Rose, "Interpreting intervention induced neuroplasticity with fMRI: the case for multimodal imaging strategies," *Neural Plasticity*, vol. 2016, 13 pages, 2016.

[17] L. Cui, X. Gong, Y. Tang et al., "Relationship between the LHPP gene polymorphism and resting-state brain activity in major depressive disorder," *Neural Plasticity*, vol. 2016, 8 pages, 2016.

[18] B. Zhang, J. Lu, J. Xia et al., "Functional insights into aberrant brain responses and integration in patients with lifelong premature ejaculation," *Scientific Reports*, vol. 7, no. 1, 2017.

[19] J. Zhao, D. Tomasi, C. E. Wiers et al., "Correlation between Traits of Emotion-Based Impulsivity and Intrinsic Default-Mode Network Activity," *Neural Plasticity*, vol. 2017, 9 pages, 2017.

[20] J. D. Schaechter, B. D. Connell, W. B. Stason et al., "Correlated change in upper limb function and motor cortex activation after verum and sham acupuncture in patients with chronic stroke," *Journal of Alternative and Complementary Medicine*, vol. 13, no. 5, pp. 527–532, 2007.

[21] P. N, "Application of ffMRI technique in evaluating electroacupuncture for ischemic stroke," *Medical Innovation of China*, vol. 16, no. 7, 2019.

[22] V. I. Müller, E. C. Cieslik, A. R. Laird et al., "Ten simple rules for neuroimaging meta-analysis," *Neuroscience & Biobehavioral Reviews*, vol. 84, pp. 151–161, 2018.

[23] M. Tahmasian, A. A. Sepehry, F. Samea et al., "Practical recommendations to conduct a neuroimaging meta-analysis for neuropsychiatric disorders," *Human Brain Mapping.*, vol. 40, no. 17, pp. 5142–5154, 2019.

[24] H. I. L. Jacobs, J. Radua, H. C. Lückmann, and A. T. Sack, "Meta-analysis of functional network alterations in Alzheimer's disease: toward a network biomarker," *Neuroscience & Biobehavioral Reviews*, vol. 37, no. 5, pp. 753–765, 2013.

[25] B. Qin, M. X. Yang, W. Gao et al., "Voxel-wise meta-analysis of structural changes in gray matter of Parkinson's disease patients with mild cognitive impairment," *Brazilian Journal of Medical and Biological Research*, vol. 53, no. 6, p. e9275, 2020.

[26] S. Cheng, G. Xu, J. Zhou et al., "A multimodal meta-analysis of structural and functional changes in the brain of tinnitus," *Frontiers in Human Neuroscience*, vol. 14, p. 28, 2020.

[27] J. Li, P. Pan, R. Huang, and H. Shang, "A meta-analysis of voxel-based morphometry studies of white matter volume alterations in Alzheimer's disease," *Neuroscience & Biobehavioral Reviews*, vol. 36, no. 2, pp. 757–763, 2012.

[28] J. Radua, D. Mataix-Cols, M. L. Phillips et al., "A new meta-analytic method for neuroimaging studies that combines reported peak coordinates and statistical parametric maps," *European Psychiatry*, vol. 27, no. 8, pp. 605–611, 2012.

[29] J. R. Dugré, J. Radua, M. Carignan-Allard, A. Dumais, K. Rubia, and S. Potvin, "Neurofunctional abnormalities in antisocial spectrum: a meta-analysis of fMRI studies on Five distinct neurocognitive research domains," *Neuroscience & Biobehavioral Reviews*, vol. 119, pp. 168–183, 2020.

[30] A. Albajes-Eizagirre, A. Solanes, M. A. Fullana et al., "Meta-analysis of voxel-based neuroimaging studies using seed-based d mapping with permutation of subject images (SDM-PSI)," *Journal of Visualized Experiments*, no. 153, 2019.

[31] W. Ping, Z. Fang, L. Yongxin et al., "Effect of acupuncture plus conventional treatment on brain activity in ischemic stroke patients: a regional homogeneity analysis," *Journal of Traditional Chinese Medicine*, vol. 37, no. 5, pp. 650–658, 2017.

[32] C. Nana, *Observation on the brain function in patients with hemiplegia treated by multiple acupuncture points*, Guangzhou

University of Traditional Chinese Medicine, Guangzhou, China, 2017.

[33] Y. Zhengfei and G. Rongai, "Effects of Yang elevating and Du meridian activating method in the treatment of stroke hemiplegia and the influence on resting - state functional brain imaging," *Journal of Sichuan of Traditional Chinese Medicine*, vol. 36, no. 8, pp. 186–188, 2018.

[34] Z. Yumei, *Effects of acupuncture on brain activity in ischemic stroke patients- an regional homogeneity analysis*, Chengdu University of Traditional Chinese Medicine, Sichuan, China, 2015.

[35] X. Ximei, W. Ping, H. Linna, and A. Junming, "FMRI research of acupuncture on brain regional homogeneity in resting-state of patients with ischemic stroke," *Liaoning Journal of Traditional Chinese Medicine*, vol. 40, no. 7, pp. 1287–1290, 2013.

[36] C. Zhihong, "A study of functional magnetic resonance imaging (fMRI) and the cinical effect in stroke patient using lifting yang to dredging du meridian manipulation," Yunnan University of Traditional Chinese Medicine, Yunnan, China, 2016.

[37] L. Lu, X.-g. Zhang, L. L. D. Zhong et al., "Acupuncture for neurogenesis in experimental ischemic stroke: a systematic review and meta-analysis," *Scientific Reports*, vol. 6, no. 1, 2016.

[38] L. Peng, C. Zhang, L. Zhou, H.-X. Zuo, X.-K. He, and Y.-M. Niu, "Traditional manual acupuncture combined with rehabilitation therapy for shoulder hand syndrome after stroke within the Chinese healthcare system: a systematic review and meta-analysis," *Clinical Rehabilitation*, vol. 32, no. 4, pp. 429–439, 2018.

[39] Y. Dauvilliers and P. Peigneux, "Ictal SPECT in patients with rapid eye movement sleep behaviour disorder," *Brain*, vol. 138, no. 11, pp. e390–e390, 2015.

[40] V. K. Neychev, X. Fan, V. I. Mitev, E. J. Hess, and H. A. Jinnah, "The basal ganglia and cerebellum interact in the expression of dystonic movement," *Brain*, vol. 131, no. 9, pp. 2499–2509, 2008.

[41] W. You, O. Yanggang, Z. Xueling, Z. Minglan, and X. Shouyong, "Effects of acupuncture on brain regional homogeneity at resting state in the patients with ischemic stroke," *Practical Geriatrics*, vol. 29, no. 12, pp. 1010–1013, 2015.

[42] C.-. Q. Lu, W. Xu, C.-. H. Zeng et al., "Altered amplitude of low-frequency fluctuation in basal ganglia correlates to pulmonary ventilation function in COPD patients: a resting-state fMRI study," *Brain and Behavior*, vol. 9, no. 7, 2019.

[43] H. Man, Y. Bi, Y. Yu et al., "Associated factors of early neurological deterioration in isolated acute lacunar infarction in basal ganglia," *Journal of Neurorestoratology*, vol. 7, no. 2, pp. 63–69, 2019.

[44] A. Primaßin, N. Scholtes, S. Heim et al., "Determinants of concurrent motor and language recovery during intensive therapy in chronic stroke patients: four single-case studies," *Frontiers in Neurology*, vol. 6, 2015.

[45] Y.-C. Chen, C. Chen, R. M. Martínez, J. L. Etnier, and Y. Cheng, "Habitual physical activity mediates the acute exercise-induced modulation of anxiety-related amygdala functional connectivity," *Scientific Reports*, vol. 9, no. 1, p. 19787, 2019.

[46] R. Leigh, K. Oishi, J. Hsu et al., "Acute lesions that impair affective empathy," *Brain*, vol. 136, no. 8, pp. 2539–2549, 2013.

[47] R. P. Dum and P. L. Strick, "Motor areas in the frontal lobe of the primate," *Physiology & Behavior*, vol. 77, no. 4–5, pp. 677–682, 2002.

[48] A. S. Oliveira, B. R. Schlink, W. D. Hairston, P. König, and D. P. Ferris, "Restricted vision increases sensorimotor cortex involvement in human walking," *Journal of Neurophysiology*, vol. 118, no. 4, pp. 1943–1951, 2017.

[49] S. Tanaka, M. Honda, and N. Sadato, "Modality-specific cognitive function of medial and lateral human Brodmann area 6," *The Journal of Neuroscience*, vol. 25, no. 2, pp. 496–501, 2005.

[50] N. Dancause, "Extensive cortical rewiring after brain injury," *The Journal of Neuroscience*, vol. 25, no. 44, pp. 10167–10179, 2005.

[51] C. M. Cirstea, W. M. Brooks, S. C. Craciunas et al., "Primary motor cortex in stroke," *Stroke*, vol. 42, no. 4, pp. 1004–1009, 2011.

[52] L. J. Volz, M. Vollmer, J. Michely, G. R. Fink, J. C. Rothwell, and C. Grefkes, "Time-dependent functional role of the contralesional motor cortex after stroke," *NeuroImage: Clinical*, vol. 16, pp. 165–174, 2017.

[53] M. F. Levin, J. A. Kleim, and S. L. Wolf, "What do motor "recovery" and "compensation" mean in patients following stroke?," *Neurorehabilitation and Neural Repair*, vol. 23, no. 4, pp. 313–319, 2009.

[54] E. MacDonald, H. Van der Lee, D. Pocock et al., "A novel phosphodiesterase type 4 inhibitor, HT-0712, enhances rehabilitation-dependent motor recovery and cortical reorganization after focal cortical ischemia," *Neurorehabilitation and Neural Repair*, vol. 21, no. 6, pp. 486–496, 2007.

[55] N. Dancause, S. Barbay, S. B. Frost et al., "Effects of small ischemic lesions in the primary motor cortex on neurophysiological organization in ventral premotor cortex," *Journal of Neurophysiology*, vol. 96, no. 6, pp. 3506–3511, 2006.

[56] S. H. Jang, "A review of the ipsilateral motor pathway as a recovery mechanism in patients with stroke," *NeuroRehabilitation*, vol. 24, no. 4, pp. 315–320, 2009.

[57] D. Tombari, I. Loubinoux, J. Pariente et al., "A longitudinal fMRI study: in recovering and then in clinically stable subcortical stroke patients," *NeuroImage*, vol. 23, no. 3, pp. 827–839, 2004.

[58] L. M. Carey, D. F. Abbott, G. F. Egan, J. Bernhardt, and G. A. Donnan, "Motor impairment and recovery in the upper limb after stroke," *Stroke*, vol. 36, no. 3, pp. 625–629, 2005.

[59] A. K. Rehme, S. B. Eickhoff, C. Rottschy, G. R. Fink, and C. Grefkes, "Activation likelihood estimation meta-analysis of motor-related neural activity after stroke," *NeuroImage*, vol. 59, no. 3, pp. 2771–2782, 2012.

37

Association between Serum Copeptin and Stroke in Rural Areas of Northern China: A Matched Case-Control Study

Hao Sun,[1] Donghui Huang,[2] Hailong Wang,[1] Bo Zhou,[1] Xiaomei Wu,[1] Bing Ma,[1] and Jingpu Shi[1]

[1]*Department of Clinical Epidemiology and Evidence-Based Medicine, Institute of Cardiovascular Diseases, The First Hospital of China Medical University, No. 155 Nanjing North Street, Heping District, Shenyang, Liaoning province 110001, China*
[2]*Department of Clinical Epidemiology, Shengjing Hospital of China Medical University, No. 36 Sanhao Street, Heping District, Shenyang, Liaoning province 110004, China*

Correspondence should be addressed to Jingpu Shi; sjp562013@126.com

Academic Editor: Ralf Lichtinghagen

Background. Copeptin has been implicated as an effective prognostic biomarker of stroke outcome; however, few studies have investigated whether copeptin could be used as an etiological factor for stroke or not. The aim of our study was to evaluate the association of serum copeptin with stroke. *Methods.* In total, 238 participants including 119 cases (87 ischemic stroke and 32 hemorrhagic stroke) and 119 controls were included in this 1 : 1 matched case-control study. Conditional multivariate logistic regression was conducted to assess the Odds Ratios (*OR*s) and 95% confidence intervals (*CI*); restricted cubic spline in logistic regression model was used to evaluate the dose-response association between serum copeptin and total stroke, ischemic stroke, and hemorrhagic stroke. *Results.* The median serum copeptin was 20.90 pmol/L, 20.90 pmol/L, 6.53 pmol/L, and 8.42 pmol/L for total stroke, ischemic stroke, hemorrhagic stroke, and healthy subjects, respectively. The corresponding *OR*s (95% CIs) for the highest compared with the lowest quartile were 1.23 (0.62–2.44) for total stroke, 4.01 (1.47–10.96) for ischemic stroke, and 0.13 (0.22–0.69) for hemorrhagic stroke. No nonlinear dose-response relationship was found between serum copeptin and total stroke ($P_{\text{nonlinear}} = 0.278$), ischemic stroke ($P_{\text{nonlinear}} = 0.362$), and hemorrhagic stroke ($P_{\text{nonlinear}} = 0.314$). Compared with the reference copeptin level, a significantly increasing trend was found between serum copeptin and ischemic stroke ($P_{\text{overall}} = 0.002$), and a decreasing trend was found between serum copeptin and hemorrhagic stroke ($P_{\text{overall}} = 0.007$). *Conclusions.* Elevated serum copeptin levels were positively associated with ischemic stroke and adversely associated with hemorrhagic stroke. Additional prospective studies with larger sample size are needed to confirm the present findings.

1. Introduction

Stroke is the second cause of death in elder people (>60 years) and the fifth leading cause of death in people aged 15 to 59 years old throughout the world [1]. In China, stroke has become the leading cause of death [2]; the incidence and prevalence are both increasing rapidly over the 30 years [3]. The National Epidemiology Survey of Stroke in China (NESS-China) has reported there was a north-to-south gradient of stroke burden in China, and the greatest stroke burden was observed in the rural areas of northern regions [3]. Therefore, the rising burden of stroke has built a serious public health problem in China, especially the rural areas of Northern China.

In China, ischemic stroke accounts for approximately 77.8% of total stroke type while the rest 22.2% is subjected to hemorrhagic stroke [3]. Early defining and categorizing of stroke are very important since the managements for ischemic stroke and hemorrhagic stroke are totally different. Currently, computed tomography (CT) and magnetic resonance imaging (MRI) cerebral imaging are most routinely used for confirming the diagnosis of stroke and distinguishing ischemic stroke from hemorrhagic stroke. However, CT and MRI scan are not available easily across all the hospitals, especially in the rural areas of China. Compared with CT and MRI, blood test is a more reliable, rapid, and cost-effective way to differentiate ischemic stroke and hemorrhagic stroke. Therefore, identifying some novel blood biomarkers to distinguish effectively and efficiently ischemic stroke from hemorrhagic stroke might help in the selection of appropriate treatment plans for stroke patients.

Arginine vasopressin (AVP), also termed as antidiuretic hormone, is a key hormone to regulate the osmoregulatory, hemodynamic, endocrinologic, and central nervous effect in human body [4]. However, AVP is hard to detect because it is extremely unstable in both *in vivo* and *ex vivo* environment and has short half-life (5–20 min) [5]. Copeptin, the C-terminal portion of provasopressin (pro-AVP), is released in a 1 : 1 ratio with AVP during precursor processing [6]. Since copeptin has a longer half-life (>90 min) and more stability *ex vivo* than AVP, it could be used as a sensitive surrogate biomarker and a valid measurement in biological fluid samples in routine clinical practice [7, 8]. Several epidemiological studies have demonstrated that copeptin might be used as a prognosis biomarker including predicting neurologic deterioration, risk stratification, and poor outcome (mortality, unfavorable outcome, and recurrence) of stroke [9–13], and the possible mechanism was the copeptin could mirror the hypothalamic-pituitary-adrenal axis as well as the sympathetic nervous system [14], which might promote pathophysiological conditions of stroke. Thus, we hypothesized that copeptin as a novel marker of neuroendocrine might also be associated with stroke risk.

Currently, little evidence was available on the role of copeptin in the patients with stroke and subtypes (ischemic and hemorrhagic) of stroke in China. To evaluate these issues, we investigated the serum copeptin levels among participants in rural areas of Northern China and assessed their relationship with stroke, ischemic stroke, and hemorrhagic stroke.

2. Materials and Methods

2.1. Study Population. Our study was a large-scale cross-sectional survey, including 11 villages covering various regions (East, South, West, North, and Middle) of Zhangwu County (Liaoning Province, China), an area with high prevalence of hypertension. A total of 6773 eligible subjects aged more than 18 years old were recruited in the survey for the questionnaires, and 6571 subjects agreed to collect blood samples, including 119 stroke patients (87 ischemic stroke and 32 hemorrhagic stroke). The ethics committee of China Medical University approved this study, and all participants offered informed consent.

2.2. Case-Control Population. This was a 1 : 1 age- and gender-matched and population-based case-control study. Eligible cases who had been diagnosed stroke were according to their medical records, which were provided by hospitals above county level. The stroke subtypes (ischemic and hemorrhagic) were determined by neurologists based on the clinical assessment and neuroimaging (CT or MRI) according to "The Diagnosis of All Type of Cerebrovascular Disease," which was adopted by the Fourth National Cerebrovascular Disease Academic Meeting in 1995 [15]. Subjects with the following diseases were excluded: (1) other cerebrovascular diseases (brain tumor, cerebrovascular malformation, or transient ischemic attack), (2) coronary heart disease, and (3) serious chronic diseases (tumor, kidney disease, endocrine disease, and immune system diseases). For each subject in the stroke group, we selected one healthy subject as matched control according to age and gender from this survey. Finally, 119 healthy subjects were included in our study.

2.3. Information Collected. The surveys were conducted at village clinics by trained interviewers (village doctors, retired medical professors, and medical students). Structured questionnaires were used to collect the following information: (1) sociodemographic information: name, age, gender, ethnicity, address, and the number of family members; (2) disease information: personal history of hypertension, stroke, and other diseases, family history of stroke; (3) stroke-related factors: smoking status, alcohol consumption, salt intake (g/day), and pickle intake (times/day); and (4) anthropometric information: weight (kg), height (cm), systolic blood pressure (SBP, mmHg), and diastolic blood pressure (DBP, mmHg). Weight, height, and blood pressure were measured twice by using the same type instruments and following standardized protocols.

In our study, hypertension was defined as SBP $\geq$ 140 mmHg and (or) DBP $\geq$ 90 mmHg or the use of antihypertensive medicine in the last two weeks [16]. Family history of stroke was defined as the presence of stroke in first degree relatives. Smokers were participants who smoked at least one cigarette per day for more than 1 year, and alcohol drinkers were those who drank alcohol more than three times a week for at least 1 year.

2.4. Blood Sample Measurements. Blood samples (5 mL venous blood) were collected from the antecubital vein in the morning after an overnight fast. The samples were centrifuged immediately, and serum samples were transported frozen to the analytical laboratory in Shenyang (Liaoning, China) and stored at −80°C for further analysis. Total cholesterol (TC), triglyceride (TG), and glucose (GLU) were measured according to standard procedures at the Clinical Laboratory, the First Hospital of China Medical University, China. Serum copeptin concentration was assessed with a commercially available enzyme-linked immunosorbent assay (ELISA) kit according to the manufacturer's instructions.

3. Statistical Analysis

Means ± standard deviations were used to express the normal distribution of continuous variables; medians and interquartile ranges were used to express the skewed distribution while counts and percentages were used to describe the categorical variable. Differences between groups were calculated by using paired *t*-test, Wilcoxon signed-rank test, Mcnemar's test, and Bowker's test. Moreover, conditional univariate logistic regression was conducted to calculate the Odds Ratios (*ORs*) and 95% confidence intervals (*CI*) of stroke-related factors.

To estimate the association of serum copeptin and stroke, serum copeptin levels were classified into tertiles based on the distribution among controls. The lowest tertile was used as reference level, and conditional univariate logistic regression and conditional multivariate logistic regression were conducted to assess the *OR* for the second and third tertiles. For the conditional multivariate logistic regression, covariates were selected and adjusted if they might be a confounder factor between serum copeptin and stroke ($P < 0.05$ in the conditional univariate logistic regression). The covariates included in the final model were as follows: (1) total stroke: personal history of hypertension, smoking status, and pickle intake; (2) ischemic stroke: BMI, personal history of hypertension, smoking status, and pickle intake; and (3) hemorrhagic stroke: none. Moreover, tests for linear trend were conducted by including serum copeptin as a continuous variable in the models. Besides, restricted cubic spline function with four knots (5th, 35th, 65th, and 95th) with reference copeptin level (25.9 pmol/L) [17, 18] in the logistic regression model was used to evaluate the dose-response association between serum copeptin and stroke, and the nonlinear effect and overall effect of the relationship were explored with the likelihood ratio test [19].

All analyses were carried out using the SAS software (version 9.1.3; SAS Institute, Cary, NC). And all statistical tests were based on two-sided probability.

4. Results

The characteristics of cases, including cases of total stroke, ischemic stroke, and hemorrhagic stroke, and their matched controls are presented in Table 1. In total, 119 stroke cases (including 87 ischemic stroke and 32 hemorrhagic stroke) and 119 controls were included in this study. The mean age was 62 years for stroke cases, 61 years for ischemic stroke cases, and 63 years for hemorrhagic stroke cases. Significant differences were found between stroke cases and controls for personal history of hypertension, smoking, and pickle intake. For ischemic stroke, BMI, personal history of hypertension, smoking status, and pickle intake were found to have significant difference between two groups. And for hemorrhagic stroke, no significant difference was found between groups.

The median levels of serum copeptin in cases and controls were also described in Table 1. The copeptin concentration was higher among stroke cases compared with that among control participants (20.90 *vs.* 8.42 pmol/L; $P < 0.001$). And in analyses stratified by stroke subtype, higher copeptin level was observed for ischemic stroke cases (20.90 *vs.* 9.55 pmol/L; $P < 0.001$) and lower copeptin level for hemorrhagic stroke cases (6.53 *vs.* 10.79 pmol/L; $P < 0.001$).

The associations between serum copeptin and total stroke, ischemic stroke, and hemorrhagic stroke by tertiles of copeptin levels are presented in Table 2. A positive association was observed between serum copeptin and total stroke ($OR_{rude} = 1.45$, 95% CI: 0.78–2.69 for tertile 3 *vs.* tertile 1; $OR_{adjusted} = 1.23$, 95% CI: 0.62–2.44 for tertile 3 *vs.* tertile 1); however, no statistical significance was found for this increasing trend ($P_{trend} = 0.052$). For ischemic stroke, a positive association was observed between serum copeptin and ischemic stroke ($P_{trend} = 0.002$). Compared with the lowest tertile (<6.478 pmol/L), the *OR* in the highest tertile (>13.599 pmol/L) was 3.99 ($OR_{rude} = 3.99$, 95% CI: 1.66–9.57); the association existed even after being adjusted for potential confounders ($OR_{adjusted} = 4.01$, 95% CI: 1.47–10.96). In contrast, we found a significantly adverse association between serum copeptin level and hemorrhagic stroke. Compared with the lowest copeptin level, the risk of hemorrhagic stroke was significantly lower in the two higher tertiles of copeptin level (tertile 2: $OR = 0.44$, 95% CI: 0.13–1.34; tertile 3: $OR = 0.13$, 95% CI: 0.22–0.69; $P_{trend} = 0.011$).

The results of dose-response relationship between serum copeptin and total stroke, ischemic stroke, and hemorrhagic stroke are shown in Table 3. In the restricted cubic spline function model with nonlinear terms, no nonlinear dose-response relationship was found between serum copeptin and total stroke ($P_{nonlinear} = 0.278$). Compared with the reference copeptin level (25.9 pmol/L), the prevalence of stroke increased with serum level of copeptin in a dose-response manner; however, no statistical significance was found for this increasing trend ($P_{overall} = 0.139$), as shown in Figure 1. For the subtype of stroke, no nonlinear dose-response relationship was found in the ischemic stroke group or hemorrhagic stroke group (ischemic stroke: $P_{nonlinear} = 0.362$; hemorrhagic stroke: $P_{nonlinear} = 0.314$). The results of dose-response relationship analysis also show that with the serum copeptin concentration increasing, the prevalence of ischemic stroke increased ($P_{overall} = 0.002$), while the prevalence of hemorrhagic stroke decreased ($P_{overall} = 0.007$), just as shown in Figures 2 and 3. The results also reported that in every 1 pmol/L serum copeptin increase, the prevalence of ischemic stroke increased 5% and the prevalence of hemorrhagic stroke decreased 8%.

5. Discussion

In this 1 : 1 matched case-control study among participants in rural areas of Northern China, we found that the increased levels of serum copeptin were significantly associated with higher risk of ischemic stroke and lower risk of hemorrhagic stroke in a dose-response manner. The prevalence of ischemic stroke increased 5% and the prevalence of hemorrhagic stroke decreased 8% for every 1 pmol/L serum copeptin increase. A positive association was observed between serum copeptin and total stroke; however, no statistical significance was found for this increasing trend. Our results suggested that copeptin might be a meaningful biomarker to discriminate the subtype of stroke and to play a potential role of the AVP system in the pathophysiology of both ischemic stroke and hemorrhagic stroke.

Our study reported the dose-response association between serum copeptin and stroke in Chinese population. To our knowledge, only three articles have reported the relationship between copeptin and stroke risk [20–22], and

Table 1: Characteristics of cases of total stroke, ischemic stroke, and hemorrhagic stroke and their matched controls[a].

	Total stroke				Ischemic stroke				Hemorrhagic stroke			
	Case ($n = 119$)	Control ($n = 119$)	P^b	OR (95% CI)[c]	Case ($n = 87$)	Control ($n = 87$)	P^b	OR (95% CI)[c]	Case ($n = 32$)	Control ($n = 32$)	P^b	OR (95% CI)[c]
Age (years)	62 (53–69)	62 (53–69)	—	—	61 (52–70)	61 (52–70)	—	—	63 (56–68)	63 (56–68)	—	—
Gender (male; n, %)	146 (61.34%)	146 (61.34%)	—	—	56 (64.4%)	56 (64.4%)	—	—	17 (53.1%)	17 (53.1%)	—	—
BMI (kg/m^2)	24.05 ± 3.85	24.84 ± 3.44	0.105	0.94 (0.88–1.01)	23.68 ± 3.74	25.02 ± 3.38	0.015	0.90 (0.82–0.98)	25.06 ± 4.03	24.37 ± 3.60	0.490	1.05 (0.92–1.19)
Personal history of hypertension (n, %)	92 (77.31%)	76 (63.87%)	0.014	2.23 (1.16–4.29)	68 (78.2%)	54 (62.1%)	0.016	2.40 (1.15–5.02)	24 (75.0%)	22 (68.8%)	0.480	1.67 (0.40–6.97)
Family history of stroke (n, %)	27 (22.69)	24 (20.17%)	0.631	1.17 (0.62–2.19)	18 (20.7%)	19 (21.8%)	0.847	0.93 (0.44–1.98)	9 (28.1%)	5 (15.6%)	0.248	2.00 (0.60–6.64)
Smoking (n, %)	65 (54.62%)	45 (37.82%)	0.002	2.82 (1.42–5.61)	53 (60.9%)	36 (41.4%)	0.003	3.13 (1.41–6.93)	12 (37.5%)	9 (28.1%)	0.317	2.00 (0.50–8.00)
Alcohol drinking (n, %)	39 (32.77%)	42 (35.29%)	0.622	0.85 (0.45–1.62)	30 (34.5%)	33 (37.9%)	0.564	0.80 (0.37–1.71)	9 (28.1%)	9 (28.1%)	1.000	1.00 (0.29–3.45)
Salt intake (≥180 g/month; n, %)	107 (88.92%)	104 (87.39%)	0.513	1.33 (0.56–3.16)	81 (93.1%)	78 (89.7%)	0.405	1.60 (0.52–4.89)	26 (81.3%)	26 (81.3%)	1.000	1.00 (0.25–4.00)
Pickle intake (times/day)			0.198				0.350				0.936	
0	30 (25.21%)	35 (29.41%)	—	1.00 (reference)	22 (25.3%)	23 (26.4%)	—	1.00 (reference)	8 (25%)	12 (37.5%)	—	1.00 (reference)
1	23 (19.33%)	28 (23.53%)	—	0.79 (0.43–1.45)	17 (19.5%)	20 (23.0%)	—	0.83 (0.42–1.65)	6 (18.8%)	8 (25%)	—	0.67 (0.19–2.36)
2	7 (5.88%)	15 (12.61%)	—	0.39 (0.14–1.08)	4 (4.6%)	12 (13.8%)	—	0.27 (0.08–0.99)	3 (9.4%)	3 (9.4%)	—	1.00 (0.14–7.10)
3	59 (49.58%)	41 (34.45%)	—	1.78 (1.07–2.97)	44 (50.6%)	32 (36.8%)	—	1.63 (0.92–2.89)	15 (46.9%)	9 (28.1%)	—	2.50 (0.78–7.97)
TC (mmol/L)	5.24 (4.48–5.75)	5.08 (4.39–5.49)	0.168	1.22 (0.92–1.61)	5.30 (4.49–5.79)	5.08 (4.38–5.40)	0.122	1.38 (0.96–2.00)	5.21 (4.47–5.63)	5.26 (4.48–5.86)	0.758	0.94 (0.75–1.18)
TG (mmol/L)	1.50 (1.02–2.38)	1.40 (0.98–2.07)	0.694	1.00 (0.82–1.20)	1.50 (1.03–2.42)	1.47 (1.01-2.11)	0.929	0.94 (0.75–1.18)	1.59 (1.07–2.35)	1.35 (0.97–1.96)	0.454	1.16 (0.79–1.68)
GLU (mmol/L)	5.00 (4.30–5.30)	4.60 (4.20–5.20)	0.107	1.15 (0.94–1.40)	5.07 (4.50–5.30)	4.70 (4.20–5.10)	0.196	1.16 (0.92–1.47)	4.80 (4.20–5.25)	4.55 (4.20–5.30)	0.388	1.11 (0.75–1.63)
Copeptin (pmol/L)	20.90 (8.65–37.40)	8.42 (5.45–15.33)	<0.001	1.02 (1.00-1.03)	20.90 (9.76–37.60)	9.55 (5.66–16.70)	<0.001	1.05 (1.02–1.08)	6.53 (4.94–9.47)	10.79 (7.28–28.87)	<0.001	0.92 (0.86–0.98)

[a]Adjusted for age and gender at sample collection. [b]Continuous variables were compared by using paired t-test and Wilcoxon signed-rank test; categorical variables were compared by using Mcnemar's test and Bowker's test. [c]The ORs and 95% CIs were derived from conditional univariate logistic regression.

TABLE 2: Association between the level of serum copeptin and total stroke, ischemic stroke, and hemorrhagic stroke.

	Level of serum copeptin Tertile 1	Tertile 2	Tertile 3
Total stroke ($n = 119$ sets)			
Copeptin range (pmol/L)	<7.256	7.256~16.440	>16.440
Number of cases/controls	37/40	28/39	54/40
OR (95% CI)	1.00 (reference)	0.77 (0.39–1.54)	1.45 (0.78–2.69)
OR (95% CI)[a]	1.00 (reference)	0.70 (0.33–1.49)	1.23 (0.62–2.44)
P_{trend}[a]		0.052	
Ischemic stroke ($n = 87$ sets)			
Copeptin range (pmol/L)	<6.478	6.478~13.599	>13.599
Number of cases/controls	17/29	15/30	55/28
OR (95% CI)	1.00 (reference)	0.82 (0.33–2.05)	3.99 (1.66–9.57)
OR (95% CI)[b]	1.00 (reference)	0.79 (0.28–2.21)	4.01 (1.47–10.96)
P_{trend}[b]		0.002	
Hemorrhagic stroke ($n = 32$ sets)			
Copeptin range (pmol/L)	<8.425	8.425~26.019	>26.019
Number of cases/controls	19/10	11/12	2/10
OR (95% CI)	1.00 (reference)	0.44 (0.13–1.43)	0.13 (0.22–0.69)
P_{trend}		0.011	

[a]The *OR* was adjusted by personal history of hypertension, smoking status, and pickle intake. [b]The *OR* was adjusted by BMI, personal history of hypertension, smoking status, and pickle intake. P_{trend}: *P* value for trend was derived from conditional logistic regression in which serum copeptin levels were used as continuous variables and adjusted by related factors.

TABLE 3: Dose-response relationship between serum copeptin and total stroke, ischemic stroke, and hemorrhagic stroke.

Serum copeptin (pmol/L)	Total stroke[a] *OR*	95% CI	Ischemic stroke[b] *OR*	95% CI	Hemorrhagic stroke *OR*	95% CI
5.9	0.92	0.48–1.74	0.34	0.15–0.75	9.17	1.96–43.01
15.9	0.76	0.48–1.20	0.44	0.25–0.80	2.21	1.11–4.38
25.9	1.00 (reference)		1.00 (reference)		1.00 (reference)	
35.9	1.30	1.04–1.62	1.70	1.26–2.30	0.69	0.37–1.26
45.9	1.67	1.03–2.70	2.34	1.24–4.42	0.61	0.13–2.87
1 pmol/L increment	1.02	1.00-1.03	1.05	1.02–1.08	0.92	0.86–0.98
$P_{nonlinear}$	0.278		0.362		0.314	
$P_{overall}$	0.139		0.002		0.007	

[a]The *OR* was adjusted by personal history of hypertension, smoking status, and pickle intake. [b]The *OR* was adjusted by BMI, personal history of hypertension, smoking status, and pickle intake.

the results were inconsistent. A population-based nested case-control study in the United States (The Northern Manhattan Study, NOMAS) found no association of serum copeptin with ischemic stroke risk [20]; another hospital-based cross-sectional study reported that plasma copeptin levels in patients with cerebral infarction, intracranial hemorrhage, and subarachnoid hemorrhage were significantly higher than that in healthy volunteers [22]. The British Regional Heart Study was a prospective study with older male participants with or without diabetes; the results demonstrated that higher serum copeptin level was independently associated with an increased risk of stroke among men with diabetes but not men without diabetes [21]. Therefore, our study might offer a robust evidence to fully evaluate the causal association between serum copeptin and stroke considering the dose-response relationship and the subtype of stroke among general population.

Since there are limited numbers of etiological studies and experimental studies involving copeptin and stroke, the possible mechanisms underlying the relationship between copeptin and ischemic stroke or hemorrhagic stroke remain unclear. According to the previous studies of copeptin, two possible mechanisms about copeptin and ischemic stroke were hypothesized. First, atherosclerotic disease caused the large majority of ischemic strokes [23]; copeptin as one of the biomarkers to reflect intima-media thickness and number of carotid plaques in carotid atherosclerosis might provide some evidences about the progression of ischemic

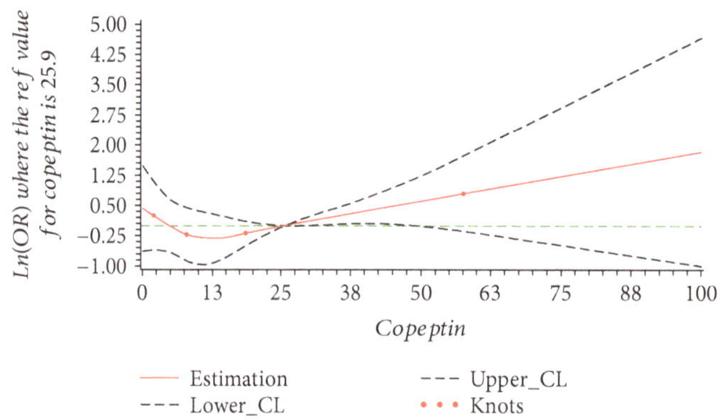

Figure 1: The plot of dose-response relationship between serum copeptin and total stroke ($P_{nonlinear} = 0.278$, $P_{overall} = 0.139$; adjusted by personal history of hypertension, smoking status, and pickle intake).

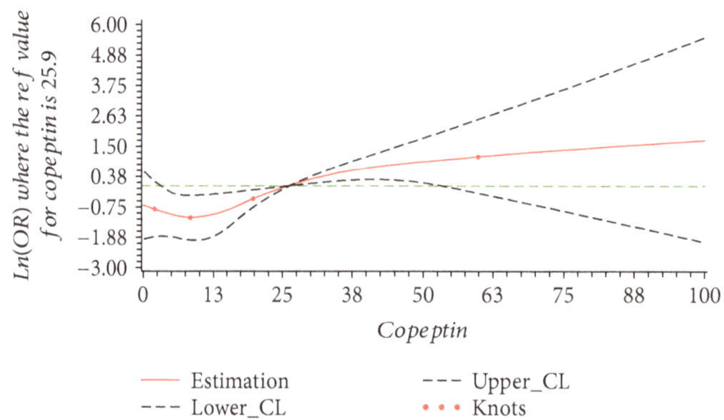

Figure 2: The plot of dose-response relationship between serum copeptin and ischemic stroke ($P_{nonlinear} = 0.362$, $P_{overall} = 0.002$; adjusted by BMI, personal history of hypertension, smoking status, and pickle intake).

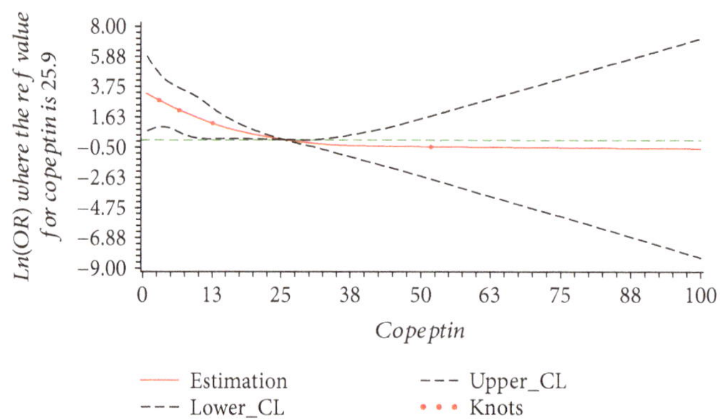

Figure 3: The plot of dose-response relationship between serum copeptin and hemorrhagic stroke ($P_{nonlinear} = 0.314$, $P_{overall} = 0.007$).

stroke [24]. Second, the antidiuretic effect of vasopressin was mediated by vasopressin 2 receptors, and this effect might increase the microalbuminuria excretion [25], suggesting copeptin might play a role for the AVP system in the development of albuminuria. A meta-analysis had proposed that microalbuminuria strongly and independently associated with the incidence of stroke and atherosclerosis might be the pathological link between microalbuminuria and stroke [26]. Regarding the hemorrhagic stroke, our results presented that higher serum copeptin level was adversely associated with hemorrhagic stroke, which was beyond our expectations. However, Faraci's study proved that endogenous AVP might play a role during hypoxia and intracranial hypertension by a negative feedback mechanism to reduce blood blow to the choroid plexus, which indicated that higher serum copeptin might be a protective factor for hemorrhagic stroke biologically plausible. Since the copeptin mostly played an indirect role in the progression of stroke in the possible mechanisms we mentioned above, cellular and molecular experiments need to be conducted in the future to explore the direct mechanisms between copeptin and ischemic stroke or hemorrhagic stroke.

In clinical practice, several studies had proved that copeptin could be applied to predict severity and outcome of stroke [9–13]. Our findings also indicated that copeptin might be used as an auxiliary biomarker to differentiate ischemic stroke and hemorrhagic stroke in clinical application, which is crucial for the immediate application of the right therapy to patients. Besides, just like the copeptin utility on suspected acute myocardial infarction, copeptin could also be used as one of combined biomarker that might improve accuracy for the early identification of different subtype of stroke. Furthermore, considering the lack of clinical characteristics that clearly differentiate stroke and stroke mimics, studies of Wendt et al. and von Recum et al. had explored whether copeptin could also be used as a potential biomarker to discriminate stroke and stroke mimics in pre-hospital stroke setting [27, 28]. Even though the results were not significant, these two studies throw light on the value of copeptin to discover noninvasive tests that aim to quickly distinguish stroke and stroke mimics and offer valuable recommendations to further studies.

Some limitations of our study must be considered. First, considering the budgets and efficiency, our study was designed as a case-control study, which was more likely to generate bias than a prospective cohort study design, and the causality of copeptin and stroke could not be inferred from the observed association. Second, the possibility of a type I error might occur in our study due to relatively small sample size; therefore, additional studies with a larger sample size are needed to confirm our findings. Third, although we considered some potential confounding factors, such as age, gender, family history of stroke, and personal history of hypertension, we could not exclude the possibility of residual confounding from inadequately measured covariates or confounders.

6. Conclusion

In summary, in this 1 : 1 age- and gender-matched and population-based case-control study, we observed that elevated serum copeptin levels were positively associated with ischemic stroke, while elevated serum copeptin levels were adversely associated with hemorrhagic stroke; no significant association was found between serum copeptin level and total stroke. Our results suggested a role of copeptin in the pathophysiological conditions of stroke; however, the confirmation of our findings in other prospective studies and further considerations of potential mechanisms are still needed.

Conflicts of Interest

All authors have no conflict of interest to disclose.

Acknowledgments

We thank all the subjects for their participation. We are also grateful to those village doctors, medical professors, medical students, and all participants in this study who had been very generous with their time and assistance.

References

[1] S. C. Johnston, S. Mendis, and C. D. Mathers, "Global variation in stroke burden and mortality: estimates from monitoring, surveillance, and modelling," *The Lancet. Neurology*, vol. 8, no. 4, pp. 345–354, 2009.

[2] Z. Wang, J. Li, C. Wang et al., "Gender differences in 1-year clinical characteristics and outcomes after stroke: results from the China National Stroke Registry," *PLoS One*, vol. 8, no. 2, article e56459, 2013.

[3] W. Wang, B. Jiang, H. Sun et al., "Prevalence, incidence, and mortality of stroke in China: results from a nationwide population-based survey of 480 687 adults," *Circulation*, vol. 135, no. 8, pp. 759–771, 2017.

[4] M. W. Dunser, V. Wenzel, A. J. Mayr, and W. R. Hasibeder, "Management of vasodilatory shock: defining the role of arginine vasopressin," *Drugs*, vol. 63, no. 3, pp. 237–256, 2003.

[5] G. Baumann and J. F. Dingman, "Distribution, blood transport, and degradation of antidiuretic hormone in man," *The Journal of Clinical Investigation*, vol. 57, no. 5, pp. 1109–1116, 1976.

[6] H. Land, G. Schutz, H. Schmale, and D. Richter, "Nucleotide sequence of cloned cDNA encoding bovine arginine vasopressin-neurophysin II precursor," *Nature*, vol. 295, no. 5847, pp. 299–303, 1982.

[7] M. Katan, N. G. Morgenthaler, K. C. Dixit et al., "Anterior and posterior pituitary function testing with simultaneous insulin tolerance test and a novel copeptin assay," *The Journal of Clinical Endocrinology & Metabolism*, vol. 92, no. 7, pp. 2640–2643, 2007.

[8] N. G. Morgenthaler, J. Struck, C. Alonso, and A. Bergmann, "Assay for the measurement of copeptin, a stable peptide derived from the precursor of vasopressin," *Clinical Chemistry*, vol. 52, no. 1, pp. 112–119, 2006.

[9] R. Zhang, J. Liu, Y. Zhang, Q. Liu, T. Li, and L. Cheng, "Association between circulating copeptin level and mortality risk in patients with intracerebral hemorrhage: a systemic review and meta-analysis," *Molecular Neurobiology*, vol. 54, no. 1, pp. 169–174, 2017.

[10] K. S. Choi, H. J. Kim, H. J. Chun et al., "Prognostic role of copeptin after stroke: a systematic review and meta-analysis of observational studies," *Scientific Reports*, vol. 5, no. 1, article 11665, 2015.

[11] X. Zeng, A. Deng, Y. Ding et al., "Copeptin and NT-proBNP as prognostic markers for recurrent ischemic cerebrovascular events in ischemic stroke patients," *Journal of the American College of Cardiology*, vol. 68, no. 24, pp. 2710-2711, 2016.

[12] X. Zhang, X. M. Lu, L. F. Huang, and H. Ye, "Copeptin is associated with one-year mortality and functional outcome in patients with acute spontaneous basal ganglia hemorrhage," *Peptides*, vol. 33, no. 2, pp. 336–341, 2012.

[13] H. Sun, T. Sun, B. Ma et al., "Prediction of all-cause mortality with copeptin in cardio-cerebrovascular patients: a meta-analysis of prospective studies," *Peptides*, vol. 69, pp. 9–18, 2015.

[14] T. Olsson, N. Marklund, Y. Gustafson, and B. Nasman, "Abnormalities at different levels of the hypothalamic-pituitary-adrenocortical axis early after stroke," *Stroke*, vol. 23, no. 11, pp. 1573–1576, 1992.

[15] Chinese Neuroscience Society, "The diagnosis of all type of cerebrovascular disease (1995)," *Journal of Clinical and Experimental Medicine*, vol. 12, no. 7, p. 559, 2013.

[16] Task Force for the Management of Arterial Hypertension of the European Society of Hypertension and Task Force for the Management of Arterial Hypertension of the European Society of Cardiology, "2013 ESH/ESC guidelines for the management of arterial hypertension," *Blood Pressure*, vol. 22, no. 4, pp. 193–278, 2013.

[17] M. Sanchez, P. Llorens, P. Herrero, F. J. Martin-Sanchez, P. Pinera, and O. Miro, "The utility of copeptin in the emergency department as a predictor of adverse outcomes in non-ST-elevation acute coronary syndrome: the COPED-PAO study," *Emergency Medicine Journal*, vol. 31, no. 4, pp. 286–291, 2014.

[18] A. A. Voors, S. von Haehling, S. D. Anker et al., "C-terminal provasopressin (copeptin) is a strong prognostic marker in patients with heart failure after an acute myocardial infarction: results from the OPTIMAAL study," *European Heart Journal*, vol. 30, no. 10, pp. 1187–1194, 2009.

[19] L. Desquilbet and F. Mariotti, "Dose-response analyses using restricted cubic spline functions in public health research," *Statistics in Medicine*, vol. 29, no. 9, pp. 1037–1057, 2010.

[20] M. Katan, Y. P. Moon, M. C. Paik et al., "Procalcitonin and midregional proatrial natriuretic peptide as markers of ischemic stroke: The Northern Manhattan Study," *Stroke*, vol. 47, no. 7, pp. 1714–1719, 2016.

[21] S. G. Wannamethee, P. Welsh, L. Lennon, O. Papacosta, P. H. Whincup, and N. Sattar, "Copeptin and the risk of incident stroke, CHD and cardiovascular mortality in older men with and without diabetes: The British Regional Heart Study," *Diabetologia*, vol. 59, no. 9, pp. 1904–1912, 2016.

[22] F. Aksu, M. Gurger, M. Yilmaz et al., "Copeptin levels in cerebral infarction, intracranial hemorrhage and subarachnoid hemorrhage," *Clinical Laboratory*, vol. 62, no. 12/2016, pp. 2387–2393, 2016.

[23] P. Amarenco, A. Cohen, M. Hommel, T. Moulin, D. Leys, and M. G. Bousser, "Atherosclerotic disease of the aortic arch as a risk factor for recurrent ischemic stroke," *The New England Journal of Medicine*, vol. 334, no. 19, pp. 1216–1221, 1996.

[24] C. Sinning, A. Kieback, P. S. Wild et al., "Association of multiple biomarkers and classical risk factors with early carotid atherosclerosis: results from the Gutenberg Health Study," *Clinical research in cardiology: official journal of the German Cardiac Society*, vol. 103, no. 6, pp. 477–485, 2014.

[25] E. Meijer, W. E. Boertien, R. Zietse, and R. T. Gansevoort, "Potential deleterious effects of vasopressin in chronic kidney disease and particularly autosomal dominant polycystic kidney disease," *Kidney & Blood Pressure Research*, vol. 34, no. 4, pp. 235–244, 2011.

[26] M. Lee, J. L. Saver, K. H. Chang, H. W. Liao, S. C. Chang, and B. Ovbiagele, "Impact of microalbuminuria on incident stroke: a meta-analysis," *Stroke*, vol. 41, no. 11, pp. 2625–2631, 2010.

[27] M. Wendt, M. Ebinger, A. Kunz et al., "Copeptin levels in patients with acute ischemic stroke and stroke mimics," *Stroke*, vol. 46, no. 9, pp. 2426–2431, 2015.

[28] J. von Recum, J. Searle, A. Slagman et al., "Copeptin: limited usefulness in early stroke differentiation?," *Stroke Research and Treatment*, vol. 2015, Article ID 768401, 4 pages, 2015.

38

Recurrent Ischemic and Hemorrhagic Stroke in Cameroon: A Case-Control Study

Jaurès Kamgang,[1] Francklin Tétinou,[1,2] Yvan Zolo,[2,3] Chee Yang Tan,[4] Christian Wambo,[5] Emerancienne J. N. Fongang,[2,6] and Ulrick Sidney Kanmounye[2]

[1]*Faculty of Medicine, Higher Institute of Health Sciences, Université des Montagnes, Bangangté, Cameroon*
[2]*Research Department, Association of Future African Neurosurgeons, Yaounde, Cameroon*
[3]*Faculty of Health Sciences, University of Buea, Buea, Cameroon*
[4]*Faculty of Medicine, University of Malaya, Kuala Lumpur, Malaysia*
[5]*Faculty of Medicine and Pharmaceutical Sciences, University of Douala, Douala, Cameroon*
[6]*Neurosurgery Unit, Laquintinie Hospital, Douala, Cameroon*

Correspondence should be addressed to Francklin Tétinou; tetinoufrancklin@gmail.com

Academic Editor: Jeff Bronstein

Introduction. Stroke recurrence accounts for a great percentage of catastrophic complications, yet no comprehensive study has analyzed the factors associated with stroke recurrence in Cameroon. We carried out this case-control study to better understand the factors associated with the stroke recurrence in Cameroon. *Methods*. We collected sociodemographic, clinical, neuroimaging, laboratory, and therapeutic data of eligible patients who consulted the neurology and cardiology department of the Yaounde Central Hospital in Cameroon. We included all patients at least five years removed from their first stroke event who consulted the authors' institution as of January 15, 2019. Wilcoxon signed-rank and Fisher's exact tests were used. Also, a Cox regression model was used to identify confounders.*Results*. We recruited 100 patients; seven out of ten patients had hypertension, while six out of 10 had a sedentary lifestyle. Half of the patients consumed alcohol regularly, while one patient out of five had diabetes. Most patients presented with their first stroke event, and a quarter had a stroke recurrence. Stroke recurrence was associated with right handedness (OR = 0.23, 95% CI = 0.16–0.33), congestive heart failure (OR = 3.45, 95% CI = 1.16–10.28), gout (OR = 4.34, 95% CI = 1.09–18.09), dysarthria (OR = 4.34, 95% CI = 1.30–14.54), and facial palsy (OR = 3.96, 95% CII = 1.49 – 10.51), as well as modifiable factors such as elevated abdominal circumference ($P < 0.01$), systolic blood pressure ($P < 0.01$), blood glucose level ($PI < I 0.01$), LDL cholesterol ($P < 0.01$), and triglyceride levels ($P < 0.01$). The mulitvariable regression model only identified laterality ($B = -1.48$, $P = 0.04$) as a statistically significant explanatory varibale for stroke recurrence. *Conclusion*. We mapped the landscape of recurrent strokes in Cameroon. There is a need to evaluate the causes of suboptimal drug adherence rates and both the role and adherence to nonpharmacologic interventions.

1. Introduction

Strokes are the second leading cause of death globally; nearly 16 million new cases and 5.7 million deaths are registered each year, 87% of which are in low- and middle-income countries (LMICs) [1]. In Cameroon, the prevalence rate of stroke is 7.3%, and its mortality rates are 26.7% during the first month and 31.7% in the first three months after the stroke event [2, 3].

Stroke recurrence is one of the most frequent and feared complications of a stroke [4]. Its prevalence varies widely. For example, in England, it is estimated at 5.6% over the first 12 months following an index stroke event [5], while in Ireland, it is almost twice the English rates (10.8%) [6]. In Cameroon, the stroke recurrence rate has been estimated at 14.5% [7]. There are several factors incriminated in stroke recurrence. These include a history of transient ischemic attack, daily alcohol consumption, smoking, age, atrial fibrillation, and diabetes [5, 8, 9]. Despite progress in preventing and treating these factors, stroke recurrence is very prevalent and deadly [7]. Recurrent strokes have higher mortality rates than index stroke events causing deaths in more than 30.6% of Senegalese patients in the first year alone [10] and 43% of Cameroonians [7].

No study has analyzed the link between sociodemographic and clinical factors on stroke recurrence in Cameroon. We carried out this case-control study to better understand the factors associated with the recurrence of stroke in Cameroon.

2. Materials and Methods

This case-control study was conducted in the neurology and cardiology departments of the Yaounde Central Hospital, Cameroon, a tertiary facility in Cameroon's capital.

2.1. Ethics. The institutional review boards of Université des Montagnes, Bangangté, Cameroon (Ref: 2019/212/UdM/PR/CIE), and the Yaounde Central Hospital (Ref: 0098/19/AR/MINSANTE/SG/DHCY/CM/SM) approved the study as part of the first author's (JK) medical thesis.

2.2. Definition of Terms. For this case-control study, recurrent stroke was defined as "clinical evidence of the sudden onset of a new focal neurological deficit with no apparent cause other than that of vascular origin (i.e., the deficit could not be ascribed to a concurrent acute illness, epileptic seizure, or toxic effect) occurring at any time after a (documented) index stroke" [4]. Patients who had suffered a recurrent stroke were defined as cases, while patients who had suffered their index stroke were defined as controls.

Medication adherence rates were defined as "the sum of the days' supply of drug therapy over (unit time) observed" [11]. Drug adherence was then classified into complete adherence (95–100% adherence rate), intermittent underexposure (>0% but <95% adherence rate), and permanent discontinuation (0% adherence rate) [12].

2.3. Data Collection. All patients at least five years (60 months) removed from their first stroke event who consulted at Yaounde Central Hospital as of January 15, 2019, were eligible. Patients without radiological confirmation of stroke were excluded from the study. The sampling was consecutive, and a minimum sample size of 48 was estimated using Cochrane's formula. The hospital prevalence of recurrent stroke in Cameroon was extracted from the work of Lekoubou et al. [7], i.e., 14.5%. Sociodemographic (age, gender, marital status, level of education, and profession), clinical (reason for consultation, vascular risk factors, comorbidities, time between the 1st episode of stroke and recurrence, and physical examination), neuroimaging, laboratory, and therapeutic data were extracted from patient charts. The authors contacted eligible patients by phone and during neurology clinics. Consent was sought during the index contact, and patients who declined consent were excluded from the study.

2.4. Data Analysis. The authors designed a five-part data collection tool administered by the first author (JK). The five parts collected sociodemographic (sex, age, marital status, level of education, urban/rural dwelling, and profession), clinical (history and presentation), workup (head computed tomography scan), therapeutic (medical and physical therapy), and follow-up data. Descriptive summary analysis was conducted for quantitative data (mean and standard deviation or median and interquartile range) and qualitative data (frequency and percentage). Wilcoxon signed-rank and Fisher's exact tests evaluated bivariable relationships between stroke recurrence status and independent variables (sociodemographic, clinical, and radiological data).

Moreover, adjusted odds ratios and *P*values were calculated for variables showing statistical significance in the bivariable analysis. Additionally, the median time from the index stroke to the second stroke was calculated for qualitative variables showing statistical significance during the bivariable analysis. These variables were then integrated into a 1000-sample bootstrap Cox regression model.

3. Results

We recruited 100 stroke patients aged 29.6 ± 11.0 years. Most patients were male (57.0%), married (64.0%), urban dwellers (64.0%), and right-handed (96.0%). 71 patients (71.0%) had hypertension, 59.0% had a sedentary lifestyle, 51.0% consumed alcohol regularly, 21.0% had diabetes, 17.0% had heart failure, and 17.0% consumed tobacco. Only 27.0% had a family history of stroke (Table 1).

Most patients (75.0%) had had a single stroke event, and 25.0% had a recurrent stroke, with one of them presenting with his third stroke event. Twenty-six patients (26.0%) had facial palsy, 19.0% had aphasia, 17.0% had alternating hemiplegia, 13.0% had dysarthria, 10% presented signs of intracranial hypertension, 3.0% had cerebellar syndrome, and 3.0% had signs of meningeal irritation.

Ischemic strokes were in the superficial (32.0%, $n = 32$), deep (15.0%, $n = 15$), and large (10.0%, $n = 10$) middle cerebral artery (MCA) territories, while nine patients (9.0%) had posterior cerebral artery (PCA) strokes. Hemorrhagic strokes were lenticular (5.0%), and four patients (4.0%) had a concomitant intraventricular hemorrhage. Five patients (5.0%) had another stroke in the same location as the index stroke event.

Most patients were taking antihypertensive medications (80.0%), 27.0% were taking acetylsalicylic acid, 17.0% were taking antidiabetics, 12.0% were taking statins, and 4.0% were taking antidepressants. In general, medication adherence rates were suboptimal (Figure 1). In addition, 18.0% of patients were treated with kinesiotherapy.

Stroke recurrence was associated with right-handedness (OR = 0.23; 95% CI = 0.16–0.33; $P = 0.02$), congestive heart failure (OR = 3.45; 95% CI = 1.16–10.28; $P = 0.03$), gout (OR = 4.44; 95% CI = 1.09–18.09; $P = 0.04$), dysarthria (OR = 4.34; 95% CI = 1.30–14.54; $P = 0.02$), and facial palsy (OR = 3.96; 95% CI = 1.49–10.51; $P = 0.01$). The association between medication observance and stroke recurrence was not statistically significant (Table 2).

The median time from the index stroke event to the second stroke was 16.0 (95% CI = 3.36–28.64) months in right-handed patients, 19.0 (95% CI = 3.76–34.25) months in patients with heart failure, and 15.0 (95% CI = 0.78–29.22)

TABLE 1: Sociodemographic characteristics of Cameroonian stroke patients.

Characteristic	Frequency (percentage)
Sex	
Female	57 (57.0)
Male	43 (43.0)
Marital status	
Married	64 (64.0)
Widow	31 (31.0)
Single	2 (2.0)
Divorced	2 (2.0)
Level of education	
Secondary education	40 (40.0)
Primary education	25 (25.0)
Tertiary education	19 (19.0)
No formal education	15 (15.0)
Residency location	
Urban	64 (64.0)
Rural	35 (35.0)
Profession	
Civil servant	31 (31.0)
Unemployed	29 (29.0)
Private formal sector	19 (19.0)
Private informal sector	16 (16.0)
Laterality	
Right handed	96 (96.0)
Left handed	4 (4.0)
Personal history	
Sedentary lifestyle	51 (51.0)
Alcohol consumption	49 (49.0)
Hypertension	29 (29.0)
Diabetes	21 (21.0)
Congestive heart failure	17 (17.0)
Tobacco consumption	17 (17.0)
Gout	9 (9.0)
Chronic kidney disease	5 (5.0)
Malignancy	2 (2.0)
Family history of stroke	27 (27.0)

months in patients with hypertension. After running the bootstrap Cox regression model, laterality was statistically significant ($B = -1.48$, $P = 0.04$). However, hypertension ($B = 0.57$, $P = 0.30$) and congestive heart failure ($B = 0.60$, $P = 0.20$) were not.

There were statistically significant differences in the abdominal circumference, heart rate, respiratory rate, systolic blood pressure, blood glucose level, hemoglobin concentration, platelet count, LDL cholesterol, triglycerides, and intraventricular hemorrhage of patients with recurrent and those without recurrent strokes ($P = < 0.01$) (Table 3).

4. Discussion

In this study, we investigated the factors associated with stroke recurrence in Cameroon. Most patients presented with their first stroke event, and a quarter of them had a stroke recurrence. Stroke recurrence was associated with modifiable factors such as elevated abdominal circumference, SBP, blood glucose level, LDL cholesterol, and triglyceride levels. Additionally, stroke recurrence was associated with laterality, congestive heart failure, gout, dysarthria, and facial palsy.

Recrudescence of old stroke deficits is common but underdiagnosed and can be confused with stroke recurrence. In our study, only 5.0% of patients had a stroke event in the same territory as the index stroke (confirmed radiologically). These findings suggest that recrudescence was very low in this population. We equally found that increased SBP and DBP were associated with stroke recurrence during bivariable analysis. However, SBP was the only statistically significant blood pressure measurement once the odds ratios were adjusted. This result indicates that DBP was a confounder. Our results are consistent with previous studies that have demonstrated that increased SBP increases the risk of stroke recurrence [13–17]. SBP measurement during the first 24 hours of stroke is a prognostic factor of stroke recurrence and has been used to identify high-risk patients [18]. The Perindopril Protection against Recurrent Stroke Study (PROGRESS) found that lowering SBP after a stroke reduced the risks of recurrent stroke among both hypertensive and nonhypertensive patients [19]. Another study showed that intensive lowering of blood pressure reduced stroke recurrence and recommended that the blood pressure target of less than 130/80 mmHg for secondary stroke prevention [20].

Diabetes was not associated with stroke recurrence in our study; however, increased casual blood glucose was statistically associated with stroke recurrence. This suggests that blood glucose control is just as important as diabetes status in preventing recurrent stroke. This finding highlights the necessity for blood glucose management and taking into consideration the low medication adherence rates. The results should be used to advocate for individual-level and public health measures that promote adherence. Our findings contradict several studies that have found a history of diabetes as an independent risk factor for an isolated stroke event and stroke recurrence. An HbA1c level ≥6.1% at admission is an independent predictor for stroke recurrence, and the risk of recurrent stroke increases with increasing HbA1c values [21–25]. In this study, we used the casual blood sugar level; however, fasting blood sugar is a better predictor of neurological outcome than casual blood sugar and HbA1c following an acute stroke event [26]. It is unclear if fasting blood glucose is a better predictor of stroke recurrence than casual blood glucose and HbA1c in this population.

Elevated LDL cholesterol and triglyceride levels were independently associated with stroke recurrence in this study. Elevated LDL is an independent predictor of stroke recurrence, and statins reduce LDL cholesterol levels and their associated recurrence risk [27]. Most patients prescribed statins in this study were observant. However, we did not find evidence that statin observance was statistically associated with decreased stroke recurrence risk. This finding warrants further investigation. Possible explanations include the dosage and LDL cholesterol target. Other lipid parameters such as triglycerides can be targeted to reduce the risk of stroke recurrence [28] and they should be studied in our setting.

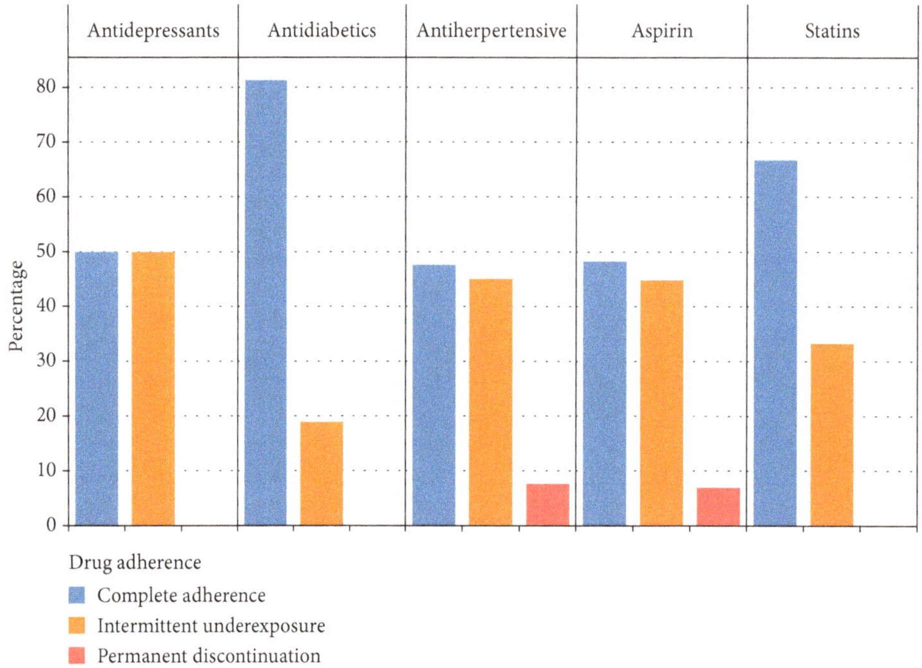

FIGURE 1: Medication adherence of Cameroonian stroke patients.

TABLE 2: Fisher's exact and odds ratios of sociodemographic, clinical, and therapeutic factors associated with stroke recurrence.

Factor	Odds ratio	95% confidence interval	*P*value
Male	0.68	0.27–1.73	0.49
Urban dwelling	1.04	0.40–2.67	0.94
Right handedness	0.23	0.16–0.33	0.02*
Personal history			
Alcohol consumption	2.26	0.89–5.77	0.11
Tobacco consumption	1.81	0.59–5.54	0.36
Sedentary lifestyle	1.28	0.50–3.28	0.65
Chronic kidney disease	0.73	0.08–6.85	0.98
Congestive heart failure	3.45	1.16–10.28	0.03*
Diabetes	2.21	0.79–6.20	0.16
Gout	4.44	1.09–18.09	0.04*
Hypertension	1.40	0.50–3.97	0.62
Family history of stroke	1.34	0.50–3.60	0.61
Presenting signs			
Alternating hemiplegia	0.91	0.27–3.09	0.98
Aphasia	0.30	0.06–1.39	0.14
Cerebellar syndrome	1.61	0.14–18.66	0.57
Dysarthria	4.34	1.30–14.54	0.02*
Facial palsy	3.96	1.49–10.51	0.01*
Intracranial hypertension	0.31	0.04–2.54	0.44
Meningeal syndrome	0.74	0.66–0.84	0.57
Medication observance			
Antidepressant	N/A	N/A	N/A
Antidiabetic	3.20	0.23–45.19	0.55
Antihypertensive	0.64	0.24–1.72	0.47
Aspirin	0.79	0.10–6.50	0.98
Statin	0.88	0.67–1.14	0.98

Recurrent strokes often affect the same brain hemisphere and location as the index stroke [5]. This tropism for the injured brain is due to altered anatomy and physiology of the injured brain [15]. An index stroke damages the cerebral blood vessels making them prone to subsequent strokes [29]. Also, risk factors that alter the function and lumen of blood vessels such as atherosclerosis increase the probability of recurrence in the same territory as the index stroke [30]. Due

Table 3: Wilcoxon ranked sum comparison of quantitative variables between Cameroonian patients with recurrent stroke and those with a first-time stroke event.

Quantitative variable	Test statistic	*P*value	Adjusted *P*value
Clinical parameters			
Age	−0.19	0.80	0.98
Abdominal circumference	9.14	<0.01**	<0.01**
Glasgow Coma Scale	1.22	0.09	0.98
Heart rate	3.87	<0.01**	<0.01**
Respiratory rate	12.30	<0.01**	<0.01**
Diastolic blood pressure	−2.05	<0.01**	0.56
Systolic blood pressure	4.75	<0.01**	<0.01**
Laboratory workup			
Blood glucose	5.17	<0.01**	<0.01**
Hemoglobin	12.20	<0.01**	<0.01**
Platelet count	8.48	<0.01**	<0.01**
HDL cholesterol	1.86	0.01*	0.98
LDL cholesterol	8.89	<0.01**	<0.01**
Triglycerides	6.91	<0.01**	<0.01**
Radiological			
Number of ventricles inundated	8.11	<0.01**	<0.01**

to the complexity of stroke recurrence, multiple studies are underway to understand better the factors surrounding lateralization of stroke recurrence [5].

We recognize a few limitations to this study. First, the study was retrospective and, therefore, prone to recall bias. We tried to mitigate this bias by carefully designing the research questions. Next, we did not evaluate adherence to nonpharmacologic measures. Given the high prevalence of stroke recurrence and its association with factors amenable to nonpharmacologic interventions, evaluating adherence to these nonpharmacologic interventions would have given a comprehensive understanding of stroke recurrence in Cameroonian patients. In addition, laterality was heavily skewed in favor of right-handedness and right-handedness seemed to be protective of stroke recurrence. Hence, our results on the role of laterality on stroke recurrence should be interpreted with caution.

5. Conclusions

We set out to understand why stroke recurrence was very high in our cohort, hypothesizing that some of the variables had a greater impact on recurrence than the others. Our study revealed insights into the landscape of recurrent strokes in Cameroon. First, they are prevalent and are associated with multiple modifiable risk factors. However, Cameroonian patients have suboptimal drug adherence rates. Future studies should evaluate the causes of suboptimal drug adherence rates and both the role and adherence to nonpharmacologic interventions. We will use the information from this study to influence department and ministry of health actions in the form of programs to improve medication adherence and research to evaluate how increased medication adherence will decrease the stroke risk.

Conflicts of Interest

The authors declare no conflicts of interest.

References

[1] K. Strong, C. Mathers, and R. Bonita, "Preventing stroke: saving lives around the world," *The Lancet Neurology*, vol. 6, no. 2, pp. 182–187, 2007.

[2] C. Nkoke, A. Lekoubou, E. Balti, and A. P. Kengne, "Stroke mortality and its determinants in a resource-limited setting: a prospective cohort study in Yaounde, Cameroon," *Journal of the Neurological Sciences*, vol. 358, no. 1–2, pp. 113–117, 2015.

[3] K.-T. Callixte, M.-N. Yacouba, G.-M. Lauriane et al., "Mortalité par Accident Vasculaire Cérébral et ses déterminants dans un Hôpital de référence de Douala (Cameroun)," *Health Sciences and Disease*, vol. 17, no. 1, 2016, https://www.hsd-fmsb.org/index.php/hsd/article/view/585.

[4] G.-R. Fu, W.-Q. Yuan, W.-L. Du et al., "Risk factors associated with recurrent strokes in young and elderly patients: a hospital-based study," *International Journal of Gerontology*, vol. 9, no. 2, pp. 63–66, 2015.

[5] T. Hillen, C. Coshall, K. Tilling et al., "Cause of stroke recurrence is multifactorial," *Stroke*, vol. 34, no. 6, pp. 1457–1463, 2003.

[6] E. Callaly, D. Ni Chroinin, N. Hannon et al., "Rates, predictors, and outcomes of early and late recurrence after stroke," *Stroke*, vol. 47, no. 1, pp. 244–246, 2016.

[7] A. Lekoubou, C. Nkoke, A. Dzudie, and A. P. Kengne, "Recurrent stroke and early mortality in an urban medical unit in Cameroon," *Journal of Stroke and Cerebrovascular Diseases*, vol. 26, no. 8, pp. 1689–1694, 2017.

[8] S. Sug Yoon, R. F. Heller, C. Levi, J. Wiggers, and P. E. Fitzgerald, "Knowledge of stroke risk factors, warning symptoms, and treatment among an Australian urban population," *Stroke*, vol. 32, no. 8, pp. 1926–1930, 2001.

[9] F. Sarfo, J. Acheampong, L. Appiah, E. Oparebea, A. Akpalu, and G. Bedu-Addo, "The profile of risk factors and in-patient outcomes of stroke in Kumasi, Ghana," *Ghana Medical Journal*, vol. 48, no. 3, pp. 127–134, 2014.

[10] D. G. Massi, J. Nyassinde, N. S. Diagne et al., "Prise en charge de l'hypertension artérielle et pronostic vital chez les patients hospitalisés pour récidive d'AVC à la clinique de neurologie du centre national hospitalier universitaire de Fann," *Revue Neurologique*, vol. 173, pp. S95–S96, 2017.

[11] B. A. Briesacher, S. E. Andrade, H. Fouayzi, and K. A. Chan, "Comparison of drug adherence rates among patients with seven different medical conditions," *Pharmacotherapy*, vol. 28, no. 4, pp. 437–443, 2008.
[12] M. Valgimigli, H. M. Garcia-Garcia, B. Vrijens et al., "Standardized classification and framework for reporting, interpreting, and analysing medication non-adherence in cardiovascular clinical trials: a consensus report from the Non-adherence Academic Research Consortium (NARC)," *European Heart Journal*, vol. 40, no. 25, pp. 2070–2085, 2019.
[13] K. M. Mohan, S. L. Crichton, A. P. Grieve, A. G. Rudd, C. D. A. Wolfe, and P. U. Heuschmann, "Frequency and predictors for the risk of stroke recurrence up to 10 years after stroke: the South London stroke register," *Journal of Neurology, Neurosurgery & Psychiatry*, vol. 80, no. 9, pp. 1012–1018, 2009.
[14] G. Xu, X. Liu, W. Wu, R. Zhang, and Q. Yin, "Recurrence after ischemic stroke in Chinese patients: impact of uncontrolled modifiable risk factors," *Cerebrovascular Diseases (Basel, Switzerland)*, vol. 23, no. 2-3, pp. 117–120, 2007.
[15] Y. Zhang, Y. Guan, Y. Zhang et al., "Recurrence rate and relevant associated factors of stroke among patients with small artery occlusion in Northern China," *Scientific Reports*, vol. 9, no. 1, p. 2834, 2019.
[16] M. Alter, G. Friday, S. M. Lai, J. O'Connell, and E. Sobel, "Hypertension and risk of stroke recurrence," *Stroke*, vol. 25, no. 8, pp. 1605–1610, 1994.
[17] S. Zheng and B. Yao, "Impact of risk factors for recurrence after the first ischemic stroke in adults: a systematic review and meta-analysis," *Journal of Clinical Neuroscience*, vol. 60, pp. 24–30, 2019.
[18] B. J. Kim, Y.-J. Cho, K.-S. Hong et al., "Trajectory groups of 24-hour systolic blood pressure after acute ischemic stroke and recurrent vascular events," *Stroke*, vol. 49, no. 8, pp. 1836–1842, 2018.
[19] PROGRESS Collaborative Group, "Randomised trial of a perindopril-based blood-pressure-lowering regimen among 6,105 individuals with previous stroke or transient ischaemic attack," *Lancet (London, England)*, vol. 358, no. 9287, pp. 1033–1041, 2001.
[20] K. Kitagawa, Y. Yamamoto, H. Arima et al., "Effect of standard vs. Intensive blood pressure control on the risk of recurrent stroke," *JAMA Neurology*, vol. 76, no. 11, pp. 1309–1318, 2019.
[21] T. Olsson, M. Viitanen, K. Asplund, S. Eriksson, and E. Hägg, "Prognosis after stroke in diabetic patients. A controlled prospective study," *Diabetologia*, vol. 33, no. 4, pp. 244–249, 1990.
[22] J. Shou, L. Zhou, S. Zhu, and X. Zhang, "Diabetes is an independent risk factor for stroke recurrence in stroke patients: a meta-analysis," *Journal of Stroke and Cerebrovascular Diseases*, vol. 24, no. 9, pp. 1961–1968, 2015.
[23] J. Han, W. Mao, J. Ni et al., "Rate and determinants of recurrence at 1 year and 5 years after stroke in a low-income population in rural China," *Frontiers in Neurology*, vol. 11, 2020.
[24] S. Zhu, L. A. McClure, H. Lau et al., "Recurrent vascular events in lacunar stroke patients with metabolic syndrome and/or diabetes," *Neurology*, vol. 85, no. 11, pp. 935–941, 2015.
[25] S. Wu, Y. Shi, C. Wang et al., "Glycated hemoglobin independently predicts stroke recurrence within one year after acute first-ever non-cardioembolic strokes onset in a Chinese cohort study," *PLoS ONE*, vol. 8, no. 11, p. e80690, 2013.
[26] J. Y. Sung, C. I. Chen, Y. C. Hsieh et al., "Comparison of admission random glucose, fasting glucose, and glycated hemoglobin in predicting the neurological outcome of acute ischemic stroke: a retrospective study," *PeerJ*, vol. 5, p. e2948, 2017.
[27] H. Naci, J. J. Brugts, R. Fleurence, and A. E. Ades, "Comparative effects of statins on major cerebrovascular events: a multiple-treatments meta-analysis of placebo-controlled and active-comparator trials," *QJM: An International Journal of Medicine*, vol. 106, no. 4, pp. 299–306, 2013.
[28] J.-H. Park, J. Lee, and B. Ovbiagele, "Nontraditional serum lipid variables and recurrent stroke risk," *Stroke*, vol. 45, no. 11, pp. 3269–3274, 2014.
[29] R. Kern, W. Steinke, M. Daffertshofer, R. Prager, and M. Hennerici, "Stroke recurrences in patients with symptomatic vs. asymptomatic middle cerebral artery disease," *Neurology*, vol. 65, no. 6, pp. 859–864, 2005.
[30] A. Ois, E. Cuadrado-Godia, E. Giralt-Steinhauer et al., "Long-term stroke recurrence after transient ischemic attack: implications of etiology," *Journal of Stroke*, vol. 21, no. 2, pp. 184–189, 2019.

Permissions

All chapters in this book were first published by Hindawi Publishing Corporation; hereby published with permission under the Creative Commons Attribution License or equivalent. Every chapter published in this book has been scrutinized by our experts. Their significance has been extensively debated. The topics covered herein carry significant findings which will fuel the growth of the discipline. They may even be implemented as practical applications or may be referred to as a beginning point for another development.

The contributors of this book come from diverse backgrounds, making this book a truly international effort. This book will bring forth new frontiers with its revolutionizing research information and detailed analysis of the nascent developments around the world.

We would like to thank all the contributing authors for lending their expertise to make the book truly unique. They have played a crucial role in the development of this book. Without their invaluable contributions this book wouldn't have been possible. They have made vital efforts to compile up to date information on the varied aspects of this subject to make this book a valuable addition to the collection of many professionals and students.

This book was conceptualized with the vision of imparting up-to-date information and advanced data in this field. To ensure the same, a matchless editorial board was set up. Every individual on the board went through rigorous rounds of assessment to prove their worth. After which they invested a large part of their time researching and compiling the most relevant data for our readers.

The editorial board has been involved in producing this book since its inception. They have spent rigorous hours researching and exploring the diverse topics which have resulted in the successful publishing of this book. They have passed on their knowledge of decades through this book. To expedite this challenging task, the publisher supported the team at every step. A small team of assistant editors was also appointed to further simplify the editing procedure and attain best results for the readers.

Apart from the editorial board, the designing team has also invested a significant amount of their time in understanding the subject and creating the most relevant covers. They scrutinized every image to scout for the most suitable representation of the subject and create an appropriate cover for the book.

The publishing team has been an ardent support to the editorial, designing and production team. Their endless efforts to recruit the best for this project, has resulted in the accomplishment of this book. They are a veteran in the field of academics and their pool of knowledge is as vast as their experience in printing. Their expertise and guidance has proved useful at every step. Their uncompromising quality standards have made this book an exceptional effort. Their encouragement from time to time has been an inspiration for everyone.

The publisher and the editorial board hope that this book will prove to be a valuable piece of knowledge for researchers, students, practitioners and scholars across the globe.

List of Contributors

Matthew A. Saxonhouse
Division of Neonatology, Department of Pediatrics, University of Florida, Gainesville, FL 32610-0296, USA

Dan Tarquinio
Division of General Pediatrics, Department of Pediatrics, University of Florida, Gainesville, FL 32610-0296, USA

Paul R. Carney
Division of Neurology, Department of Pediatrics, University of Florida, Gainesville, FL 32610-0296, USA

Jeff Bennett
Department of Radiology, University of Florida, Gainesville, FL 32610-0296, USA

Amy Smith
Division of Hematology/Oncology, Department of Pediatrics, University of Florida, Gainesville, FL 32610-0296, USA

Stephen P. Hunger
Section of Pediatric Hematology/Oncology/Bone Marrow Transplantation and Center for Cancer and Blood Disorders, The Children's Hospital, University of Colorado, Denver School of Medicine, Aurora, CO 80045, USA

James D. Geyer
Division of Neurology and Sleep Medicine, Department of Internal Medicine, College of Community Health Sciences, University of Alabama, Tuscaloosa, AL 35487, USA

Vineet Gupta
Department of Medicine, University of California SanDiego (UCSD), San Diego, CA 92103, USA

Naveen Dhawan
Nova Southeastern University, 3301 College Avenue, Fort Lauderdale, FL 33314, USA

Jaya Bahl
Florida International University (FIU), 11200 SW 8th Street, Miami, FL 33174, USA

A. Williams
Department of Neurosurgery, Derriford Hospital, Plymouth, PL6 8DH, UK

M. Sittampalam and A. Mohd Nor
Department of Neurology, Derriford Hospital, Plymouth, PL6 8DH, UK

N. Barua
Department of Neurosurgery, Frenchay Hospital, Bristol, BS16 1LE, UK

Guillaume Cassourret, Bertrand Prunet, Julien Bordes, Olga Maurin and Henry Boret
Intensive Care Unit, Sainte-Anne Hospital, Boulevard Sainte Anne, 83000 Toulon, France

Fabrice Sbardella
Department of Radiology, Sainte-Anne Hospital, 83000 Toulon, France

Jose Irazuzta
Division of Pediatric Critical Care Medicine, University of Florida Health Science Center at Jacksonville and The Wolfson Children's Hospital, 800 Prudential Drive, Jacksonville, FL 32207, USA

Kevin J. Sullivan
Division of Pediatric Critical Care Medicine, University of Florida Health Science Center at Jacksonville and The Wolfson Children's Hospital, 800 Prudential Drive, Jacksonville, FL 32207, USA
Department of Anesthesia, Mayo Clinic Rochester, Rochester, MN 55905, USA

Hussein Assallum, Mohammad Alkayem and Nehad Shabarek
Department of Internal Medicine, Lincoln Medical and Mental Health Center, 234 E 149th Steet, Bronx, NY 10451, USA

Kavitha Gopalratnam, Kevin Andrew Woodson, Jigarkumar Rangunwala, Kanaga Sena and Manisha Gupta
Bridgeport Hospital-Yale New Haven Health, 267 Grant St, Bridgeport, CT 06610, USA

Saira Chaughtai, Zeeshan Chaughtai, Muhammad Shaheryar Haider, Hasnan M. Ijaz, Sarah Elmedani, Mohamed Bakr, Mohammad A. Hossain and Arif Asif
Department of Medicine, Jersey Shore University Medical Center, Hackensack Meridian Health, Neptune, NJ 07753, USA

Charles Donohoe
Department of Neurology Chair, Truman Medical Center, 2301 Holmes St, Kansas City, MO 64108, USA

Nooshin Kiani Nia
Department of Neurology, Truman Medical Center, 2301 Holmes St, Kansas City, MO 64108, USA

Patricia Carey and Vamsi Vemulapalli
University of Missouri-Kansas City School of Medicine, 2411 Holmes St, Kansas City, MO 64108, USA

Bertram K. Woitok, Shawki Bahmad and Gregor Lindner
Department of General Internal and Emergency Medicine, Buergerspital Solothurn, Solothurn, Switzerland

Prudence Plummer
Division of Physical Therapy, Department of Allied Health Sciences, The University of North Carolina at Chapel Hill, 3020 Bondurant Hall, Campus Box No. 7135, Chapel Hill, NC 27599, USA

Raymond M. Villalobos, Moira S. Vayda, Myriam Moser and Erin Johnson
New England Rehabilitation Hospital, Woburn, MA 01801, USA

Jens Minnerup, Ilka Kleffner, Heike Wersching, Julian Zimmermann, Wolf-Rüdiger Schäbitz and Rainer Dziewas
Department of Neurology, University of Münster, Albert-Schweitzer Straße 33, 48149 Münster, Germany

Thomas Niederstadt
Department of Clinical Radiology, University of Münster, Albert-Schweitzer Straße 33, 48149 Münster, Germany

Rafael R. Lima, Luana N. S. Santana, Rafael M. Fernandes, Ana Carolina A. Oliveira, Luanna M. P. Fernandes and Enio Mauricio N. dos Santos
Institute of Biological Sciences, Laboratory of Functional and Structural Biology, Federal University of Pará, 66075-900 Belém, PA, Brazil

Elder M. Nascimento, Patrycy Assis N. Tavares, Ijair Rogério dos Santos, Adriano Gimarães-Santos and Walace Gomes-Leal
Institute of Biological Sciences, Laboratory of Experimental Neuroprotection and Neuroregeneration, Federal University of Pará, 66075-900 Belém, PA, Brazil

Muhammad U. Siddiqui
Department of Medicine, Marshfield Clinic, Rice Lake, WI 54701, USA

David Scalzitti
Department of Biostatistics, George Washington University, Washington, DC 20052, USA

Zunaira Naeem
Department of Medicine, Marshfield Clinic, Chippewa Falls, WI 54721, USA

Aleksandra Jotic, Katarina Lalic, Tanja Milicic, Milija Mijajlovic, Ljiljana Lukic, Milorad Civcic, Marija Macesic, Jelena P. Seferovic, Sandra Aleksic and Nebojsa M. Lalic
Clinic for Endocrinology, Diabetes and Metabolic Disorders, Clinical Centre of Serbia, Faculty of Medicine, University of Belgrade, Dr Subotica 13, 11000 Belgrade, Serbia

Nadezda Covickovic Sternic and Vladimir S. Kostic
Clinic for Neurology, Clinical Centre of Serbia, Faculty of Medicine, University of Belgrade, Dr Subotica 6, 11000 Belgrade, Serbia

Emina Colak
Institute of Medical Biochemistry, Clinical Centre of Serbia, Pasterova 2, 11000 Belgrade, Serbia

Vistasp J. Daruwalla and Hassan Tahir
ConemaughMemorial Hospital/Temple University, USA

Keyur Parekh, Jeremy D. Collins and James Carr
Department of Cardiovascular Radiology, Northwestern University Feinberg School of Medicine, USA

Halim Yilmaz, Gulten Erkin and Lutfiye Nalbant
The Department of Physical Medicine and Rehabilitation, Konya Education and Research Hospital, 42040 Konya, Turkey

Haluk Gumus
The Department of Neurology, Konya Education and Research Hospital, 42040 Konya, Turkey

Hitesh Gupta and Alakananda Banerjee
Max Healthcare, Saket, New Delhi 110017, India

Sebastiaan Velthuis, Martin J. Swaans, Benno J.W. M. Rensing, Lucas V. A. Boersma and Martijn C. Post
Department of Cardiology, St. Antonius Hospital, 3435 CM Nieuwegein, The Netherlands

Johannes J.Mager
Department of Pulmonology, St. Antonius Hospital, 3435 CM Nieuwegein, The Netherlands

Raghvendra Ramdasi, Amit Mahore, Abhijeet Kulkarni, Vithal Rangarajan and Manoj Patil
Department of Neurosurgery, King Edward Memorial Hospital and Seth Gordhandas Sunderdas Medical College, Parel, Mumbai 400012, India

Juhi Kawale
Department of Medicine, King Edward Memorial Hospital and Seth Gordhandas Sunderdas Medical College, Parel, Mumbai 400012, India

Karine Berthet and Marie-Germaine Bousser
Department of Neurology, Lariboisière Hospital, Assistance Publique Hôpitaux de Paris and University Paris 7 Diderot, 2 rue Ambroise Paré, 75475 Paris Cedex 10, France

Anne Claire Lukaszewicz and and Didier Payen
Department of Anesthesiology & Critical Care Medicine, Lariboisière Hospital, Assistance Publique Hôpitaux de Paris and University Paris 7 Diderot, 2 rue Ambroise Paré, 75475 Paris Cedex 10, France

Hugo P. Aben
Department of Neurology, Elisabeth Tweesteden Hospital, Tilburg, Netherlands
Department of Neurology, Brain Center Rudolf Magnus, University Medical Center Utrecht, Utrecht, Netherlands

Yael D. Reijmer and Geert Jan Biessels
Department of Neurology, Brain Center Rudolf Magnus, University Medical Center Utrecht, Utrecht, Netherlands

Johanna M. A. Visser-Meily
Department of Rehabilitation Medicine, Brain Center Rudolf Magnus, University Medical Center Utrecht, Utrecht, Netherlands

Jacoba M. Spikman
Department of Clinical and Experimental Neuropsychology, University of Groningen, Groningen, Netherlands

Paul L. M. de Kort
Department of Neurology, Elisabeth Tweesteden Hospital, Tilburg, Netherlands

John P. O'Laughlin and Gautam Verma
Department of Internal Medicine, New York Methodist Hospital, 506 6th Street, Brooklyn, NY 11215, USA

Iosif Gulkarov
Department of Cardiothoracic Surgery, New York Methodist Hospital, 263 7th Avenue, Brooklyn, NY 11215, USA
Department of Cardiothoracic Surgery, Weill Cornell Medicine, 68th Street M404, New York, NY 10021, USA

Fan Ye and Christopher L. Bray
College of Medicine, University of Central Florida, Orlando, FL 32827, USA
Department of Medicine and Graduate Medical Education, North Florida Regional Medical Center, Gainesville, FL 32605, USA

Burton V. Silverstein, Matheen A. Khuddus and Arthur C. Lee
North Florida Regional Medical Center, The Cardiac and Vascular Institute, Gainesville, FL 32605, USA

Deborah Osafehinti and Kaveh Zivari
Department of Internal Medicine, Maimonides Medical Center, Brooklyn, NY, USA

Sofie Søndergaard Mørch
Department of Anaesthesiology and Intensive Care, Bispebjerg Hospital, Bispebjerg Bakke 23, 2400 København NV, Denmark

Johnny Dohn Holmgren Andersen
Department of Anaesthesiology and Intensive Care, Hvidovre Hospital, Kettegård Alle 30, 2650 Hvidovre, Denmark

Morten Heiberg Bestle
Department of Anaesthesiology and Intensive Care, Nordsjællands Hospital, Dyrehavevej 29, 3400 Hillerød, Denmark

Kyaw Kyaw, Sammy San Myint Aung and Chanwit Roongsritong
Institute for Heart and Vascular Health, Renown Regional Medical Center, 1500 E. 2nd St. No. 302, Reno, NV 89502, USA

Htun Latt
Department of Internal Medicine, University of Nevada-Reno, School of Medicine, 1155 Mill St. No. W11, Reno, NV 89502, USA

Osayi Lawani
University of Houston College of Medicine/HCA Houston Healthcare, USA

Edward Baptista
Vital Heart & Vein, USA

Nurbanu Gurbuzer, Eren Gozke and Zeliha Ayhan Basturk
Department of Neurology, FSM Teaching and Research Hospital, E-5 Uzeri, Bostanci, 34744 Istanbul, Turkey

Archit Bhatt, Adnan Safdar, Dhara Chaudhari, Diane Clark, Amber Pollak, Arshad Majid and Mounzer Kassab
Providence Brain and Spine Institute, Portland, OR 97225, USA

Antonino Sant'Angelo, Sergio Bagnato, Cristina Boccagni and Giuseppe Galardi
Rehabilitation Department, Fondazione Istituto "San Raffaele-G. Giglio", 90015 Cefalù (PA), Italy

Vincenzo Guardabasso
Azienda Policlinico-Vittorio Emanuele, University of Catania, 95123 Catania, Italy

Theresa M. Smith
Department of Occupational Therapy, Texas Woman's University, 6700 Fannin Street, Houston, TX 77030, USA

Monique R. Pappadis
Division of Rehabilitation Sciences, School of Health Professions, University of Texas Medical Branch, 301 University Blvd, Galveston, TX 77555, USA
Sealy Center on Aging, University of Texas Medical Branch, 301 University Blvd, Galveston, TX 77555, USA

Shilpa Krishnan
Department of Rehabilitation Medicine, Division of Physical Therapy, Emory University, School of Medicine, 1462 Clifton Road, Atlanta, GA 30322, USA

Timothy A. Reistetter
Division of Rehabilitation Sciences, School of Health Professions, University of Texas Medical Branch, 301 University Blvd, Galveston, TX 77555, USA
Sealy Center on Aging, University of Texas Medical Branch, 301 University Blvd, Galveston, TX 77555, USA
Department of Occupational Therapy, School of Health Professions, University of Texas Medical Branch, Galveston, 301 University Blvd, Galveston, TX 77555, USA

Ki-Woong Nam, Tae Jung Kim, Sang Joon An, Sang-Bae Ko and Byung-Woo Yoon
Department of Neurology, Seoul National University Hospital, Seoul, Republic of Korea

Chi Kyung Kim and Kyungmi Oh
Department of Neurology, Korea University Guro Hospital and Korea University College of Medicine, Seoul, Republic of Korea

Hyo Geun Choi
Department of Otorhinolaryngology-Head & Neck Surgery, Hallym University College of Medicine, Anyang, Republic of Korea

So Young Kim
Department of Otorhinolaryngology-Head & Neck Surgery, CHA Bundang Medical Center, CHA University, Seongnam, Republic of Korea

Vânia A. M. Goulart
Department of Biochemistry and Immunology, Federal University of Minas Gerais, Belo Horizonte-MG, Brazil
Department of Chemistry, Federal University of Minas Gerais, Belo Horizonte-MG, Brazil

Marcelo M. Sena
Department of Chemistry, Federal University of Minas Gerais, Belo Horizonte-MG, Brazil
National Institute of Science and Technology in Bioanalytics, Campinas-SP, Brazil

Thiago O. Mendes
Institute of Learning and Research Santa Casa de BH, Belo Horizonte-MG, Brazil

Helvécio C. Menezes, Zenilda L. Cardeal and Maria J. N. Paiva
Department of Chemistry, Federal University of Minas Gerais, Belo Horizonte-MG, Brazil

Valéria C. Sandrim
Institute of Learning and Research Santa Casa de BH, Belo Horizonte-MG, Brazil

Mauro C. X. Pinto
Department of Pharmacology, Federal University of Goiás, Goiânia-GO, Brazil

Rodrigo R. Resende
Department of Biochemistry and Immunology, Federal University of Minas Gerais, Belo Horizonte-MG, Brazil

Qiuyi Lv, Xing Chen, Lan Jiang and Yihuai Zou
Department of Neurology and Stroke Center, Dongzhimen Hospital, The First Affiliated Hospital of Beijing University of Chinese Medicine, Beijing, China

Guixing Xu
The Acupuncture and Tuina School/The 3rd Teaching Hospital, Chengdu University of Traditional Chinese Medicine, Chengdu, China

Yuxin Pan
Institute of Neuroscience, Chinese Academy of Sciences, Shanghai, China

Tongtong Liu
Guang'anmen Hospital, China Academy of Chinese Medical Sciences, Beijing, China

Xiaodong Liu, Yingjia He and Rong Zhang
Beijing University of Chinese Medicine, Beijing, China

Linqing Miao
Beijing Institute of Technology, Beijing, China

Jie Chen
School of Life Science, Peking University, Beijing, China

Hao Sun, Hailong Wang, Bo Zhou, Xiaomei Wu, Bing Ma and Jingpu Shi
Department of Clinical Epidemiology and Evidence-Based Medicine, Institute of Cardiovascular Diseases, The First Hospital of China Medical University, No. 155 Nanjing North Street, Heping District, Shenyang, Liaoning province 110001, China

Donghui Huang
Department of Clinical Epidemiology, Shengjing Hospital of China Medical University, No. 36 Sanhao Street, Heping District, Shenyang, Liaoning province 110004, China

Jaurès Kamgang
Faculty of Medicine, Higher Institute of Health Sciences, Université des Montagnes, Bangangté, Cameroon

Francklin Tétinou
Faculty of Medicine, Higher Institute of Health Sciences, Université des Montagnes, Bangangté, Cameroon
Research Department, Association of Future African Neurosurgeons, Yaounde, Cameroon

Yvan Zolo
Research Department, Association of Future African Neurosurgeons, Yaounde, Cameroon
Faculty of Health Sciences, University of Buea, Buea, Cameroon

Chee Yang Tan
Faculty of Medicine, University of Malaya, Kuala Lumpur, Malaysia

Christian Wambo
Faculty of Medicine and Pharmaceutical Sciences, University of Douala, Douala, Cameroon

Emerancienne J. N. Fongang
Research Department, Association of Future African Neurosurgeons, Yaounde, Cameroon
Neurosurgery Unit, Laquintinie Hospital, Douala, Cameroon

Ulrick Sidney Kanmounye
Research Department, Association of Future African Neurosurgeons, Yaounde, Cameroon

Index

O

P

R

S

T

U

V

W

www.ingramcontent.com/pod-product-compliance
Lightning Source LLC
LaVergne TN
LVHW082222200926
848484LV00008B/2292